Nonunion of the Long Bones

Diagnosis and treatment with compression-distraction techniques

Redento Mora (Ed.)

Nonunion of the Long Bones

Diagnosis and treatment with compression-distraction techniques

Foreword by Dror Paley

Springer

Redento Mora
Department of Orthopaedics
and Traumatology
University of Pavia
Città di Pavia Institute
Pavia, Italy

Library of Congress Control Number: 2005936344

ISBN 10 88-470-0408-X Springer Milan Berlin Heidelberg New York
ISBN 13 978-88-470-0408-5 Springer Milan Berlin Heidelberg New York

Springer is a part of Springer Science+Business Media
springer.com

Printed in Italy

Cover design: estudio Calamar, Barcelona, Spain
Typesetting: Graphostudio, Milan, Italy
Printing: Grafiche Porpora, Cernusco s/N (MI), Italy

Foreword

Professor Mora's book on pseudoarthrosis is a comprehensive text, based on his carrer's interest and expertise in this field. While previous texts have focused on internal fixation methods, this new one also details the use of external fixation methods, in particular those introduced by Professor Gavril Abramovitch Ilizarov. Methods of compression, distraction, and bone transport of the pseudoarthrosis have added to the armamentarium and success of treatment of this frequently unsolved orthopaedic problem. These newer methods have greatly reduced the need for amputation as the final solution for this disease.

This text has three parts. The first part deals with present-day knowledge of the mechanisms of fracture healing and the features and diagnosis of nonunions. The second presents indications, surgical methods, and technical details for treatment of noninfected and infected nonunions. In the third part, the first chapters discuss several important subjects connected with the nonunion problem, and the final chapters, dedicated to computer-assisted surgery and documentation systems, explore future perspectives of compression-distraction techniques in the management of nonunions.

With a wide range of diagrams, x-rays, and photogaphs, Professor Mora's book guides the reader through the classification, strategy of treatment and methodology. Throughout twenty-two chapters, this new publication, offers the most exhaustive overview on this subject since Weber and Cech brought out their research three decades ago.

Dror Paley
Director, Rubin Institute for Advanced Orthopaedics
Co-Director, International Center for Limb Lengthening
Sinai Hospital of Baltimore

Preface

Expressions such as "compression-distraction techniques", "transosseous osteosynthesis methods", and "circular external fixation", born in past decades in the former Soviet Union, are interchangeable and will be used in this book without distinguishing between them. Moreover, the term "screw" is used throughout this volume instead of "fiche", as established in the Instructional Courses "External Fixation in Italy" which took place in the 1990s.

These methods, almost unknown in Western countries until 30 years ago, have a very ancient past. Indeed, the description of a circular external fixation system for the purpose of reducing and immobilizing leg fractures dates back to Hippocrates, about 2,400 years ago. It was not until the twentieth century, however, that both the theory and practice of circular external fixation was further developed to a greater extent. The American surgeon Bittner, in 1934, had the idea of a circular external fixation system so perfect that it can be considered the real precursor of today's systems. At the same time the Italian surgeon Della Mano, in 1938, described a ring apparatus which he successfully used to treat leg fractures. However, the German surgeon Wittmoser was credited with recognizing the advantages of external circular fixation based on two or more crossed wires on a single ring plane.

Unfortunately, these systems only met with little success in Western countries. The concepts, devices, and applications for circular external fixation were highly developed in the former Soviet Union, though, mainly thanks to the work and colloboration of G.A. Ilizarov in Kurgan, M. Volkov and O. Oganesian in Moscow, and V. Kalnberz in Riga. From there, these methods gradually began to spread to Western Europe and America in the 1980s. This somewhat disordered and uncontrolled diffusion produced two unfavorable consequences: the conviction that these techniques were "miraculous" (being the remedy for all problems, that is, any orthopaedic and traumatological pathology) and "easy", and that a rapid and superficial knowledge of wire and screw application sites was sufficient to employ the technique. That inevitably produced treatment indication errors (first an excess of indications and then in the kinds of defects) and insufficient treatment (mainly postoperative), and led many specialists away from this area of orthopaedics and traumatology.

In the orthopaedic literature, many good treatises on fracture nonunions and excellent texts on compression-distraction systems have been published, but scientific papers concerning the treatment of nonunions with external fixation techniques are poorly represented, and most of all, they rarely address the main problem: specify the indications. That is the aim of the present work.

It must be undercored that all the photographs refer to clinical and radiographic features of patients treated in the Orthopaedic Department of the University of Pavia – "Città di Pavia" Institute, and that all the preparations and microphotographs of biological specimens were performed at the research laboratories of the same department.

This text is based on knowledge gained over almost 30 years, starting with a long stay in the former Soviet Union in 1978 and 1979 and extended by an ever-increasing intensive collaboration with the Central Institute of Orthopaedics and Traumatology of Moscow and with the Latvian Institute of Traumatology and Orthopaedics of Riga, and on the continuous practice and development of the devices and the operative techniques of compression-distraction. This has resulted in about 3,000 patients personally treated both in the former Soviet Union and in Italy for orthopaedic and traumatological pathologies.

This work aims to debunk many still existing myths concerning circular external fixation methods, to specify the indications, and to show exactly the limitations of these techniques.

We do not dwell on preconstituted and, in general, hardly useful assembly schemes (also because the choice of the best assembly always depends on the orthopaedic surgeon), and instead focus on and describe the technical details that experience makes more important and interesting.

I extend warm thanks to the international and Italian colleagues who, with some fundamental chapters, collaborated with me and gave of their precious experience to write this book.

I sincerely thank all my assistants, who patiently and competently helped me prepare texts and images for each chapter.

Finally, I would like to thank our publisher Springer-Verlag for the competent collaboration to achieve the best presentation of this work.

Redento Mora

Contents

Section V Future Directions

Contributors

BARBARA BERTANI
Assistant Surgeon
Department of Orthopaedics
and Traumatology
of the University of Pavia
Città di Pavia Institute
Pavia, Italy

GIOVANNI BATTISTA GALLI
Orthopaedic Fellow
University of Pavia
School of Medicine
Pavia, Italy

STEFANO GILI
Orthopaedic Fellow
University of Pavia School of Medicine
Pavia, Italy

ANNA MACCABRUNI
Professor of Infectious Diseases
University of Pavia School of Medicine
Department of Infectious Diseases of
the University of Pavia
Policlinico San Matteo
Pavia, Italy

MILENA MICELI
Orthopaedic Fellow
University of Pavia School of Medicine
Pavia, Italy

REDENTO MORA
Professor of Orthopaedic Surgery
University of Pavia
School of Medicine
Director of the Department of
Orthopaedics and Traumatology of the
University of Pavia
Città di Pavia Institute
Pavia, Italy

LUISELLA PEDROTTI
Chief Assistant Surgeon
Department of Orthopaedics
and Traumatology of the University of
Pavia, Città di Pavia Institute
Pavia, Italy

FABRIZIO QUATTRINI
University of Pavia School of Medicine
Pavia, Italy

PIER PAOLO RAGUZZI
Sales and Applications Engineer
BrainLAB AG
Munich, Germany

LEONID N. SOLOMIN
Head of External Fixation Department
R.R. Vreden Russian Research Institute
of Traumatology and Orthopaedics
St. Petersburg, Russia

Gabriella Tuvo
Assistant Surgeon
Department of Orthopaedics
and Traumatology
of the University of Pavia
Città di Pavia Institute
Pavia, Italy

Section I
Fracture Healing

Diaphyseal Fracture Repair

Redento Mora, Luisella Pedrotti, Gabriella Tuvo

Introduction

A description of the process of fracture repair can be found in many orthopaedic surgery textbooks', but a careful evaluation of the literature easily shows important differences in opinions about the aspects and phases of this process [1–3].

The gradual evolution of ideas about the biology of fracture healing, which took place over the course of the past 30 years, and the enormous increase in knowledge about the regulation of bone cell activity have gradually extended interest from a cellular basis to a molecular basis and to the genetics of bone consolidation: "...consolidation needs much more than osteoblasts" [4].

In light of current knowledge, bone consolidation must be considered as a complex recruitment and cellular differentiation process, led by local mediators that send particular physical and chemical signals to the cells.

A fracture is a break in the continuity of a bone (and a disruption of the blood supply to the bone) and the healing process begins as soon as the bone is broken, provided that the fundamental principles of fracture treatment (reduction and immobilization) are respected.

Fracture repair must be considered a regenerative process rather than a healing process, because the injured part is replaced by the formation of new bone tissue (callus) instead of scar tissue. The callus formed outside the bone is termed external callus; the callus in the medullary cavity is termed internal callus.

If a fracture is not displaced and stable, only a cast or a brace may be necessary to maintain immobilization (with a small amount of interfragmentary motion): in this case bone callus forms "under natural conditions". For unstable or displaced fractures operative treatment with an internal or external fixation is required. Operative treatment modifies the process of fracture repair: in this case a different kind of process (callus formation "after operative treatment") is observed.

Callus Formation Under Natural Conditions

Fracture healing proceeds through a number of stages:

- Inflammation (hematoma formation followed by local inflammation reaction);
- Soft callus (or primary callus);
- Hard callus (stage of consolidation);
- Bone remodeling.

Inflammation

Inflammation represents the opening phase and lasts about 2–3 weeks. As a consequence of the fracture and the vascular interruption not only is the bone broken but the periosteum is also torn, the marrow is ruptured, and the surrounding soft tissues are damaged. Therefore, the periosteal and endosteal vascular complex is interrupted, and the interruption of blood supply provokes necrosis (of varying degrees according to the trauma severity and complexity) at the ends of the bone fragments: the necrosis is histologically explained by the empty aspect of the osteocytic gaps.

The resulting cellular injury induces chemotactic cytokine production. The vascular damage even provokes bleeding of the fragments and of the surrounding soft tissues, forming a hematoma.

The hematoma has great importance in the consolidation process, as experimentally demonstrated by Mizuno et al. [5]: they observed that fracture hematoma transplant in subperiosteal and muscular site triggers bone production only at the periosteal site on the second postoperative day and bone production at both sites on the fourth day. Therefore, they came to the conclusion that on the fourth day the hematoma has osteogenic power.

Acute inflammation then arises in tissues which surround the fracture, with invasion by histiocytes and macrophages.

At this moment, the "regional acceleratory phenomenon" (RAP), caused by unknown signals and which has been described by Frost [3], starts. It consists of a complex process of cellular recruitment, migration, multiplication, osteoblast and osteoclast differentiation, mineralization control, and remodeling control.

Cellular Recruitment

Osteoblast progenitor recruitment takes place almost certainly by osteogenic induction on undifferentiated cells: in the bone marrow and in the periosteal deep layer mesenchymals cells develop an osteogenic potential in the presence of adequate stimulus. The osteoclasts seem to originate from hemopoietic cells deposited in bone marrow.

Migration

The recruited osteoprogenitor cells migrate towards the fracture focus, stimulated by chemotactic factors (cytokines) released by the necrotic cells.

Proliferation

Osteoprogenitor cells proliferate and give origin to cellular colonies: they are called colony forming unit fibroblasts (CFU-F) or mesenchymal stem cells (MSC) [6]. This proliferation is stimulated by mitogen agents released by cells damaged by fracture trauma, in particular platelet-derived growth factor (PDGF) and transforming growth factor-β (TGF-β), secreted by the blood platelets.

Differentiation

The differentiation takes place because of systemic or local osteoinductive factors that orientate towards different cell groups (osteoblasts and osteocytes, osteoclasts).

Osteoblasts

Osteoblasts form a layer of polyhedral cells covering the bone surfaces (Fig. 1). They show a marked cytoplasmic basophilia, and alkaline phosphatase is present in osteoblasts which are actively forming bone and in the adjacent tissue.

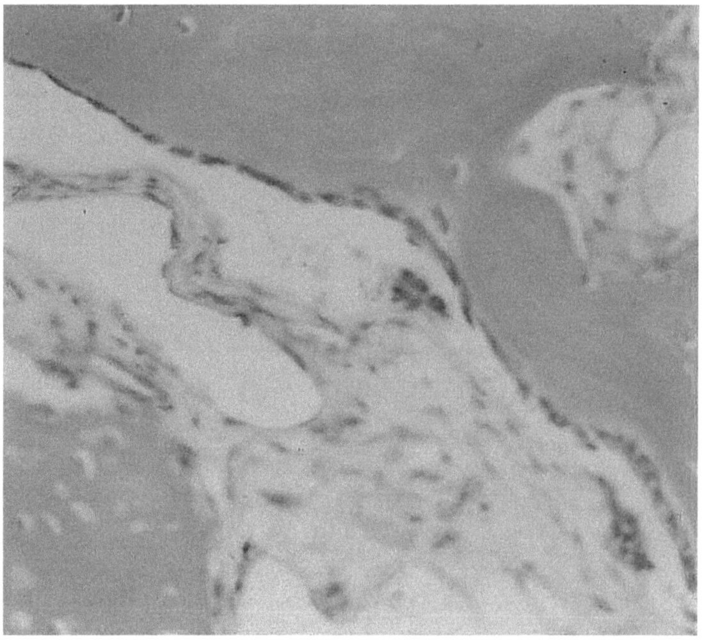

Fig. 1. Osteoblasts forming an epithelial-like structure at the bone surface (Hematoxylin and Eosin, original magnification: x 125)

The ultrastructural appearance of an osteoblast shows abundant rough endoplasmic reticulum, free ribosomes, a well-developed Golgi zone, numerous mitochondria, and an acentric nucleus. The cell surface has a small number of microvilli.

Osteocytes

Osteocytes are formed by the incorporation of osteoblasts in bone matrix (Fig. 2). Osteocytes are small cells surrounded by mineralized bone matrix (with the exception of a limited space which forms the so-called osteocyte "lacuna". Osteocytes have several long cytoplasmic processes which fill narrow spaces called "canalicula" [7].

Ultrastructurally these cells show small nuclei and sparse organelles with few mitochondria, a small Golgi apparatus, and little rough endoplasmic reticulum.

Osteocyte lacunae were classified into four different types by Baud and Auil [8]:

- Inactive: small lacunae with smooth borders;
- Osteolytic: large lacunae with irregular borders;
- Osteoplastic: large lacunae with recently formed matrix;
- Empty: lacunae only containing cellular debris.

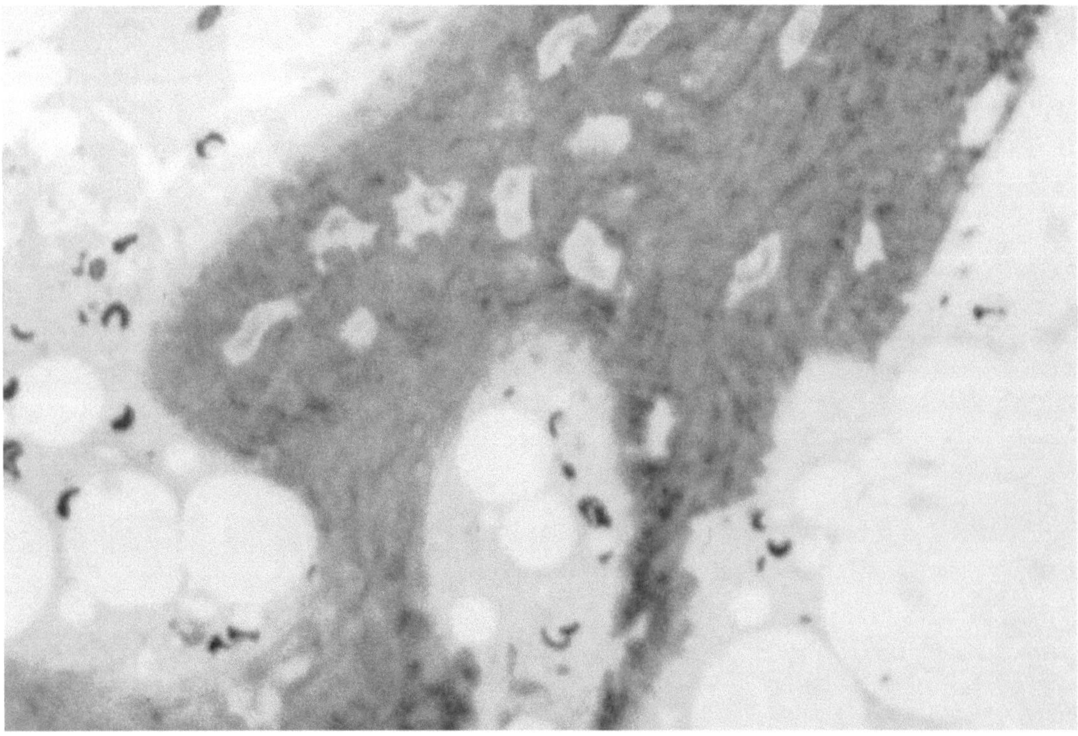

Fig. 2. Osteocytes located in lacunae surrounded by mineralized bone matrix (semi-thin section, Rosenqvist silver stain, original magnification: x 1250)

Osteoclasts

Osteoclasts are multinucleated giant cells observed singly or in small groups on the inner surfaces of trabecular and compact bone (Fig. 3). The cytoplasm is moderately acidophilic and the nuclei are round or oval. Bone resorption is identified by the presence of osteoclasts in resorption lacunae (so-called Howship lacunae) at the bone surfaces. A striated border can be observed at the surface in contact with the bone.

Ultrastructural studies show deep invaginations of the cell membrane at the ruffled border of the cell which is adjacent to bone.

Osteoclasts show different structural features, depending on their function. The moving, resting, resorbing, and dying osteoclasts show typical structural features: this series of cellular events is called the "resorption cycle" [9]. Resting osteoclasts accumulate a large number of acidic vesicles inside the cytoplasm. Resorbing osteoclasts show a ruffled border adjacent to bone: At the end of the resorption cycle, multinucleated osteoclasts undergo the final phase of the life cycle (programmed cell death by apoptosis).

Mineralization Control

Systemic regulatory factors include calcium and phosphorus regulatory hormones:

- Growth hormone (GH): hypophysiectomy provokes delayed unions; GH administration prevents this effect [10]. According to Northmore-Ball et al. this action is present only in the initial stages of the consolidation [11].

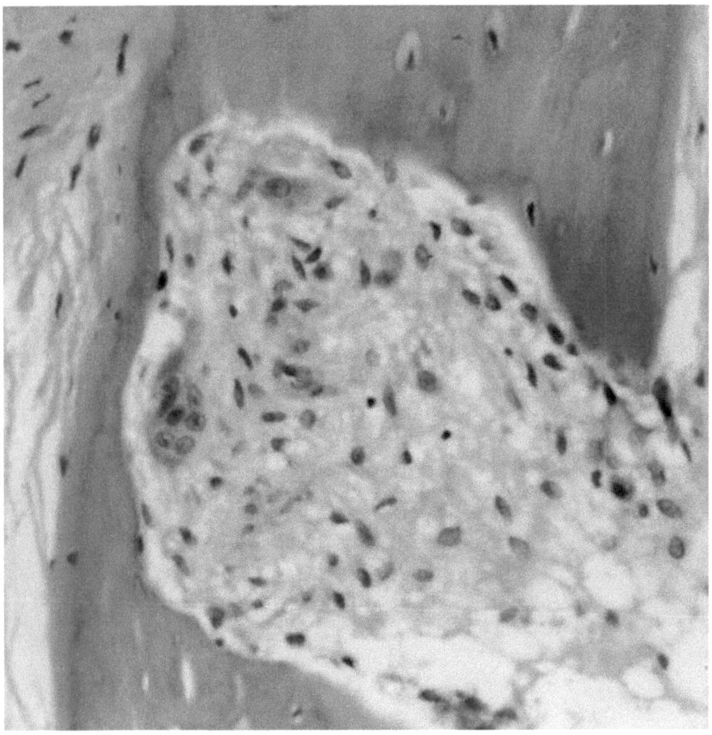

Fig. 3. Osteoclasts situated on the surface of the trabecular bone (Hematoxylin and Eosin, original magnification: x 125)

- Tyroxin: this stimulates the consolidation [12].
- Adrenocorticotropic hormone (ACTH; and hydrocortisone): supplied at high doses, it may reduce or stop the consolidation [13].

Local regulatory factors (of chemical nature) include growth factors that act as agonists and antagonists among themselves and stimulate bone formation or resorption by cell proliferation and biosynthetic activity. These polypeptides affect osteogenesis at the level of recruitment, proliferation, differentiation, and collagen production. They are present in the bone matrix and are synthesized by the osteoblasts but also by other cellular elements; they are named after their origin or their actions [14].

The growth factors are one of the functional categories into which the cytokines (proteins secreted by different cells which are involved in regulating the inflammatory response) are grouped; other functional categories include interferons, colony stimulating factors, and interleukins [15] (Table 1).

Table 1. Growth factors involved in bone formation

Growth factors	Source	Action on the skeleton
TGF-β	Platelets Inflammatory cells Chondrocytes Osteoblasts	Progenitor cell stimulation
BMPs	Chondrocytes Osteoblasts	Cartilage formation Recruitment, proliferation, differentiation, and enhancement
FGF	Inflammatory cells Chondrocytes Osteoblasts	Mesenchymal cell proliferation enhancement Neovascularization stimulation
PDGF	Platelets Inflammatory cells Endothelial cells	Stimulation of type I collagen synthesis Mesenchymal cell proliferation enhancement
IGF	Chondrocytes Osteoblasts	Production of type I collagen Stimulation

TGF-β, transforming growth factor-beta; *BMP*, bone morphogenetic protein; *FGF*, fibroblast growth factor; *PDGF*, platelet-derived growth factor; *IGF*, insulin-like growth factor

Local regulatory factors (of a physical nature) include mechanical factors, which greatly affect the fracture repair (influence of stability, instability, and micromotion are well known) and biophysical phenomena (bioelectricity, bioelectromagnetism, and ultrasound) [16].

Due to the action of all these different regulatory factors, osteoprogenitor cells gradually differentiate, creating different cellular groups.

Granulation Tissue Formation

The hematoma evolves towards a fibrovascular granular tissue rich in type II collagen, which fills the interfragmentary space. It is constituted by newly formed vessels, cellular elements (mainly fibroblasts), and extracellular matrix.

Soft Callus (Primary Callus)

After 2 weeks (in human beings) bone fragments are linked by a bridge surrounded by a fibrous membrane (which corresponds to the external layer of the periosteum).

Osteoprogenitor cells differentiate into two different cellular types, which are distinct according to their site. At a distance of some millimeters from the fracture site at the level of each fragment, the cells differentiate into osteoblasts, which in turn produce organic matrix (an osteoid substance which contains collagen fibers without a spatial direction). The osteoid substance rapidly mineralizes to form an immature bone tissue (so-called woven bone), nonoriented, whose organization is linked to the irregular growth of the capillaries.

At the fracture site, osteoprogenitor cells differentiate into chondrocytes, which produce cartilaginous matrix (a chondroid substance).

As the focus solidity increases, the cartilaginous cells hypertrophize and the cartilage progressively mineralizes by endochondral ossification.

In contact with the periosteal covering, a bone lamina forms that links the fragments as in a bridge, and the mineralization progresses from the immature bone bridge towards the focus. Soft callus turns into hard callus.

Hard Callus

Initially, hard callus is formed by immature bone, but, when the interfragmentary bridge is strong enough, the immature bone turns into primary lamellar bone, which gradually grows in many directions. This transformation commences in the 4th week and finishes around the 16th week.

Remodeling

Remodeling slowly restores normal bone structure, passing through stages of primary lamellar bone (with osteons with multidirectional orientation) to secondary lamellar bone (with osteons with longitudinal orientation).

Remodeling is based on the action of special units known as bone modeling units (BMU) described by Frost in 1989 [3]. Each unit, in which new bone resorption and apposition are co-ordinated in time and space, is histologically constituted by a "head" that covers a capillary vessel shaped like a bonnet and formed by osteoclasts which actively re-absorb the bone (Figs. 4, 5).

The growth pattern of the capillary follows that of the osteoclastic head and it is accompanied by osteoblasts. They produce new bone in concentric lamellae on the reabsorption channel walls, creating in this way a Haversian structure. The remodeling stage is remarkably long (more than a year) [17].

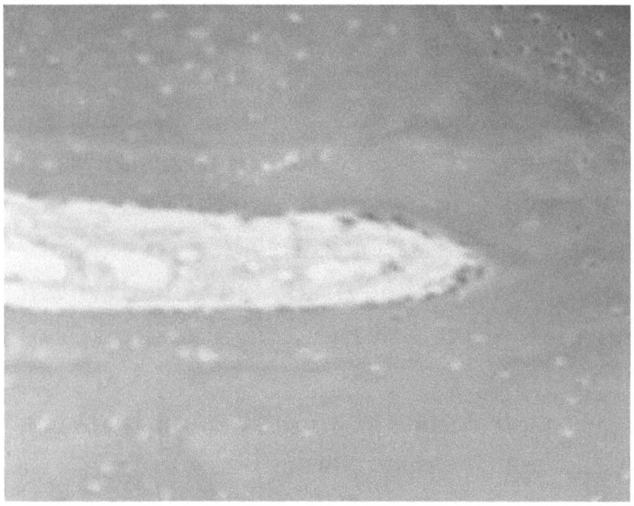

Fig. 4. A typical remodeling unit with osteoclasts located in the "head" and osteoblasts situated on the lateral walls (Hematoxylin and Eosin, original magnification: x 125)

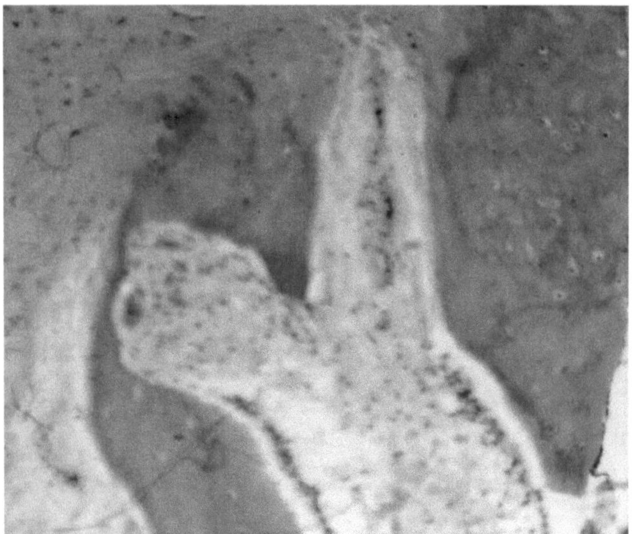

Fig. 5. A remodeling unit where capillaries follow the osteoclastic double "head" (Hematoxylin and Eosin, original magnification: x 125)

Callus Formation After Operative Treatment

After operative treatment osteosynthesis remarkably modifies bone healing.

Studies of this kind of callus formation have often shown controversial results, depending on the method of fracture treatment.

Internal Fixation: Parosteal Synthesis

Plate fixation, characterized by remarkable stability and rigidity, implies two aspects of surgery that are particularly deleterious in fracture repair: hematoma removal and the periosteal wound (more or less serious).

As a consequence, periosteal callus (or external callus or peripheral callus), whose formation is stimulated by moderate mobility of the fracture focus, is not present in case of stable fixation whereas it can be observed on the opposite side of the plate: cartilaginous tissue areas can be seen inside it, as a sign of a certain degree of instability.

The periosteal callus ossifies around the 12th week in the form of primary bone, initially not directed longitudinally but in all spatial directions.

The fundamental role of marrow callus, whose importance was neglected for a long time, has recently been acknowledged by different authors [2, 18–21]. In particular, McKibbin [2] underlined its importance in the substitution of missing tissue mainly in the filling of the fracture gap. The marrow callus does not have the mechanical characteristics of periosteal callus but is fundamental for cortical callus formation. The marrow callus has the appearance of a double-concave disk, which peripherically adheres to the endosteum.

After 6 weeks the callus that is formed by immature bone completely occupies the marrow channel at the fracture site. From this stage on, vessels are observed which, starting from the marrow, penetrate the cortical gap. Around the vessels granulation tissue develops first and then osteoid substance, which turns into woven bone. Woven bone appears to be continuous with the marrow callus and proceeds from the marrow towards the external bone area [2, 4]. The immature bone becomes lamellar around the 12th week.

This cortical callus formation (gap healing or gap repair) can be observed as described above in cases of stable osteosynthesis, in which an interfragmentary space is present. In cases of osteosynthesis with perfect contact among the fragments, the healing is produced by the direct passing of osteons (contact healing or primary fracture healing or direct fracture healing).

As described by Danis [22] and by Schenk [19], at the fracture line the so-called "cutterheads" cross into the opposite fragment, imitating the remodeling process (generally occurring in the diaphyseal cortex); this takes place according to the ARF scheme (activation, resorption, formation). In conclusion, this process does not strictly correspond to callus formation (because new bone production is not observed) but rather to remodeling.

Bone is remodeled thanks to many BMU in which the osteoclastic destructive activity is more rapid and livelier than in the lamellar new bone setting by the osteoblasts. This triggers a temporary characteristic spongy aspect of the cortical bone, which should not be considered a structural modification but rather as the final rebuilding stage.

Internal Fixation: Intramedullary Osteosynthesis

Fractures treated with intramedullary nailing consolidate mainly by forming an abundant external callus. There are two explanations for this: (1) the fixation is not rigid and the nail allows movement at the fracture site; and (2) during reaming in preparation for nailing, the hematoma is extruded under pressure in and around the fracture site with osteoprogenitor cells and other osteoinductive factors without the need for migratory agents. As a consequence, a rich new periosteal bone formation is induced [23].

External Fixation

Taking into account the extreme variety of devices that can be grouped into external axial fixation and external circular fixation, both the biologic process of fracture repair with abundant periosteal cells and the process of gap and contact healing type can be seen with external fixation.

New periosteal bone usually forms when less rigid fixation is applied, whereas bone healing of both the gap and the contact type can be observed if the external fixation device configuration is made more elastic [24, 25].

References

1. Ham AW, Harris WR (1971) Repair and transplantation. In: Bourne GH (ed) Biochemistry and physiology of bone. Academic Press, New York, pp 57–74
2. McKibbin B (1978) The biology of fracture healing in long bones. J Bone Joint Surg Br 60:150–162
3. Frost HM (1989) The biology of fracture healing. Clin Orthop Relat Res 248:283–309
4. Meyrueis JP, Cazenave A (2004) Consolidation des fractures. Encycl Méd Chir 14-031-A-20:1-17, Elsevier, Paris
5. Mizuno K, Mineo K, Tachibana T et al (1990) The osteogenic potential of fracture haematoma. Subperiosteal and intramuscular transplantation of the haematoma. J Bone Joint Surg Br 72:822–829
6. Bruder SP, Jaiswal N, Ricalton NS et al (1998) Mesenchymal stem cells in osteobiology and applied bone regeneration. Clin Orthop Relat Res 355 [Suppl]:247–256
7. Revell P (1986) Pathology of bone. Springer, Berlin Heidelberg New York
8. Baud CA, Auil E (1971) Osteocyte differential count in normal human alveolar bone. Acta Anat 78:321–327

9. Vaananen HK, Salo J, Lehenkari P (1996) Mechanism of osteoclast-mediated bone resorption. J Bone Miner Metab 14:187–192
10. Tylkovsky CM, Wezeman FA, Ray RD (1976) Hormonal effects on the morphology of bone defect healing. Clin Orthop Relat Res 115:274–285
11. Northmore-Ball MD, Wood MR, Meggitt BF (1980) A biomechanical study of the effects of growth hormone in experimental fracture healing. J Bone Joint Surg Br 62:391–396
12. Ray RD (1973) The role of pituitary and thyroid in the healing of standard bone defects. J Bone Joint Surg Br 55:442–447
13. Sissons HA, Hadfield GJ (1954) The influence of cortisone on the repair of experimental fractures in the rabbit. Br J Surg 38:172–176
14. Lieberman J, Daluiski A, Einhorn TA (2002) The role of growth factors in the repair of bone: biology and clinical applications. J Bone Joint Surg Am 84:1032–1044
15. Cho TJ, Gerstenfeld LC, Barnes GL (2001) Cytokines and fracture healing. Curr Opin Orthop 12:403–408
16. Einhorn TA (1994) Enhancement of fracture healing by molecular or physical means: an overview. In: Brighton CT, Friedlander GE, Lane JM (eds) Bone formation and repair. AAOS, Rosemont (Illinois), pp 223–238
17. Alberts B, Bray D, Lewis J et al (1983) Molecular biology of the cell. Garland, New York
18. Rhinelander FW (1974) Tibial blood supply in relation to fracture healing. Clin Orthop Relat Res 105:34–81
19. Schenk R (1986) Histopathology of bone remodelling and bone repair. In: Lin OC, Chao EY (eds) Perspectives on biomaterials. Materials Science Monographs, vol 33, Elsevier, Paris
20. Ilizarov G (1989) The tension-stress effect on the genesis and growth of tissues. Clin Orthop Relat Res 238:249–281
21. Markel M, Wikenheiser MA, Chao EY (1991) Formation of bone in tibial defects in a canine model. Histomorphometric and biomechanical studies. J Bone Joint Surg Am 73:914–922
22. Danis R (1949) Théorie et pratique de l'ostéosynthèse. Masson, Paris
23. Oni OO (1996) Callus formation during diaphyseal fracture repair. Orthopaedics 4:269–277
24. Ilizarov G, Green SA (1992) Transosseous osteosynthesis. Springer, Berlin Heidelberg New York
25. Volkov MV, Oganesian O (1978) Treatment of lesions of bones and joints by the devices of Authors. Meditsina, Tashkent

Assessment of Fracture Healing

Luisella Pedrotti, Barbara Bertani, Redento Mora

Introduction

Markel and Chao [1] underlined that long bone fractures consolidate without complications in most patients. Moreover, in patients in whom the use of complex monitoring techniques of fracture healing was indicated, these techniques were often in an experimental stage and hardly available, and their use was limited to the study of some selected bone segments.

For these reasons the techniques most commonly employed to assess fracture repair until a few years ago included: subjective criteria (patient's evaluation of pain), objective criteria (manual examination of the fracture stability), temporal criteria (simple passage of time), and instrumental criteria (radiographic evidence of consolidation).

In brief, if bone healing conditions are normal, traditional methods of monitoring are considered adequate. In particular, radiographic investigation is the most important method because it is the simplest, it provides continuous information, and it is easily used for iterative interpretations [2].

Radiographic Evaluation

Radiographic criteria of consolidation generally include these features: in the first month you can see demineralization, with broadening of the fracture line and sometimes a shadow showing the fibrous callus formation (Fig. 1). In the second month, you notice the appearance of peripheral callus and little bone bridges, whereas the solution of continuity begins to fade. In the third month (or even later) the bone trabeculae extend from one fragment to the other, the solution of continuity dissolves, and the callus formation is completed (Fig. 2).

Clearly, many variations of this scheme can be observed, according to kind and place of the fracture and the different treatments.

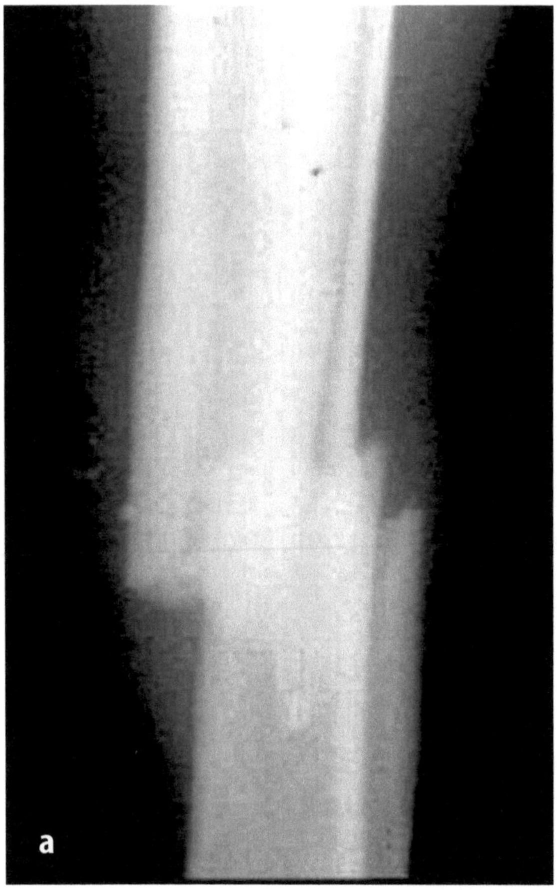

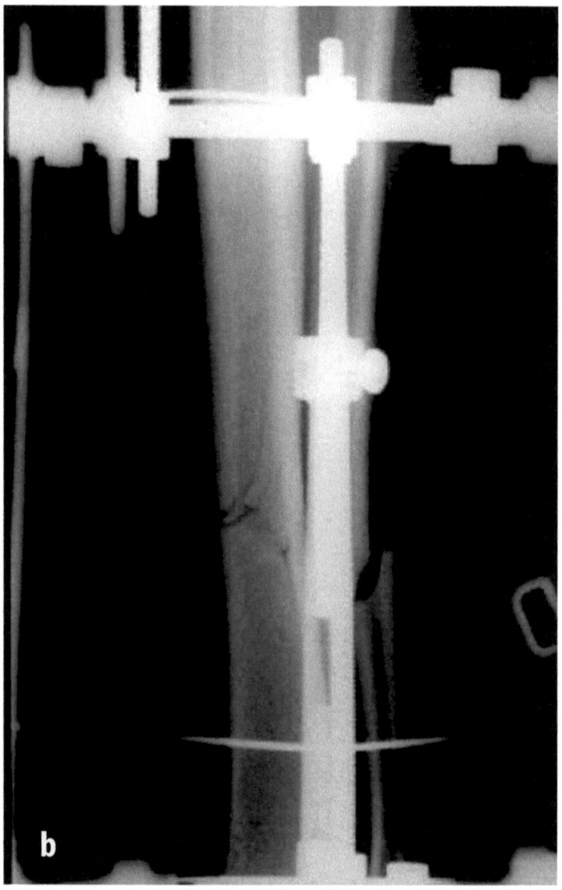

Fig. 1a, b. X-ray of a fresh fracture of the leg (**a**) after reduction and stabilization with an Ilizarov external fixation device (**b**)

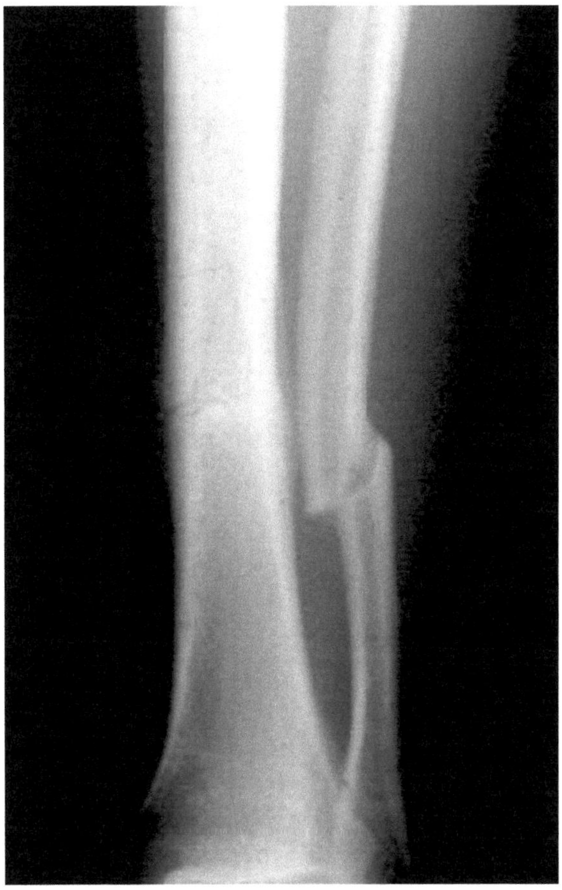

Fig. 2. Same case as in Fig. 1. X-ray at the end of treatment with complete formation of bone callus

Alternative Methods

Conversely, in cases where the consolidation process is abnormal, alternative methods of instrumental investigation can provide more useful information and are necessary to make quick decisions about treatment changes, too. To sum up, noninvasive techniques for fracture healing assessment have some important advantages [1]:

- Prediction of normal and abnormal consolidation;
- They can help make a decision about the beginning of weight bearing;
- Evaluation of timing of fixation device removal.

The ideal characteristics of these noninvasive techniques should be as follows [1]:

- The ability to quantify the state of bone union and to detect abnormal bone healing early in the course of fracture treatment;
- The ability to quantify the real state of bone healing in patients with radiographic and clinical signs of delayed union;
- The ability to evaluate the quality of the gap tissue in patients with established nonunion.

To date, the most commonly used techniques for the noninvasive assessment of fracture healing are: ultrasound (US) evaluation, which provides morphological qualitative information, and extensimetric monitoring, which in contrast, provides functional-quantitative information.

US Evaluation

The US evaluation of bone callus formation has the double advantage of reducing the total amount of radiographic examinations carried out during the treatment (since US can periodically be used instead) and of indicating the early stages of the callus formation during the first 4 weeks, during which the radiographic examination cannot provide useful information [3–6].

In fact, the cortex of long bones is a linear structure which is extremely important in US images: it represents the target of the scanning and splits the echographic image into a superficial zone, which is represented by the soft tissues, and a deep zone, namely, the artifacts' zone, in which it is possible to point out reverberations with longitudinal morphology which simulate a second cortical bone.

Some echographic phases in the evolutionary morphology of the bone callus in a long bone fracture treated by external fixation can be distinguished [7]:

- The first phase (7–10 days): an evident gap is demonstrated between the two cortices with clear-out margins; sometimes a hypoechogenic area with shading margin may be seen related to the hematoma (Fig. 3).

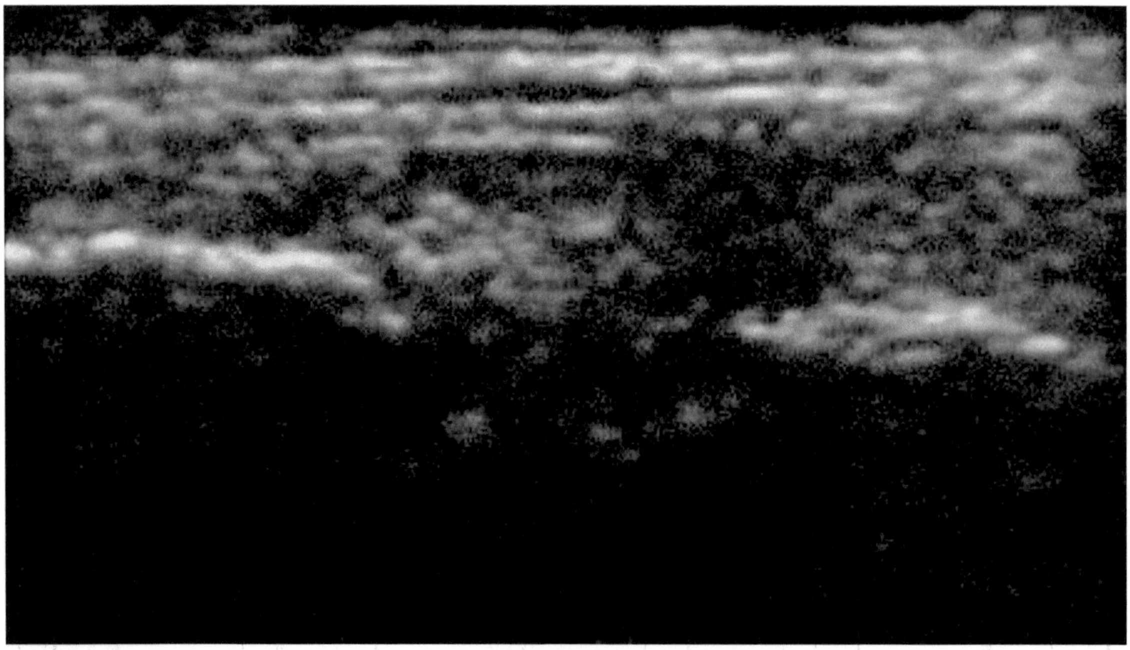

Fig. 3. Ultrasonographic evaluation of bone callus: first phase

- The second phase (10–25 days): two kinds of formations can be observed related to the periostal collars that tend to meet from the two sides of the fracture filling the gap. If the fracture has an ideal strain, a global formation is evident; in overstressed fractures or in inadequately fixed ones, a cuspidal structure can be observed (Fig. 4).

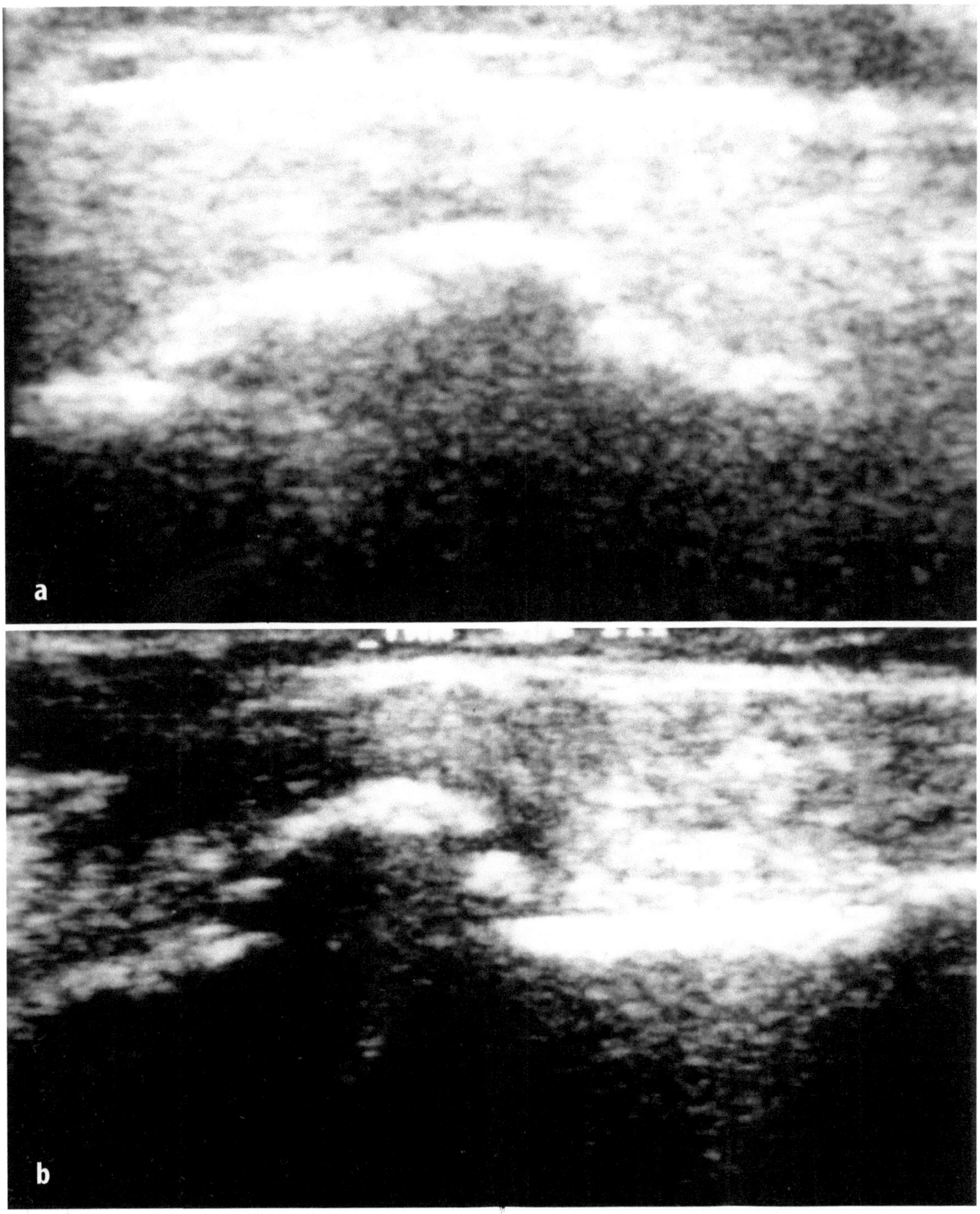

Fig. 4a, b. *Ultrasonographic evaluation of bone callus: second phase.* a Global structure. b Cuspidal structure

- The third phase (25–35 days): the echo reflected by the focus increases in intensity according to the initial callus calcification; the collars meet in one hyperecogenic convex, bridge-shaped structure on the fracture gap.
- The fourth phase (35–50 days): the hyperecogenic structure represents a clear obstacle to the ultrasounds, and an acoustic shadow appears below the newly formed periosteal callus according to its progressive calcification (Fig. 5a).
- The fifth phase (50–90 days): the cortex is being rebuilt. In the deep area the reverberation artifacts reappear parallel to the cortical bone which is the scanning object.

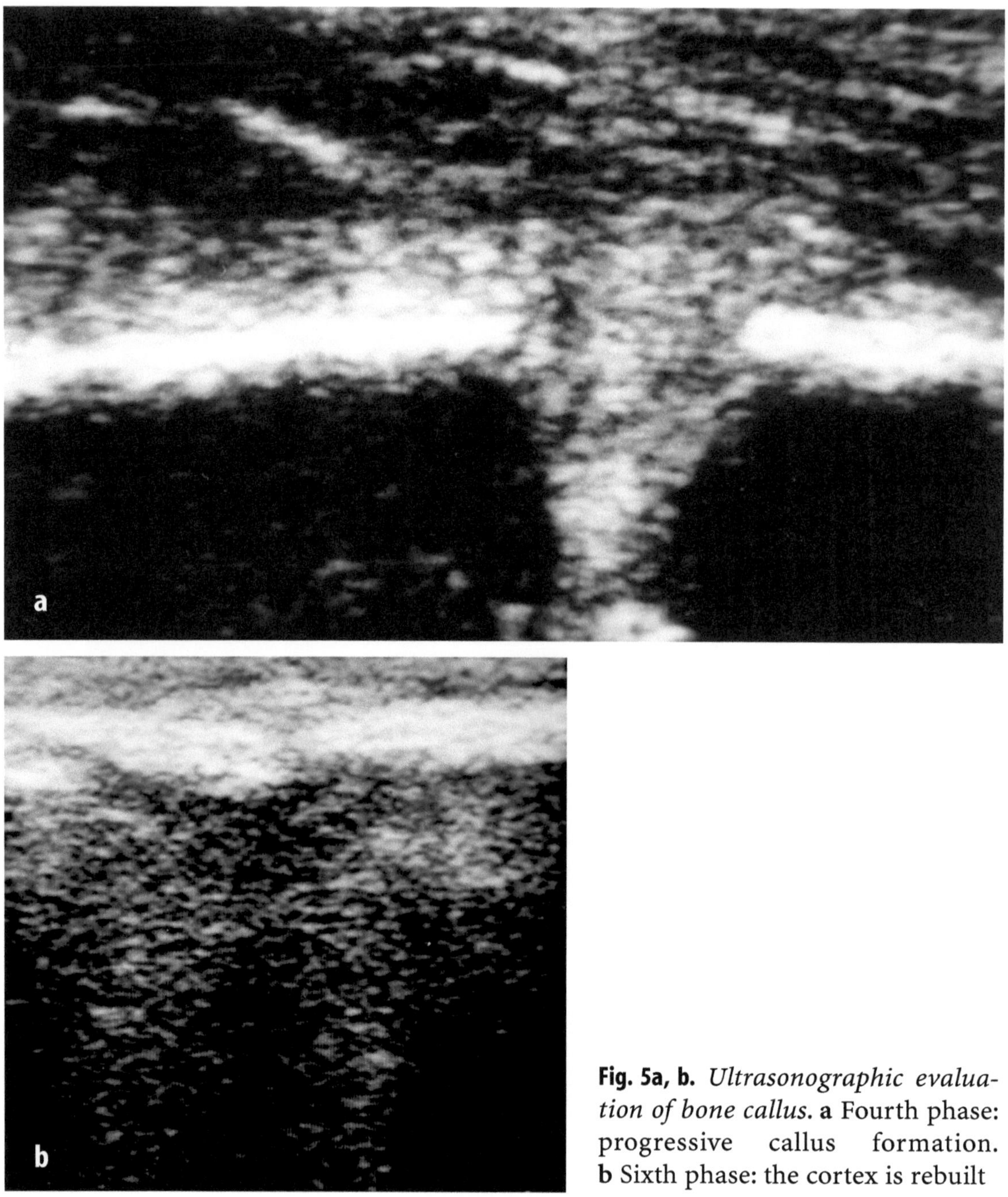

Fig. 5a, b. *Ultrasonographic evaluation of bone callus.* **a** Fourth phase: progressive callus formation. **b** Sixth phase: the cortex is rebuilt

- The sixth phase (90–140 days): the bone callus image is clearly outlined and appears reduced in volume (Fig. 5b).

Extensimetric Monitoring

The echographic controls described provide information on the morphologic aspects and on the biological state of the bone tissue but they allow only an indirect evaluation of its mechanical strength. Furthermore, it is often difficult to choose the right moment for fixation device removal when assessing the solidity of the skeletal segment being treated. Removing the fixation device too early, in fact, represents the risk of new fracture or collapsing of the newly formed tissue, but removing it too late would be risky as well because of the excessive bone stresses by the fixation device, which may cause a new fracture.

Extensimetric monitoring has been developed to help solve this problem. A further aim is finding out how to restore the mechanical resistance of the fracture focus and that of the bone regeneration site in order to detect any possible delay or consolidation problem beforehand.

Should external osteosynthesis be used, extensimetric monitoring quantifies the mechanical properties of the callus by measuring the deformities of the bone-fixator system at different moments of the consolidation [8]. During the early stages of the treatment, alterations of the fixation device, which has been too elastic or too rigid, might be indicated, whereas in the following stages it is useful to monitor the correct progress of the bone formation.

After the beginning of the rehabilitation up to weight-bearing, extensimetric monitoring quantifies the fracture site strength some days before and after weight bearing is permitted. Determining the allowed load is, in fact, the most difficult decision in treatment with external fixation and its effect is important for the the consolidation process. Therefore, weight-bearing must be allowed at the right moment, extensimetric monitoring providing early and reliable information about the callus and regenerated bone resistance.

The principle on which the extensimetric method is based is well known: the deformation of the external fixation device can be considered as the witness of the callus or bone regenerate deformation. Progressively during treatment, the bone participates in the system resistance even more and the registered deformations become less and less important. The machine functions on the electric resistance variation stress.

In monitoring fractures treated by circular external fixation devices, first of all, a flexion-extension test of the distal joint is carried out, then the " bending" test takes place (deformation when the limb is lifted), and at the end the marching test (regular deambulation allowing the maximum load) is performed [9–11].

In addition to the information about solidity of the bone union, these tests, regularly repeated during the treatment, also provide useful information about the evolutionary stage of the callus and regenerated bone consistency.

In fact, by analyzing the greatest deformation graphic, five stages of treatment, each mechanically different and corresponding to a specific biologic stage, can be identified and a "deformation curve" created (Fig. 6):

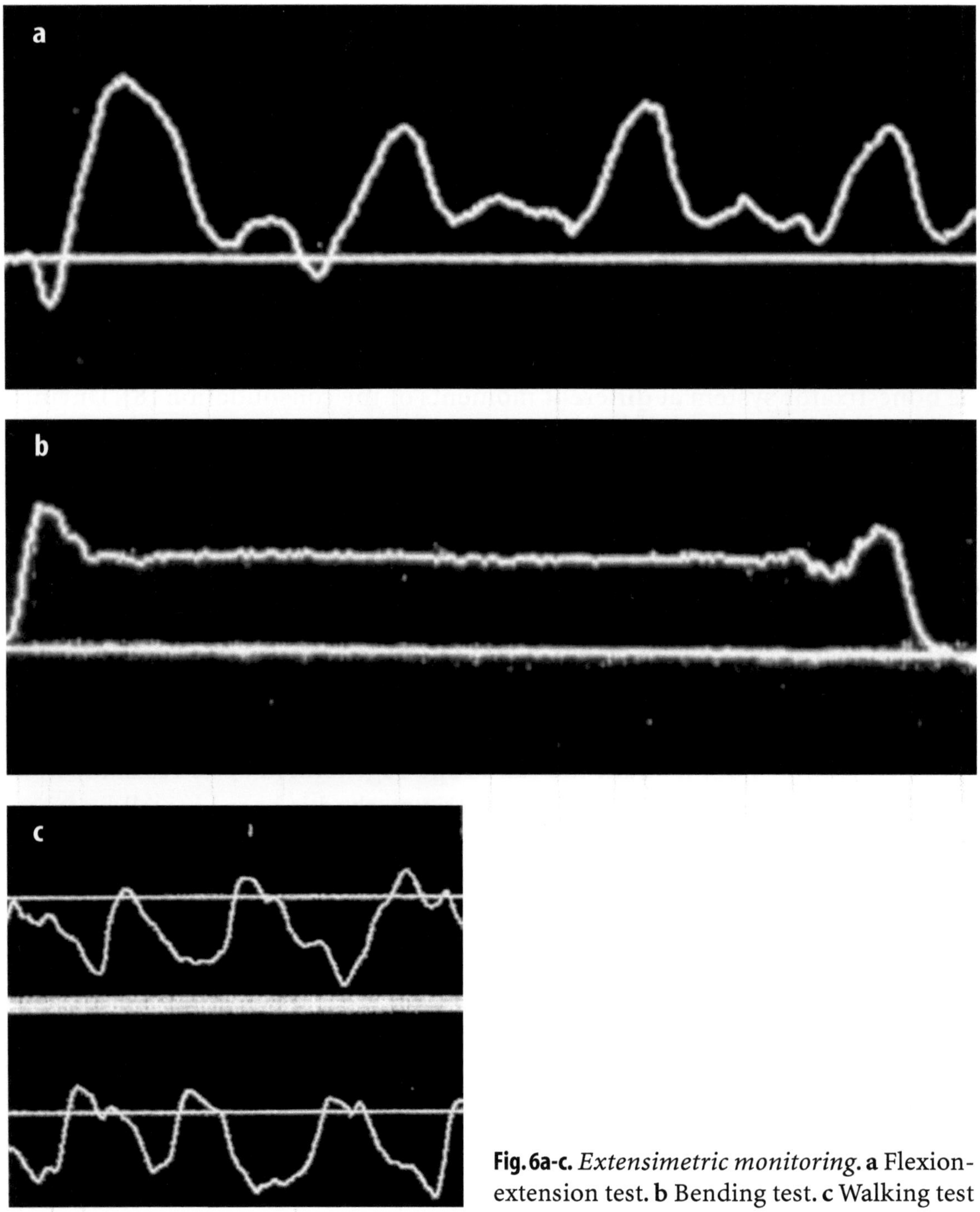

Fig. 6a-c. *Extensimetric monitoring.* **a** Flexion-extension test. **b** Bending test. **c** Walking test

- Initial stage of solidity diminuition (of varying importance and lasting according to the kind of treatment carried out);
- Greatest deformability stage of the system (when the regenerating bone or the procallus, partially calcified, is in an extremely plastic biomechanical condition);
- Rapid reduction stage of the deformability (thanks to the progressive calcification of the regenerated tissue or that of the procallus osteoid trabeculae;
- Mechanical stability stage (with the least deformation values);
- Elasticity reestabilished stage (with deformation levels higher than those registered in the previous stage, probably related to the bone reshaping phenomenon).

If the morphologic-qualitative information (radiographic and echographic tests) correspond to the functional-quantitative ones (exstensimetric data), once the fourth stage is reached, the removal of the external fixation device can usually be planned.

References

1. Markel MD, Chao EY (1993) Noninvasive monitoring techniques for quantitative description of callus mineral content and mechanical properties. Clin Orthop Relat Res 293:37–45
2. Massare C, Evrard J (1976) Critères de consolidation des fractures des os longs de l'adulte. Rev Chir Orthop 62[Suppl. 2]:177–186
3. Abendschein W, Hyatt GW (1970) Ultrasonics and selected physical properties of bone. Clin Orthop Relat Res 69:294–301
4. Gerlanc M, Haddad D, Hyatt GW et al (1975) Ultrasonic study of normal and fractured bone. Clin Orthop Relat Res 111:175–180
5. Dzene II, Dzenis VV, Petukhova LI et al (1980) Human tibia in the presence of coxarthrosis and fracture using exponential ultrasonic concentrators. Mekhanika Kompozitnykh Materialov 6:1081–1087
6. Carlini C, Aldegheri R (1982) Studio sperimentale del callo osseo mediante ultrasuoni. Chir Organi Mov 68:33–39
7. Ricciardi L, Perissinotto A, Dabalà M (1993) Mechanical monitoring of fracture healing using ultrasound imaging. Clin Orthop Relat Res 293:71–76
8. Burny F (1968) Étude par strain gauges de la consolidation des fractures en clinique. Acta Orthop Belg 34:917–925
9. Ceffa R, Perissinotto A (1995) Strain analysis. In: Bianchi Maiocchi A (ed) Advances in Ilizarov apparatus assembly. Medicalplastic, Milan, pp 15, 16
10. Ceffa R, Bombelli M, Boero S et al (1997) Extensimetric monitoring of healing in the treatment with the Ilizarov apparatus–a multicenter clinical trial. Bull Hosp Joint Dis 56:41–45
11. Mora R (2000) Tecniche di compressione-distrazione. Amplimedical, Milano

Section II
Nonunions: General Features

Failure of Union

Redento Mora, Luisella Pedrotti, Giovanni Battista Galli

Definitions of Delayed Union and Nonunion

"Despite the improvement in the understanding of fracture repair and treatment techniques...delayed unions and nonunions occur all too frequently in our violent society..." [1].

Delayed union is a mainly clinical diagnosis, "a clinical entity of a slowly healing fracture" [2]. It is defined as the failure of a fracture to heal in the usual period of time, depending on the type and site of fracture and on the bone and soft tissue damage. Upon physical examination generally some tenderness and mild movement are observed; x-ray findings highlight a certain degree of callus formation but radiolucency at the fracture site.

Nonunion is defined as the failure of a fracture to heal in twice the usual period of time (at least 6 months after trauma); the fracture gap is bridged by fibrous tissue or fibrocartilage instead of bone tissue. The main clinical signs are tenderness and presence of micromotion. Radiographic signs include: persistent fracture line, bone end sclerosis, hypertrophic callus formation or atrophic bone resorption, and possibly radiolucency around osteosynthetic devices.

Pseudoarthrosis (or synovial pseudoarthrosis) is defined as a fracture that has failed to heal and in which a cleft is observed between the bone ends. This cavity is fluid-filled and lined by a membrane. Radiographic examination very often shows a typical "mortar and pestle" bone configuration.

Epidemiology

About 70 million trauma injuries occur annually in the United States. Most of these involve the musculoskeletal system, and lower extremity injuries account for 31% of the total [3, 4].

Only a small percentage of fractures (between 2% and 7%) [5] result in delayed unions or nonunions. Heppenstall [6] reported that of the 2 million long bone fractures sustained each year in the United States, about 100,000 resulted in nonunions and an even larger number in delayed unions.

The distribution among the long bones has changed over the years: Boyd et al. [7] reported a similar distribution among the tibia, femur, humerus, and forearm. In the series of Connolly [8] the tibia was the predominant location (62% of cases). Weitzel and Esterhai [1] also reported a location predominance in the tibia (45% of cases).

The incidence of delayed union and nonunion is higher in open diaphyseal fractures. The reported rate of delayed union in lower grade open tibial shaft fractures (Gustilo types I, II and IIIA) varies from 16% to 60% and in higher grade open tibial shaft fractures (Gustilo types IIIB and IIIC) [9] ranges from 43% to 100% [10, 11].

Classification

Many types of nonunion classifications have been proposed. Unfortunately these classifications have a common defect: they are based on morphological or topographical appearance and not on the reason for the pathological condition.

The preliminary and most important classification is obviously the classification into noninfected and infected nonunions, based on the presence or not of infection.

Noninfected Nonunions

Noninfected nonunions were classified by Judet et al. [12] and later by Weber and Cech [13] into hypertrophic/hypervascular and atrophic/avascular by radiographic, scintigraphic, and histologic appearance, according to the viability of the ends of the fragments.

Scintigraphic studies show a rich blood supply in the hypertrophic types and a poor blood supply in the ends of fragments in the atrophic types. Hypertrophic/hypervascular nonunions are further subdivided by Weber and Cech [13] as follows:

- Elephant foot nonunions: highly hypertrophic and rich in callus. They occur after unstable fixation or premature weight-bearing.
- Horse hoof nonunions: mildly hypertrophic and poor in callus. They typically occur after a moderately unstable immobilization.
- Oligotrophic nonunions: not hypertrophic with absence of callus. They generally occur after fracture displacement or distraction of the fragments.

Atrophic/avascular nonunions are subdivided as follows:

- Torsion wedge nonunions: characterized by the presence of an intermediate fragment with decreased blood supply;
- Comminute nonunions: characterized by the presence of one or more intermediate necrotic fragments;
- Defect nonunions: characterized by the loss of a diaphyseal fragment. These types are observed after open fractures or sequestration in osteomyelitis;
- Atrophic nonunions: final result when intermediate fragments are missing; the ends of the fragments are osteoporotic and atrophic.

The Paley classification of tibial nonunions [14] is based on bone loss, fracture laxity, deformity, and shortening. These parameters are then employed as a guide for treatment with the Ilizarov method. According to this classification:

Type A nonunions have less than 1 cm of bone loss and are subdivided into:

- A-1: lax nonunions
- A-2: stiff nonunions
- A-2-1: stiff nonunions without deformity
- A-2-2: stiff nonunions with deformity

Type B nonunions have more than 1 cm of bone loss and are subdivided into:

- B-1: nonunions with bone defect but not shortening
- B-2: nonunions with shortening but no bone defect
- B-3: nonunions with shortening and bone defect.

Infected Nonunions

Infected nonunions are generally classified according to the infection extent and the bone stability.

Cierny et al. [15] divided osteomyelitis into four anatomic types, based on the local extent of the infection:

- Type 1: medullary osteomyelitis
- Type 2: superficial osteomyelitis
- Type 3: localized osteomyelitis
- Type 4: diffuse infection

Each type is further subdivided into three physiologic classes, based on systemic characteristics:

- A: hosts physiologically normal
- B: hosts with local or systemic compromise to wound and fracture healing
- C: hosts with high risk of complications in case of surgical treatment.

Umiarov's classification [16] divides infected nonunions into four types, based on the viability of bone ends, the presence of limb shortening, the presence of bone, and soft tissue defect.

- In the first type the nonunion is normotrophic without shortening
- In the second type the nonunion is hypertrophic with shortening
- In the third type the nonunion is atrophic with shortening
- In the fourth type the nonunion is atrophic with bone and soft tissue defect, in general as a result of an open fracture, with extensive soft tissue damage, complicated by infection and loss of bone substance.

May et al. [17] proposed a classification of post-traumatic osteomyelitis of tibia (based on the size of the tibial defect and the conditions of the fibula) into five types. Types III, IV, and V involve nonunions.

- Type III: tibial defect of 6 cm or less with intact fibula
- Type IV: tibial defect larger than 6 cm with intact fibula
- Type V: tibial defect larger than 6 cm with no usable fibula.

Pathogenesis

Multiple systemic or local adverse factors, singly or in combination, can influence fracture repair and cause nonunion [18, 19], and every effort to minimize the impact of these factors must be made during the fracture treatment. Systemic factors include:

- Age
- Nutritional status
- Systemic diseases
- Corticosteroid therapy
- Metabolic bone diseases
- Tumors
- Antineoplastic drugs

Local factors include:

- Vascular supply
- Fracture level
- Reduction (distraction, compression)
- Immobilization
- Injury to the soft tissues
- Local radiation therapy
- Infection.

To this day, the precise etiology of a nonunion is often unclear, especially when an adequate treatment, with reduction and immobilization of the fracture, has been carried out.

Histology

Microscopic investigations of delayed unions and nonunions in humans are surprisingly rare; therefore, recently conducted studies have improved our knowledge of this subject.

On light microscopic investigations, delayed unions show callus formation and interfragmentary fibrous or fibrocartilaginous tissue, with slow progression towards fracture repair [1].

Andrew et al. [20] observed an inactive and avascular histologic pattern, correlated with the radiologic finding of a sclerotic end cap across the medullary canal, in both radiologically atrophic and hypertrophic nonunions. They concluded that there is not any consistent difference in the histologic appearance of the tissue in the fracture gap.

However, in the opinion of most authors, atrophic and hypertrophic types of nonunions show important histologic differences.

On light microscopy, atrophic nonunions show bundles of disorganized fibrous tissue, collagen fibers, and abundant fibroblasts within the fracture gap. Areas of fibrocartilage can also be observed [1, 21] (Figs. 1, 2).

On electron microscopic studies, the fibroblast-like cells show abundant mitochondria and endoplasmic reticulum within the fibrous tissue; the extracellular matrix is rich in collagen fibrils oriented in all directions [22]. In fibrocartilaginous areas, chondroblasts are surrounded by a matrix rich in collagen fibers, where many dense, nonmineralized vesicles are observed.

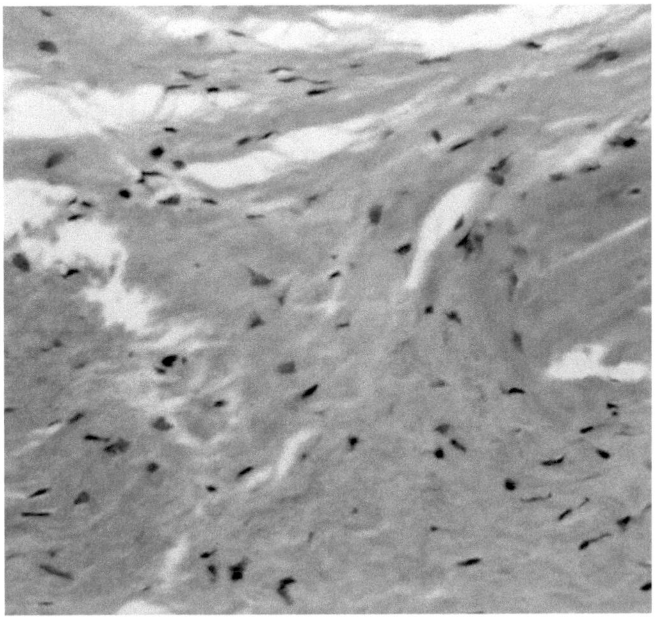

Fig. 1. Microscopic picture of an atrophic nonunion with disorganized fibrous tissue (Hematoxylin and Eosin, original magnification: x 125)

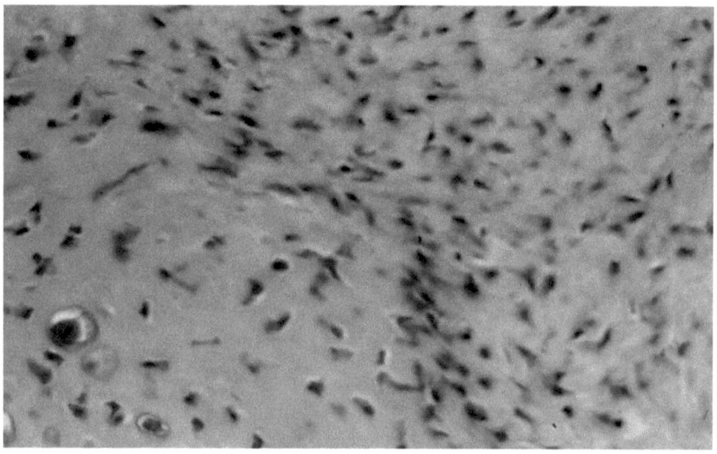

Fig. 2. Atrophic nonunion: the microscopic picture shows an area of cartilaginous tissue (Hematoxylin and Eosin, original magnification: x 125)

In hypertrophic nonunions, fibrocartilaginous tissue with a remarkable tendency towards matrix mineralization (endochondral ossification) is seen on light microscopy. In this tissue osteoid trabeculae are frequently observed. Capillary vessels in the fibrocartilaginous tissue are constantly empty and some of them are clearly closed [23, 24] (Figs. 3, 4).

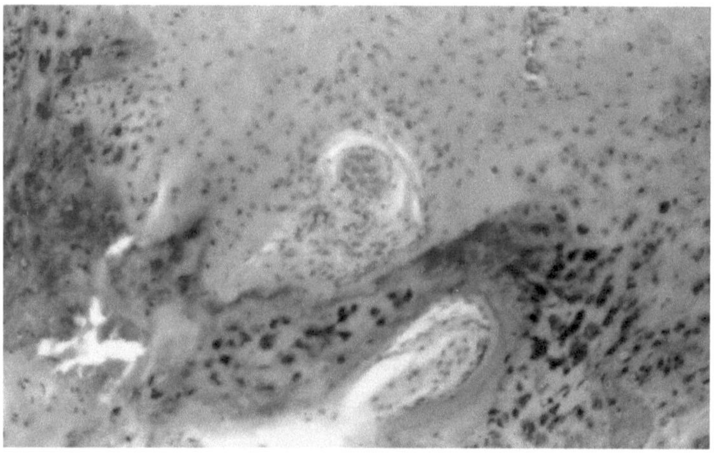

Fig. 3. Histologic feature of a hypertrophic nonunion. In the fibrocartilaginous tissue some osteoid trabeculae are seen (Hematoxylin and Eosin, original magnification: x 125)

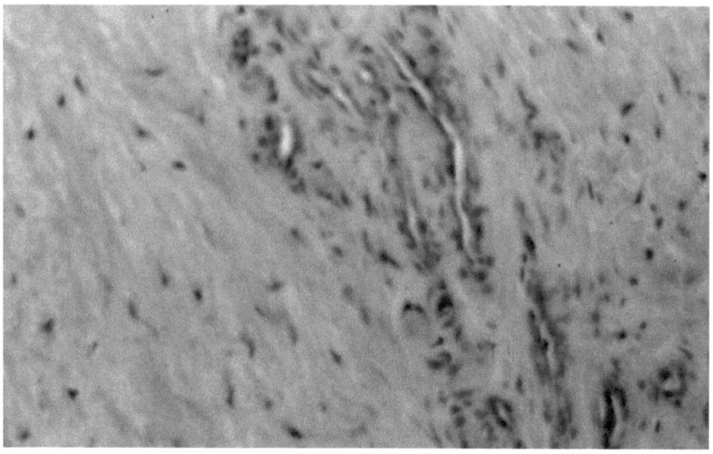

Fig. 4. Hypertrophic nonunion: microscopic feature. Capillary vessels are clearly empty (Hematoxylin and Eosin, original magnification: x 125)

On electron microscopy chondroblasts in mineralized areas show a large cytoplasm with abundant mitochondria and endoplasmic reticulum. Within the matrix numerous dense vesicles, partially containing hydroxyapatite crystals, are seen [22].

Synovial pseudoarthroses may be a late manifestation of more mobile nonunions that progressively tear apart, although in some cases pseudoarthroses may exist from the start.

Microscopic examination shows cleft-like spaces filled with synovial fluid within the soft tissues of the nonunion. True synovial lining cells are absent, but fronds similar to synovial villi are sometimes observed [2, 25].

In infected nonunions, microscopic investigation reveals an acute inflammatory cell exudate within intertrabecular myeloid tissues and trabecular resorption due to necrosis. Vascular local edema, leukocyte activity, and changes in pH all contribute to the bone necrosis [26] (Fig. 5).

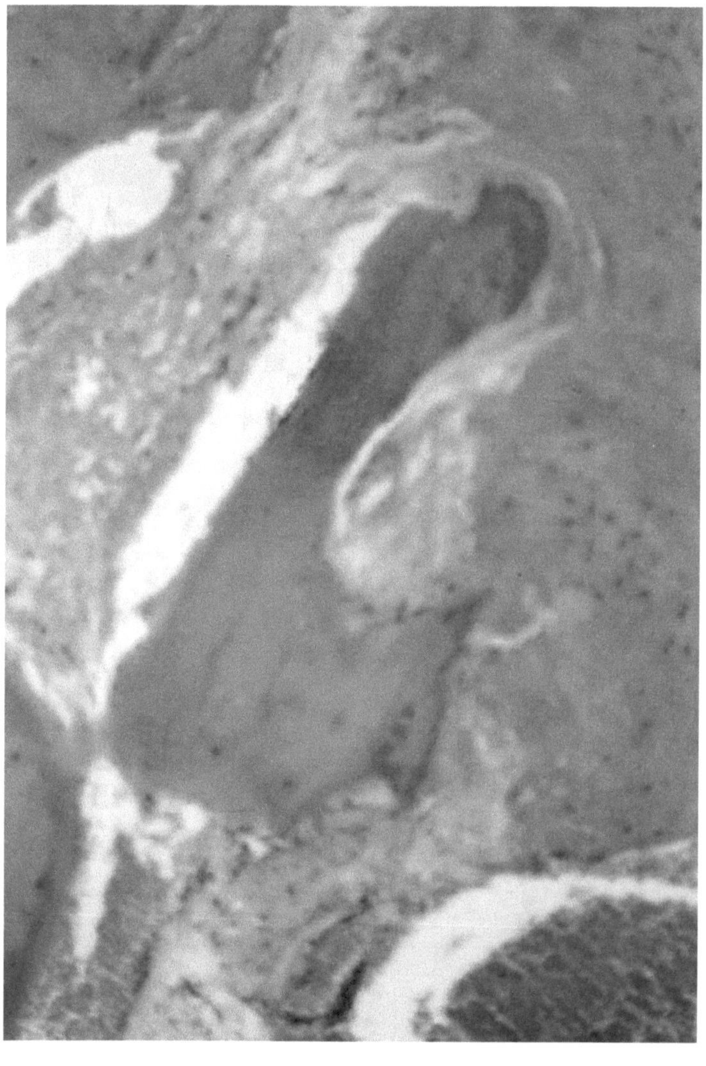

Fig. 5. Histologic feature of an infected nonunion shows inflammatory tissue with trabecular resorption related to bone necrosis (Hematoxylin and Eosin, original magnification: x 125)

Psychological Impact

Evaluation of the patient and of his strength to withstand a complex and long duration of treatment is a matter of utmost importance but often neglected: generally little attention is directed to treating the patient's psyche [27]. Patients often experience depression, analgesic drug addiction, and also altered sexuality as a consequence of complex orthopaedic problems that require prolonged care such as multiple hospitalizations, repeated operations, and prolonged periods of immobilization. The patients need to be treated by the orthopaedic surgeon as a "whole person" instead of an "ununited fracture".

In the preliminary interviews, it is necessary that the patient gains (with the help of drawings or photographs) a full comprehension and acceptance of the kind, length, and inconveniences of the treatment and of the kind of rehabilitation. Only a conscious and motivated patient can profit from the treatment: as a consequence, the orthopaedic team also must have the right psychological attitude. This attitude has to be complemented by two other qualities, especially if the treatment consists of compression-distraction techniques (i.e., a dynamic treatment that requires frequent adjustments): plenty of time (in connection with the need for clinical controls and device adjustments) and experience (interpreted as complete knowledge of the surgical instruments and techniques and full knowledge of one's own limitations, in order to avoid starting a treatment which is beyond one's ability, and as a source of ideas in order to improve particular techniques or particular treatment guidelines).

Cost Analysis

Analysis of the costs associated with common treatment for fractures, delayed unions, and nonunions confirms that nonunions are costly to treat, requiring multiple procedures and delaying a return to work. The literature concerning this subject is poor, but some interesting publications can help us understand the problem complexity.

It must be emphasized that an exact cost analysis of orthopaedic trauma injuries includes clinical outcomes (such as survival, rates of union or nonunion, and short-term morbidity) and functional outcomes (more difficult to quantify than clinical ones), which can not be defined by clinical examination and radiographic findings (e.g., lost wages, quality of life, return to work, and emotional well-being). Moreover, a cost analysis of orthopaedic trauma injuries must also consider two factors: direct costs (associated with all aspects of treatment) and indirect costs (associated with lost productivity).

A study of the literature shows that indirect costs are not as well documented as direct costs [5]. Furthermore, few studies report cost analyses of traumatic injuries to the long bones: for example, the costs of femoral neck fractures treatment are better documented than costs of long bone diaphyseal fractures in the international literature. It is noteworthy that the elderly incur the highest direct costs, and people between 45 and 64 years incur the highest amount of indirect costs.

Heckman and Sarasohn-Kahn [28] estimated the direct and indirect costs of closed or grade I open tibial shaft fractures treated conservatively by means of cast immobilization or operatively by means of intramedullary nailing in a study aiming to demonstrate that pulsed low-intensity ultrasound therapy shortened the healing time and reduced the incidence of delayed unions. Average costs of conservative treatment were estimated at 27,000 US$, those for operative treatment at 58,000 US$.

Toivanen et al. [29] calculated conservative and operative treatment direct and indirect costs for closed tibial shaft fracture treatment. Average costs were 24,000 US$ for conservative and 17,000 US$ for operative treatment (1/6 direct and 5/6 indirect cost).

Laughlin et al. [30] estimated direct costs in open tibial shaft fracture grade IIIB and IIIC treated with limb salvage. The average initial hospital costs were 33,000 US$; the average costs for additional procedures to achieve union was 15,000 US$ (total 48,000 US$).

Beaver et al. [31] examined the direct costs of tibial nonunion : the average result was 11,000 US$ per patient.

Williams [32], in a very interesting publication, compared the costs of tibial nonunions, infections, and bone defects treated by the Ilizarov method and those treated by amputation:

- Cost of limb reconstruction (~ 59,000 US$)
- Cost of amputation (~ 30,000 US$)
- + long-term cost of prosthetic usage and fabrication (~ 403,000 US$).

These studies are not well comparable because the composition of their cohorts is not in perfect agreement and economic evaluations are different according to the country in which the study was developed. However, they are very interesting because they confirm that costs vary according to the fracture severity. Moreover, in severe, infected nonunions with bone and soft tissue loss, a complete cost analysis clearly demonstrates that the long and difficult reconstructive treatments by means of compression-distraction methods appear to be much less expensive than the easier and apparently cheaper management by amputation.

References

1. Weitzel PP, Esterhai JL (1994) Delayed union, non-union and synovial pseudoarthrosis. In: Brighton CT, Friedlander GE, Lane JM (eds) Bone formation and repair. AAOS, Rosemont (Illinois), pp 505–527
2. Milgram JW (1991) Nonunion and pseudoarthrosis of fracture healing. A histopathologic study of 95 human specimens. Clin Orthop Relat Res 268:203–213
3. Sackett DL, Straus SE, Richardson WS et al (eds) (2000) Evidence-based medicine: how to practice and teach EBM. Churchill Livingstone, London
4. McKenzie EJ, Cushing BM, Jurkovich GJ et al (1993) Physical impairment and functional outcomes six months after severe lower extremity fractures. J Trauma 34: 528–538
5. Saleh KJ, Hak DJ, Nierengarten MB (2001) Socioeconomic burden of traumatic tibial fractures: non union or delayed union. MedScape Orthopaedics Clinical updates, pp 1–22
6. Heppenstall RB (ed) (1980) Fracture treatment and healing. Saunders, Philadelphia
7. Boyd HB, Anderson LD, Johnston DS (1965) Changing concepts in the treatment of non-union. Clin Orthop Relat Res 43:37–54
8. Connolly JF (ed) (1991) Tibial non-union. Diagnosis and treatment. AAOS, Park Ridge (Illinois)
9. Gustilo RB (1989) Orthopaedic infection. Saunders, Philadelphia
10. Sanders R, Jersinovich I, Anglen J et al (1994) The treatment of open tibial shaft fractures using an interlocked intramedullary nail without reaming. J Orthop Trauma 8:504–510
11. Riemer BL, DiChristina DG, Cooper A et al (1995) Nonreamed nailing of tibial diaphyseal fractures in blunt polytrauma patients. J Orthop Trauma 9:66–75
12. Judet R, Judet J, Roy Camille R (1958) La vascularisation des pseudarthroses des os longs d'après une étude clinique expérimentale. Rev Chir Orthop 44:5–14
13. Weber BG, Cech O (eds) (1976) Pseudoarthrosis. Huber, Berne
14. Paley D (1990) Treatment of tibial non-union and bone loss with the Ilizarov technique. Instr Course Lect 39:185–197
15. Cierny G, Mader JT, Penninck JJ (1985) A clinical staging system for adult osteomyelitis. Contemp Orthop 10:17–37
16. Umiarov GA (1986) Classification of nonunions of the long bones complicated by infection, and principles of treatment. Sborn Trud CITO 30:5–9
17. May JW Jr, Jupiter JB, Weiland AJ et al (1989) Clinical classification of post-traumatic tibial osteomyelitis. J Bone Joint Surg Am 71:1422–1428
18. Heiple KG, Herndon CH (1965) The pathologic physiology of non-union. Clin Orthop Relat Res 43:11–21
19. Rodriguez-Merchan EC, Forriol F (2004) Nonunion: general principles and experimental data. Clin Orthop Relat Res 419:4–12
20. Andrew G, Marsh D, Freemont A et al (1995) Histological and radiological appearances of non-union. J Bone Joint Surg Br 77[Suppl. 1]:92
21. Rhinelander FW (1974) Tibial blood supply in relation to fracture healing. Clin Orthop Relat Res 105:34–81
22. Caterini R, Farsetti P, Tudisco C, Bellocci M (1996) Studio istologico ed ultrastrutturale della pseudoartrosi nell'uomo. Giorn Ital Ortop Traumatol 22:109–117
23. Dell'Orbo C, Quacci D, Bartolozzi P et al (1988) Aspetti morfologici del tessuto di pseudoartrosi. Atti SOTIMI 51:93–97
24. Mora R (2000) Tecniche di compressione-distrazione. Amplimedical, Milano
25. Esterhai JL, Brighton CT, Heppenstall RB et al (1981) Detection of synovial pseu-

doarthrosis by 99mTC scintigraphy: application to treatment of traumatic non-union with constant direct current. Clin Orthop Relat Res 161:15–22
26. Revell P (1986) Pathology of bone. Springer, Berlin Heidelberg New York
27. Mora R, Pedrotti L, Benazzo F, Ceciliani L (2000) Stimolazione meccanica della consolidazione nelle pseudoartrosi ipertrofiche mediante osteosintesi in distrazione. Giorn Ital Ortop Traumatol 26:3–8
28. Heckman JD, Sarasohn Kahn J (1997) The economics of treating tibia fractures. The cost of delayed unions. Bull Hosp Joint Diseases 56:63–72
29. Toivanen JA, Hirvonen M, Auvinen O et al (2000) Cast treatment and intramedullary locking nailing for simple and spiral wedge tibial shaft fractures – a cost benefit analysis. Ann Chir Gynaecol 89:138–142
30. Laughlin RT, Smith KL, Russell RC et al (1993) Late functional outcome in patients with tibia fractures covered with free muscle flaps. J Orthop Trauma 7:123–129
31. Beaver R, Brinker MR, Barrack RL (1997) An analysis of the actual cost of tibial nonunions. J La State Med Soc 149:200–206
32. Williams MO (1994) Long term cost comparison of major limb salvage using the Ilizarov method versus amputation. Clin Orthop Relat Res 301:156–158

Section III
NONUNIONS: DIAGNOSIS

Diagnosis

Redento Mora, Luisella Pedrotti, Gabriella Tuvo, Stefano Gili

The differential diagnosis of a fracture that does not show signs of healing includes delayed union, nonunion, synovial pseudoarthrosis, infection, and unrecognized pathological fracture [1]. History, physical examination, laboratory tests, imaging studies, and bone biopsy can give important information about this.

History

A detailed history of the patient with a diaphyseal fracture nonunion must be taken, including: patient nutritional status, systemic diseases, weight, and fracture history (including bone involved, damage to soft tissues, mechanism of fracture, type and duration of treatment, physiologic loading, pain, motion at the fracture site, soft tissue swelling, neurovascular limb compromise, and presence of infection).

Physical Examination

Physical examination contributes information about tenderness, instability (motion, crepitus), pain, functional loss, and possible signs of infection such as swelling, warmth, drainage, and erythema (Fig. 1).

Laboratory Tests (in Noninfected Nonunions)

Laboratory tests including determination of serum albumin levels, total lymphocyte count, and electrolyte values can give indications of nutritional deficiencies. The Westergren erythrocyte sedimentation rate can remain elevated for several months after a fracture.

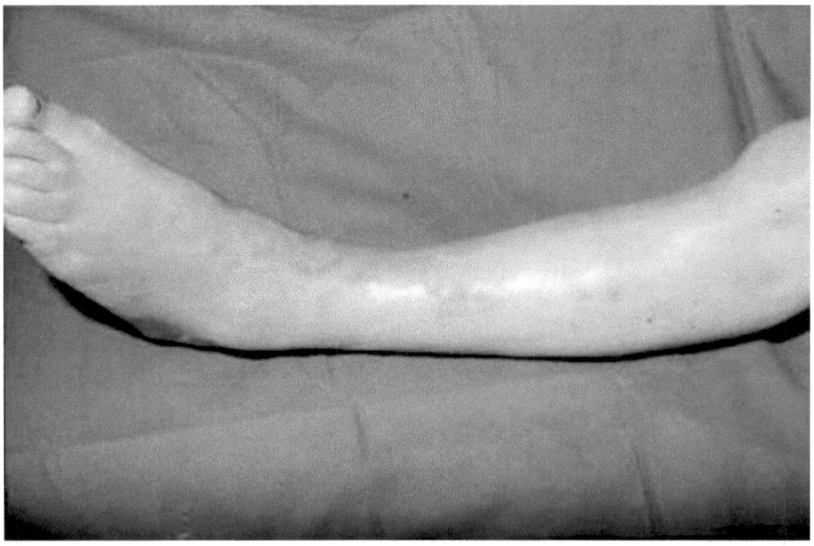

Fig. 1. Clinical feature of a tibial nonunion with deformity and instability at the nonunion site

Imaging Studies (in Noninfected Nonunions)

X-Ray Studies

Four radiographic views (anteroposterior, lateral, and both oblique) are needed to assess long bone nonunion. Furthermore, stress view roentgenograms (obtained during application of varus-valgus or anterior-posterior force to the limb) and fluoroscopic examination are often employed to demonstrate micromovements at the fracture site (Fig. 2).

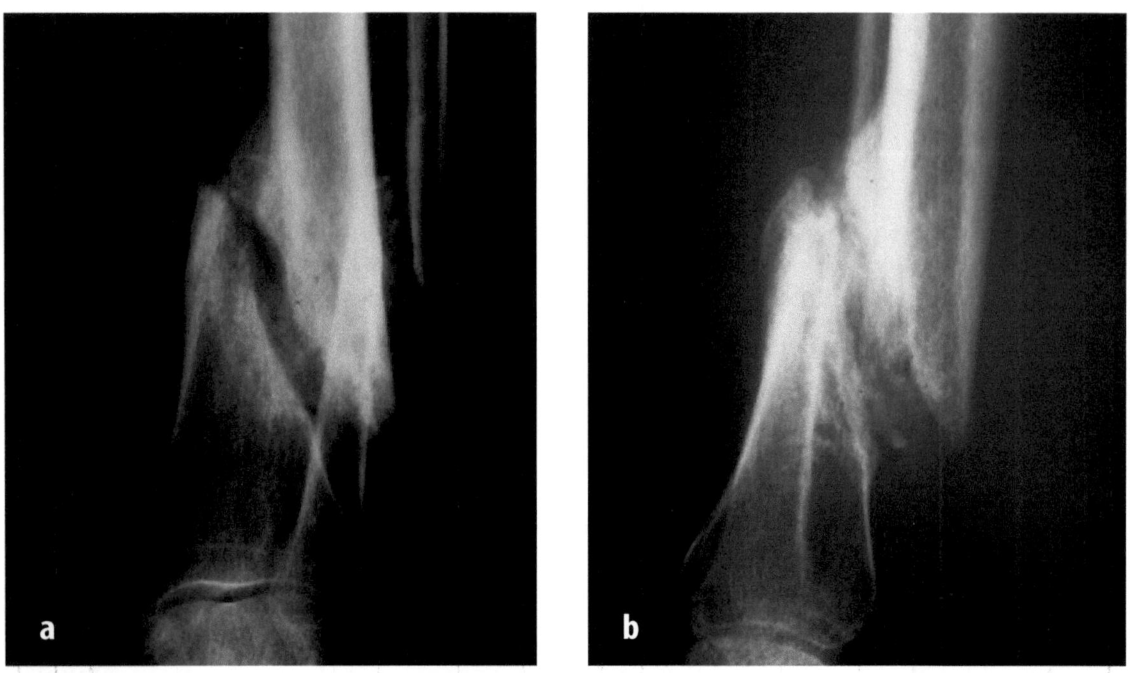

Fig. 2a, b. Anteroposterior (**a**) and lateral (**b**) x-rays of a tibial hypertrophic nonunion

Osteomedulloangiography

Osteomedulloangiography is employed to evaluate whether the medullary circulation at the site of a fracture has been reestablished. Contrast medium is injected, by intraosseous phlebography, into the medullay canal distal to the fracture site and a fluoroscopic examination shows whether it flows across the fracture. If intraosseous veins do not cross the fracture, delayed union or nonunion is very likely [1, 4].

Nuclear Medicine

In cases of noninfected nonunions, technetium methylene diphosphonate scintigraphy has been used to detect the presence of synovial pseudoarthrosis with a high sensitivity: in these cases a cold cleft between two areas of high uptake is generally seen [1]. Furthermore, scintigraphy has gained increased importance in the "functional diagnosis" of nonunion.

Due to the relationship that exists between local bone metabolism (osteogenic activity) and deposition and remodeling of bone tissue [5], scintigraphy is employed to assess nonunion biological activity.

Finally, scintigraphy is a particularly useful technique to distinguish between biologically active and nonresponsive nonunions because this distinction is often clinically and radiographically difficult (Fig. 3).

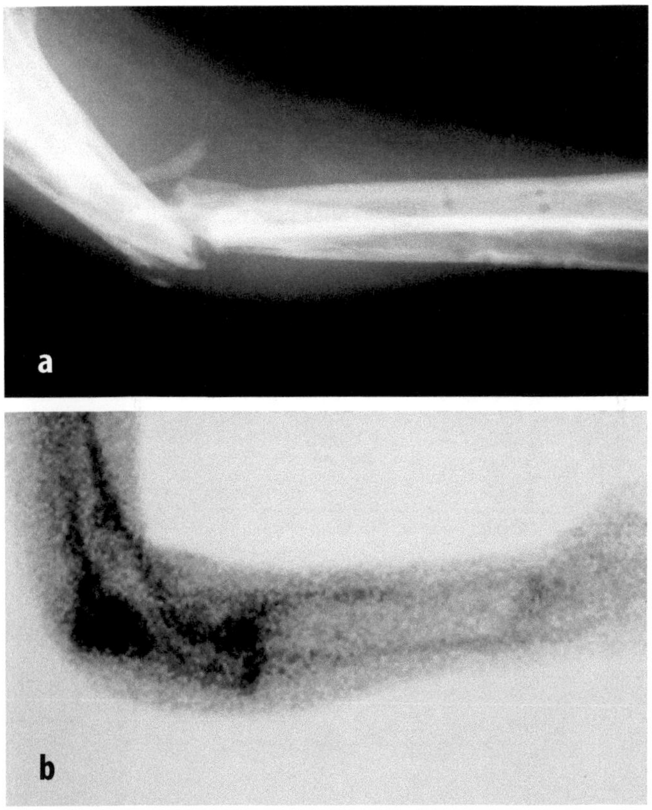

Fig. 3a, b. **a** X-ray of a forearm nonunion where the biological activity at the nonunion site is difficult to assess. **b** TC [99] scintigraphy is very useful to show biological activity

Computed Tomography

In particular cases CT scans can find fracture lines where standard radiogram cannot show persistence of fracture signs, for instance in oblique or spiroid fractures [6].

At the same time this kind of investigation can show the persistence of a fracture line in cases of hypertrophic nonunion with callus abundance (Fig. 4).

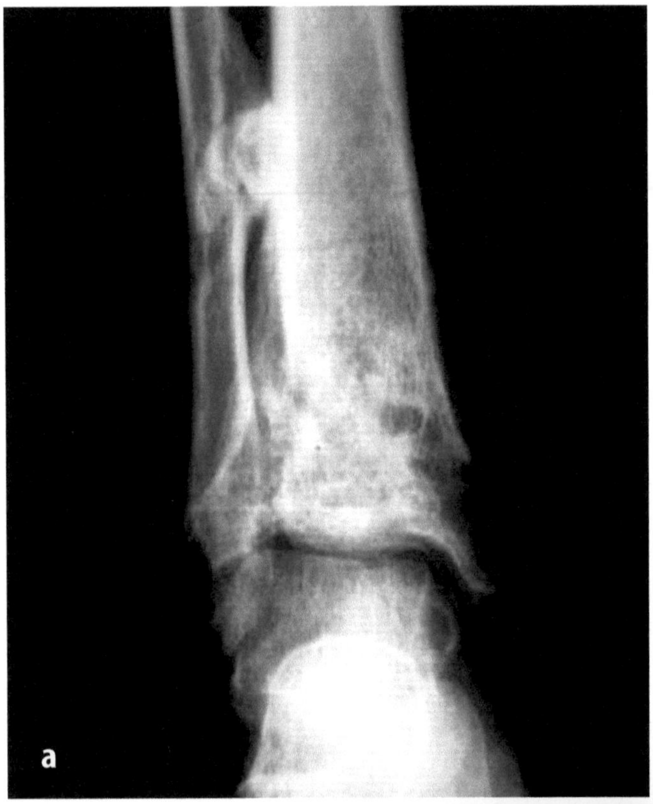

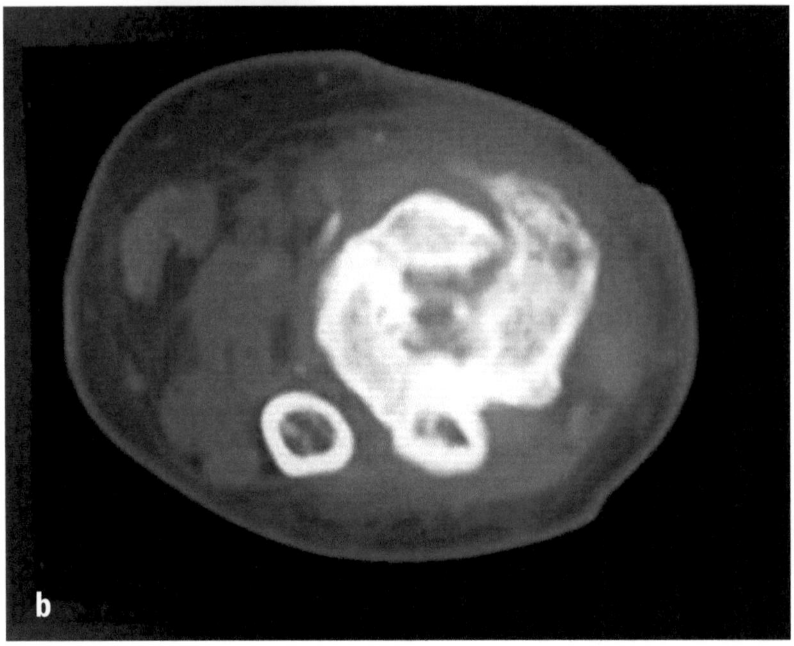

Fig. 4a, b. Combination of x-ray and CT scan of a distal tibial nonunion shows persistence of fracture signs

Magnetic Resonance Imaging

In noninfected nonunion, MRI can accurately visualize the vascular supply of the long bones, thus providing an indication of bone end viability and contributing to making a correct treatment choice [6].

In certain instances, MRI can be enhanced by the injection of an intravenous contrast agent, such as gadolinium (Gd).

Bone Biopsy

A closed or open bone biopsy is sometimes indicated for differential diagnosis of infected or noninfected nonunions, neoplasm, and systemic diseases.

Noninfected hypertrophic nonunions show a rich vascular plexus invading the external callus. Into the fracture gap fibrous or fibrocartilaginous tissue with void capillaries is seen (Fig. 5).

In noninfected atrophic nonunions, fibrous tissue within the fracture is disorganized, and some areas of fibrocartilage are seen (Fig. 6).

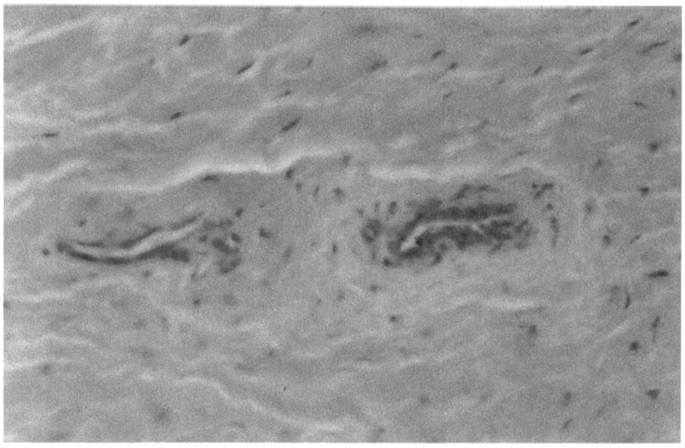

Fig. 5. Histologic feature of a noninfected hypertrophic nonunion: rare and void capillaries are seen into the fracture gap (Hematoxylin and Eosin, original magnification: x 125)

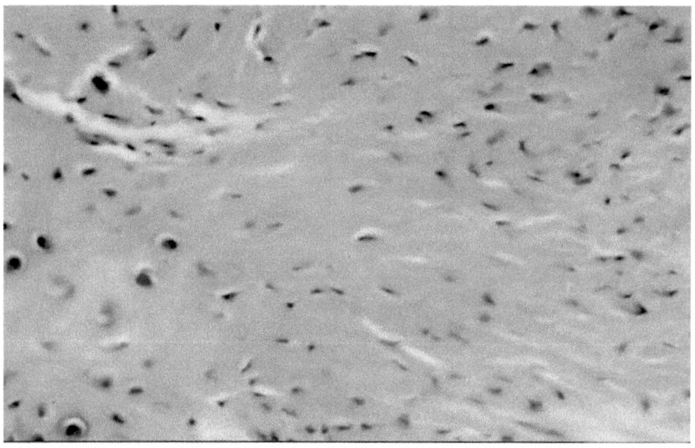

Fig. 6. Microscopic feature of an atrophic nonunion where fibrous tissue with an area of cartilaginous tissue can be observed (Hematoxylin and Eosin, original magnification: x 125)

Infected nonunions show signs of inflammation and trabecular resorption due to necrosis. If infection is suspected, multiple samples must be obtained, but it is often difficult to determine whether a nonunion is infected (Fig. 7). If microbiological investigations are negative or uncertain, histological analysis of specimens taken from the nonunion site are of particular use: a highly inflammatory infiltrate is strongly suggestive of infection [7].

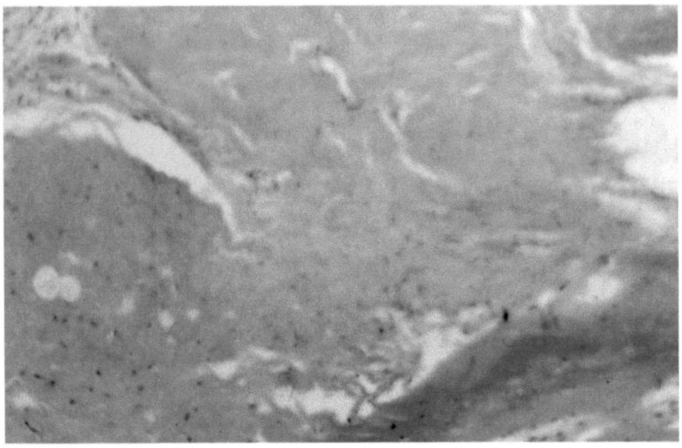

Fig. 7. Microscopic feature of an infected nonunion with sign of inflammation and trabecular bone resorption (Hematoxylin and Eosin, original magnification: x 125)

References

1. Connolly JF (1991) Tibial non-union. Diagnosis and treatment. AAOS, Park Ridge (Illinois)
2. Hammer R, Edholm P, Lindholm B (1984) Stability of union after tibial shaft fracture: analysis by a non-invasive technique. J Bone Joint Surg Br 66:529–534
3. Carrata A, Rampini C, Failoni S (1988) Stato attuale della radiologia in tema di pseudoartrosi diafisaria. Apparato locomotore 2:43–49
4. Puranen J, Punto L (1981) Osteomedulloangiography: a method of estimating the consolidation prognosis of tibial shaft fractures. Clin Orthop Relat Res 161:8–14
5. Weber BG, Cech O (eds) (1976) Pseudoarthrosis. Huber, Berne
6. Weitzel PP, Esterhai JL (1994) Delayed union, non-union and synovial pseudoarthrosis. In: Brighton CT, Friedlander GE, Lane JM (eds) Bone formation and repair. AAOS, Rosemont (Illinois), pp 505–527
7. Simpson AH, Wood MK, Athanasou NA (2002) Histological assessment of the presence or absence of infection in fracture non-union. Injury 33:151–155

Diagnosis of Infection

Anna Maccabruni, Redento Mora

"Awareness of the infection and knowledge of the event of bone compromised by it are important to the surgeon weighing treatment alternatives and forms of actives intervention" [1].

However, infection developing in fractures is often difficult to diagnose and all the useful diagnostic means must be employed.

History

The patient history should include detailed fracture history and assessment of potential presence of infection.

Physical Examination

The patient must be evaluated for signs of infection: fever, chills, diaphoresis, skin and soft tissue status, erythema, warmth, swelling, exudates, and drainage as well as for signs of instability such as motion, crackling, pain, tenderness, and functional loss [strength, range of motion (ROM) of the joint, weight-bearing status].

In particular, the skin often shows the results of multiple previous operations, with scarring and avascularity of the environment around the non-union site; a sinus tract indicates either a dead bone or sequestrum; and limited joint ROM is often observed as a consequence of prolonged immobilization or repeated previous surgical procedures (Fig. 1).

Some of these infections can be diagnosed easily by the patient history and physical examination, but instrumental diagnostic tests are often needed for a complete diagnosis. These studies have been grouped into five classes [2]: (1) serologic; (2) imaging; (3) histological; (4) cell culture; (5) molecular.

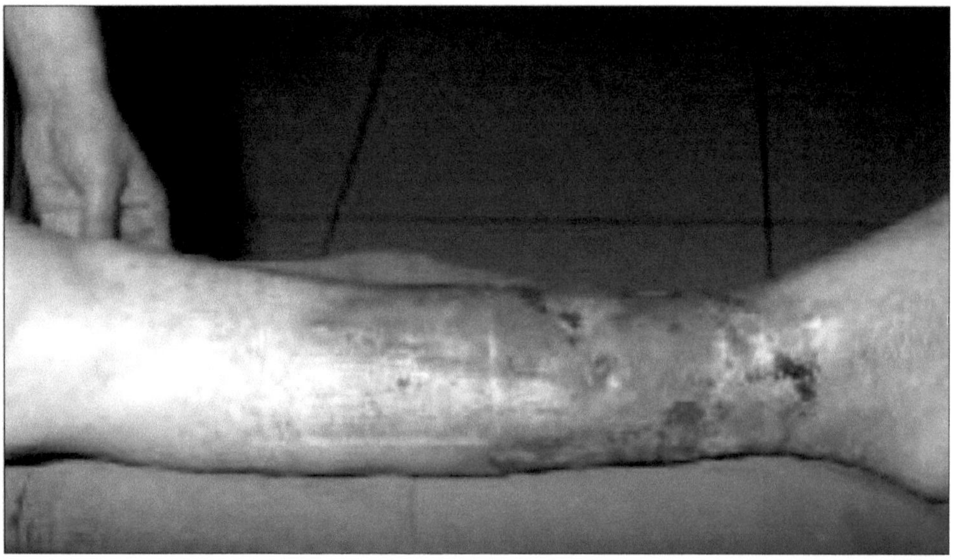

Fig. 1. External signs of infection (erythema, swelling, and drainage) in a patient with infected nonunion

Laboratory Tests

The most useful hematologic parameters are white blood cell (WBC) count and inflammatory indicators: erythrocyte sedimentation rate and C-reactive protein (CRP) [3]. The leukocyte count is often normal. Erythrocyte sedimentation rate and CRP elevations are usually found, but they are not very sensitive. Erythrocyte sedimentation rate can be normal, but a low level does not exclude the diagnosis of infection.

These laboratory values can be useful in monitoring the therapeutic response: the success of a treatment is defined not only by total clinical resolution, but even by erythrocyte sedimentation rate and CRP normalization [4] – hence the importance of monitoring inflammatory indicators before beginning the treatment and during and after the end of treatment.

Particular laboratory tests can be useful to monitor nutritional status (serum albumin level), comorbidities (blood glucose level for patients with diabetes), and drug toxicity (liver function tests) [5].

Imaging Studies

A multimodality approach is often needed to establish the diagnosis, including plain radiography, ultrasound, computed tomography (CT) scan, magnetic resonance imaging, radionuclide imaging, and positron emission tomography.

Plain Radiography

Conventional radiographs represent the basic examination: they are important for the diagnosis, staging, and evaluation of progression of the infection [6] (Fig. 2).

Plain radiographs of the bone are of relatively little value during the first weeks; in this phase they often do not reveal the presence of infection in a nonunion [7].

The earliest alterations can be observed on radiographic images only some weeks after the septic process has started and consist of a radiotransparency area in relation to osteopenia, sometimes followed by a nonspecific periosteal reaction. In fact, the bone alterations depend on the inflammatory state during the early stages (with hyperemia and osteopenia) rather than on the bone tissue damage. In later phases, an impoverishment of bone matrix is clear, and the possible presence of sequestration can be detected.

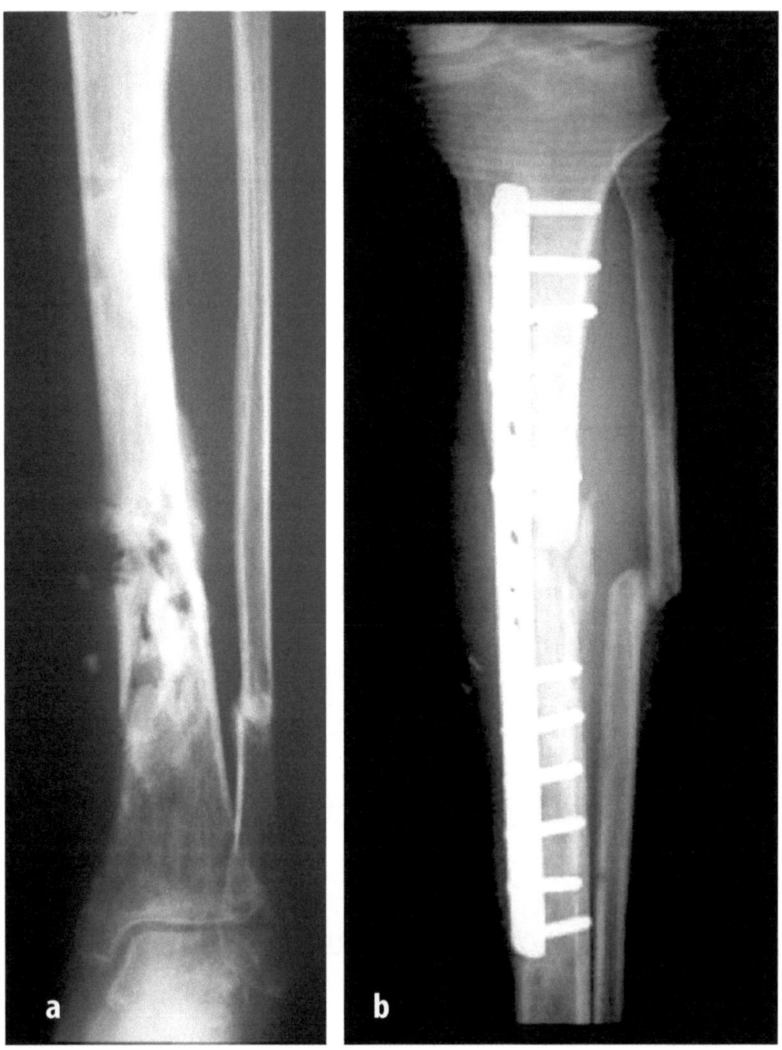

Fig. 2a, b. Radiographic evidence of infected nonunion of two tibial fractures (**a**) after repeated surgical procedures in an open fracture, (**b**) after internal fixation of a closed fracture

Ultrasound

Osseous structures are not well imaged by ultrasound, which cannot directly show a bone infection. However, it can identify the presence of soft tissue alterations and, in case of bone infection, it can accurately identify the presence of fluid directly in contact with bone [8, 9].

Computed Tomography

CT scanning can be useful to identify the presence of bone destruction, fluid or hemorrhagic mass, and sinus tracts [10, 11]. It is particularly useful to identify infections too small to be detected by plain radiographs and cortical or medullary sequestra.

Magnetic Resonance Imaging

Magnetic resonance imaging (MRI) can be useful in diagnosing bone and soft tissue infection. In these cases, the normal fat in the normal bone marrow cavity is replaced by cells and fluid in the inflammatory exudates. The changes in concentration of mobile protons result in significant alterations of the signal intensity of the bone marrow.

Thanks to its multiplanar imaging capability and high resolution, MRI can offer a very precise definition of the spatial extent and localization of the inflammatory process in the bone. Moreover, MRI can distinguish between bone and soft tissue infection and can easily identify the sinus tracts.

MRI has some limitations: in particular, it lacks specificity because the aspects of infection are similar to those produced by trauma or tumors in bone and soft tissue, but a study of osteomyelitis complicating fractures, performed by Mason et al. [12], showed a sensitivity of 100%, specificity of 63%, and accuracy of 93%.

Radionuclide Imaging

Nuclear medicine is useful in detecting infection associated with a nonunion.

Infection-specific scintigraphy is carried out with a variety of radiopharmaceuticals [6, 13]. Currently used radiopharmaceuticals include: 99mTc methylene diphosphonate, gallium-67 citrate, indium-^{111} or ^{99m}Tc-labeled leukocytes, and immunoscintigraphy with ^{99m}Tc-labeled monoclonal antigranulocytic antibodies.

Evaluation with triple-phase technetium and gallium scans is not very useful in differentiating osteomyelitis from soft tissue infection in the presence of nonunion: the accuracy reported in a study of Merkel et al. [14] is only 50%–60%.

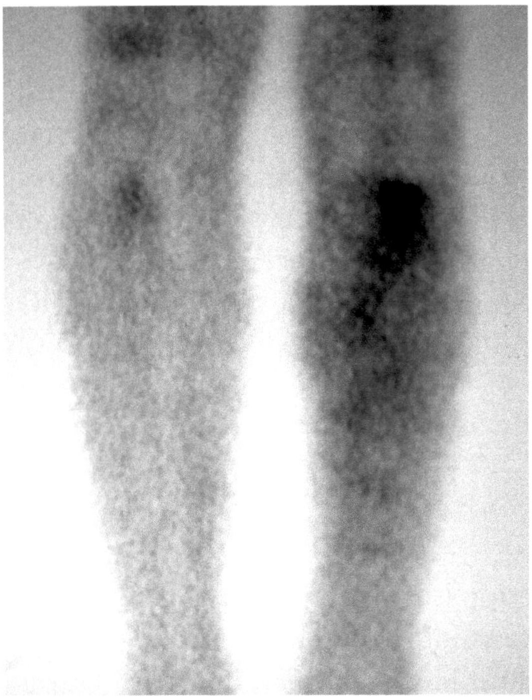

Fig. 3. Indium^{111}-labeled leukocyte imaging clearly shows localization at the site of the nonunion in the left tibia

Indium^{111} labeled leukocyte imaging detects skeletal infections with a sensitivity of 83%, specificity of 86%, and accuracy of 89% [14]. This high sensitivity seems lower if infections complicate the nonunion [15] (Fig. 3).

Immunoscintigraphy has the advantage of the simplicity of the labeling process of ^{99m}Tc with the antibodies [6].

A limitation of radionuclide scans is that they often overestimate the extent of the process because of increased blood flow and bone metabolism in adjacent structures.

Positron Emission Tomography

Positron emission tomography (PET) measures function rather than analyzing the anatomic structure: in this way it is possible to measure local metabolic velocity, blood flow, and protein-synthesis velocity.

PET with F18-fluorodeoxyglucose (FDG) is very sensitive in imaging an infection because the FDG uptake is elevated in inflammatory cells such as leukocytes, granulocytes, and macrophages due to the improved glucose metabolism by inflammatory cells as compared to normal cells [16, 17].

Images are interpreted according to qualitative criteria, comparing areas of altered uptake with areas of basal activity.

This newly developed diagnostic tool enhances diagnostic accuracy when compared with both scintigraphy and MRI [18].

Histological Studies

Tissue specimens obtained for histopathology as frozen sections are useful because the presence of abundant neutrophils is indicative of infection: it has been observed that more than five neutrophils per high-power field indicates infection with a specificity of 93%–97 % [19]. In paraffin sections, a high level of inflammatory infiltrate is highly suggestive of infection [20].

As previously described in the section "Bone Biopsy" in Chapter 4, classic microscopic investigation in infected nonunions shows signs of inflammation and trabecular resorption due to necrosis.

Culture Studies

The critical moment in the diagnosis of infection is isolation of pathogens in cultures from the bone lesion. If possible, cultures should be collected before beginning the antibiotic treatment or 24–48 h after it has been interrupted [5]. Aerobic and anaerobic bacteria, mycobacteria, and mycetes should be searched for.

Cultures of specimens from sinus tracts have a poor sensitivity and are not reliable for predicting which organism will be isolated from infected bone [21]. Other noninvasive diagnostic methods, such as needle biopsy, have a low predictive value. Only with cultures of bone taken at the time of *débridement* or deep bone biopsies can allow to perform an accurate isolation and a definitive diagnosis of infecting organisms be ensured.

It is important to collect the specimen under aseptic conditions in order to minimize the risk of blood sample pollution. The sample must immediately be sent to the microbiological laboratory and kept in sterile containers in saline solution in order to avoid desiccation.

Staphylococcus aureus is by far the most commonly involved organism; however, gram-negative bacilli and anaerobic organisms are also frequently isolated.

Once the etiologic agent and its antibiogram have been identified, the minimal inhibiting concentration (MIC) and the minimal bactericidal concentration (MBC) of the proper antibiotic must be determined.

Direct communication between the orthopaedic surgeon and the microbiology laboratory regarding patient history and risk factors, antibiotic therapy, and precise culture site may aid in directing the appropriate workup in the laboratory [22].

Molecular Studies

This class of diagnostic procedures targets specific macromolecules unique to infecting pathogens and can provide rapid results with high accuracy [2].

Two groups of molecular diagnostic techniques can be identified: amplified and nonamplified. Amplified methods include: polymerase chain reaction (PCR), reverse transcriptase polymerase chain reaction (RT-PCR), ligase chain reaction, and branched chain reaction. Nonamplified methods include: monoclonal antibodies, direct detection of rRNA, and hybridization of rRNA.

Polymerase chain reaction is the most frequently employed method: it is not sufficiently specific to serve as a screening test, but may be useful in confirming skeletal infection.

References

1. Connolly JF (ed) (1991) Tibial non-union. Diagnosis and treatment. AAOS, Park Ridge (Illinois)
2. Hoeffel DP, Hinrichs SH, Garvin KL (1999) Molecular Diagnostic for the Detection of Musculoskeletal Infection. Clin Orthop Relat Res 360:37–46
3. Roesgen M, Hierholzer G, Hax PM (1989) Post-traumatic osteomyelitis. Arch Orthop Trauma Surg 108:1–9
4. Schulak DJ, Rayhack JM, Lippert F 3rd et al (1982) The erythrocyte sedimentation rate in orthopaedic patients. Clin Orthop Relat Res 167:197–202
5. Lazzarini L, Mader J, Calhoun J (2004) Osteomyelitis in long bones. J Bone Joint Surg Am 86:2305–2318
6. Gross T, Kaim A, Regazzoni P et al (2002) Current concepts in posttraumatic osteomyelitis: a diagnostic challenge with new imaging options. J Trauma 52:1210–1219
7. Tumeh S, Allabadi P, Weissman B et al (1987) Disease activity in osteomyelitis: role of radiography. Radiology 165:781–784
8. Abiri M, Kirpekar M, Ablow M (1989) Osteomyelitis: detection with US. Radiology 172:509–511
9. Concia E, DeLalla F, DiPerri G et al (2003) Orientamenti diagnostico-terapeutici nella gestione delle infezioni osteoarticolari. Pharma Project Group Edizioni Scientifiche, Saronno
10. Ochsner PE, Sokhegyi A, Petralli C (1990) The value of computerized tomography in the assessment of chronic osteomyelitis: a radiological, histological and clinical correlation study. Z Orthop 128:313–318
11. Vasiliev A, Bulanova T, Onishcenko MP (2003) Spiral computed tomography in the diagnosis of limb osteomyelitis. Vestn Rentgenol Radiol 6:44–49
12. Mason M, Zlatkin M, Esterhai J et al (1989) Chronic complicated osteomyelitis of the lower extremity: evaluation with MR imaging. Radiology 175:355–359
13. Lew D, Waldvogel F (2004) Osteomyelitis. Lancet 364:369–379
14. Merkel KD, Brown ML, Dewanjee MK et al (1985) Comparison of Indium-labeled leukocyte imaging with sequential Technetium-Gallium scanning in the diagnosis of low grade musculoskeletal sepsis. A prospective study. J Bone Joint Surg Am 67:465–476
15. Schauwecker D, Park H, Mock B et al (1984) Evaluation of complicating osteomyelitis with Tc-99m MDP, In-111 granulocytes and Ga-67 citrate. J Nucl Med 25:849–853
16. Sugawara Y, Braun D, Kison P et al (1998) Rapid detection of human infections with fluorine-18 fluorodeoxyglucose and positron emission tomography: preliminary results. Eur J Nucl Med 25:1238–1243

17. Stumpe K, Dazzi H, Schaffner A et al (2000) Infection imaging using whole body FDG-PET. Eur J Nucl Med 27:822–832
18. Robiller FC, Stumpe KD, Kossmann T et al (2000) Chronic osteomyelitis of the femur: value of PET imaging. Eur Radiol 10:855–858
19. Abdul-Karim FW, McGinnis MG, Kraay M et al (1998) Frozen section biopsy assessment for the presence of polymorphonuclear leukocytes in patients undergoing revision of arthroplasties. Mod Pathol 11:427–431
20. Simpson AH, Wood MK, Athanasou NA (2002) Histological assessment of the presence or absence of infection in fracture non-union. Injury 33:151–155
21. Perry GR, Pearson RL, Miller GA (1991) Accuracy of cultures of material from swabbing of the superficial aspect of the wound and needle biopsy in the preoperative assessment of osteomyelitis. J Bone Joint Surg Am 73:745–749
22. Gustilo R (1989) Orthopaedic infection. Saunders, Philadelphia

Section IV
Nonunions: Treatment

Prevention

Redento Mora, Luisella Pedrotti, Giovanni Battista Galli, Stefano Gili, Anna Maccabruni

Introduction

Prevention of nonunions is based on complete understanding of both biological and mechanical aspects of bone callus formation; it requires a good control of fracture treatment technique, which has to be most accurate from the start following the classic rules of reduction and immobilization [1]. Prevention is also based on accurate soft tissue reconstruction (in fractures with soft tissue loss), functional loading as soon as possible, and infection risk control by all necessary means (and disregarding all unnecessary ones) because surgical site infection is the leading complication of surgery [2]. It has been reported that the operative treatment of a closed fracture elevates infection risk by 1.2% [3] (Figs. 1–4).

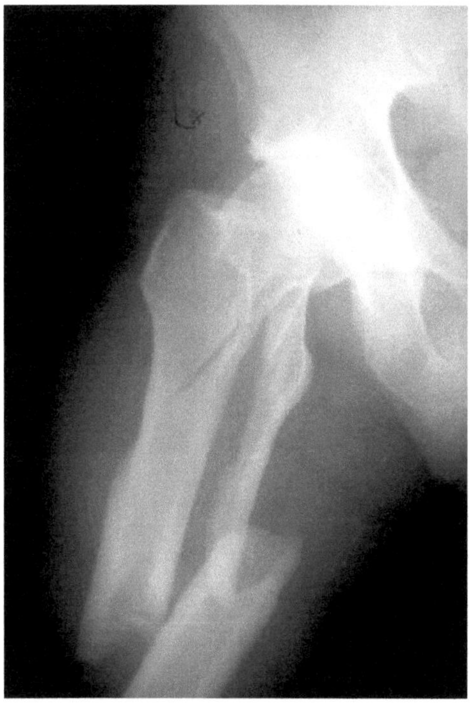

Fig. 1. X-ray of a closed fracture of the right femur

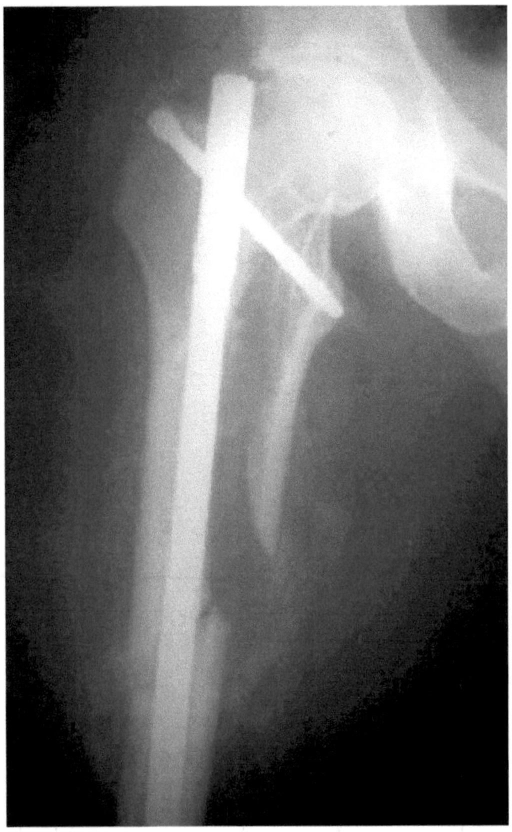

Fig. 2. Same case as in Fig. 1. Management of the fracture with internal osteosynthesis (intramedullary nailing)

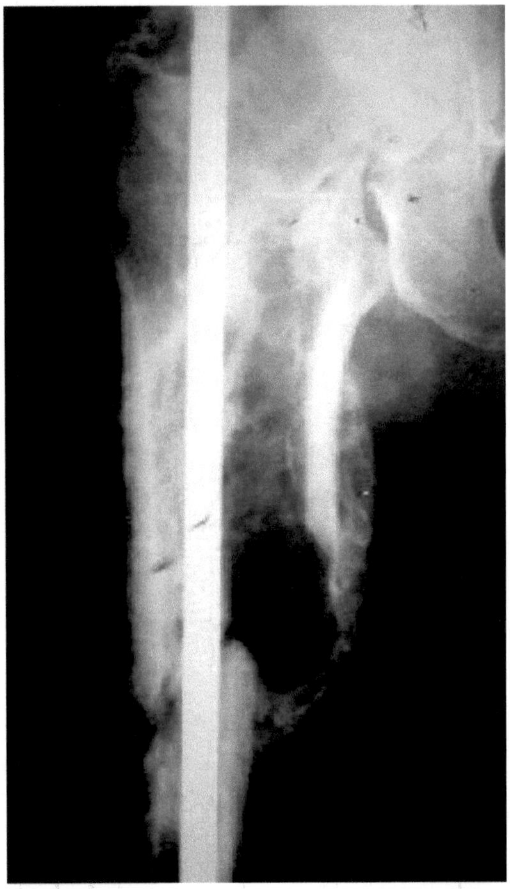

Fig. 3. Same case as in Fig. 1. Massive infection developed 4 months after surgery

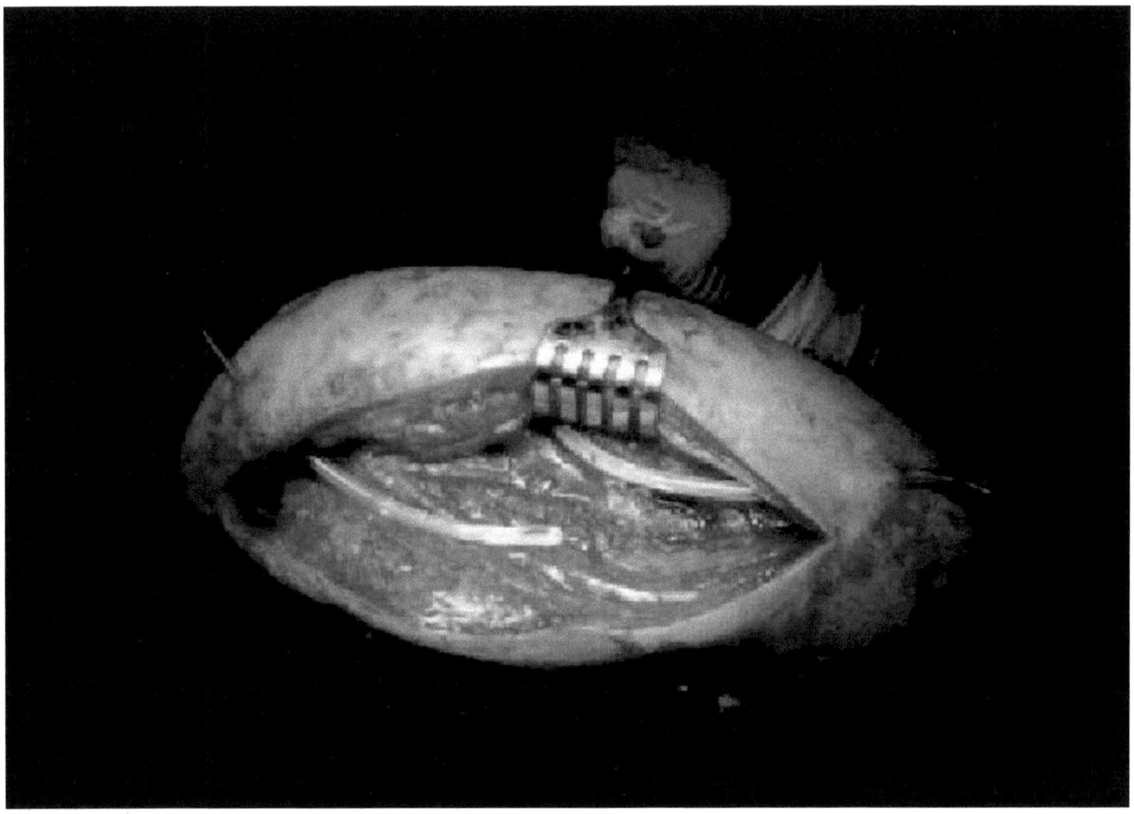

Fig. 4. Same case as in Fig. 1. Radical *débridement* and application of an irrigation system

In particular, closed tibial fractures treated by intramedullary nailing have a risk of infection of up to 1.5%, elevated 4.4% in Gustilo type IIIA and to 15% in Gustilo type IIIB [4]. In another series, the reported infection rate after operative treatment in open tibial fractures "up to grade IIIA" was 7% [5]. Cordero [6] reported that the incidence of infection in tibial intramedullary nailing is different, depending on the soft tissue damage: 2% in closed fractures, 4% in Gustilo II fractures, 6% in Gustilo IIIA fractures, and up to 18% in Gustilo IIIB type fractures.

Open and Closed Fractures

The difference between closed and open fractures is sometimes blurred and it is important to try and elucidate the real differences between them. In each diaphyseal fracture both bone and surrounding soft tissues are involved [7], including the skin, the subcutaneous tissue, fascia, muscles, tendons, ligaments, periostium, vessels, and nerves [8]. Skin lesions appear as excoriations, blister, sharp-edged injury (from stab wound), contused-edges injury (from stab wound and compression), suprafascial detachment, or necrosis; muscular injuries can involve muscles or tendons; and vascular injuries include arterial, venous, and lymphatic injuries.

A careful evaluation of soft tissue involvement is mandatory in both exposed and closed fractures due to the fact that the extent and severity of the soft tissue involvement and its possible evolution represent the main criteria for prognosis and treatment (Fig. 5).

It is of some interest, in this respect, to be reminded of the evolution of the classification systems for fractures. In general, they are too complicated or too detailed [9], neglecting the trauma mechanism and considering only the anatomical structures that have been involved.

In 1957 Cauchoix presented a classification of open fractures into three types according to the extent of the cutaneous injury [10]. Anderson in 1971 proposed a classification into three types based on the extent of the skin lesion and the extent of contamination and necrosis of the wound [11]. During the same period Allgower's classification [12] was also published, dividing injury into three grades according to the extent of soft tissue involvement.

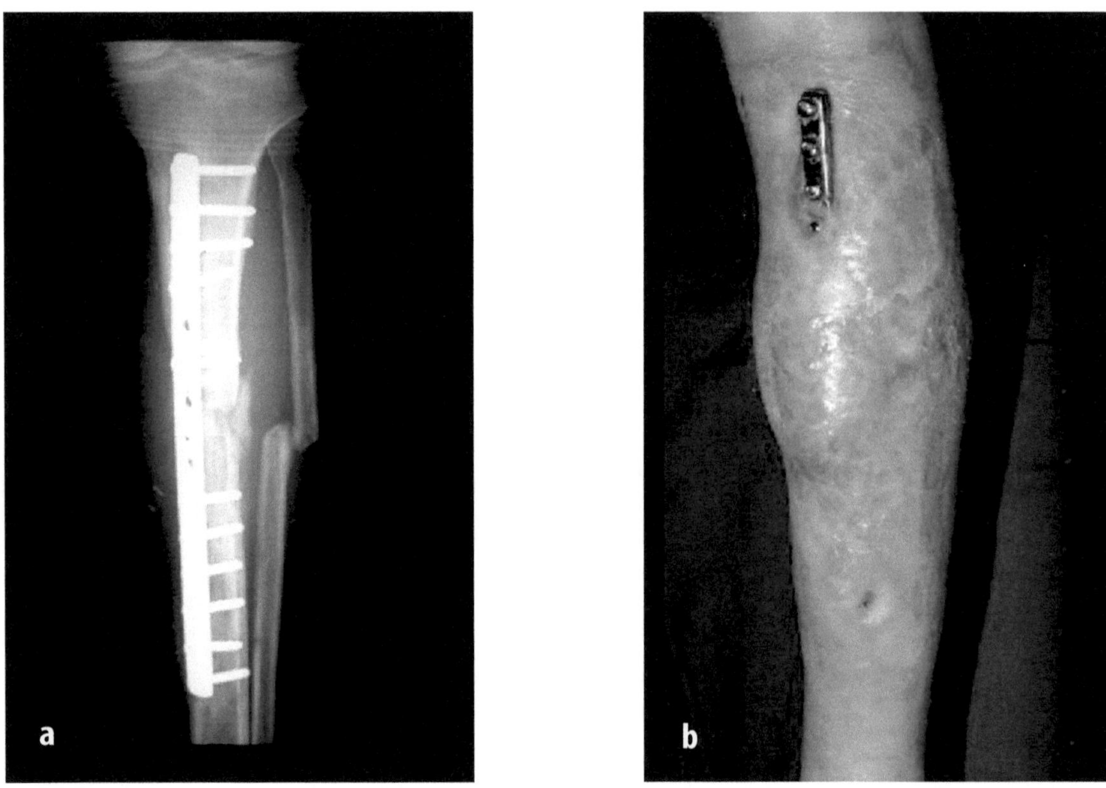

Fig. 5a, b. **a** X-ray of a tibial closed fracture with soft tissue damage treated by plating. **b** Clinical picture of the leg with exposure of the proximal part of the plate

Subsequently, the effect of soft tissue injury on the consolidation of a fracture became more evident, and in 1976 Gustilo's classification into three types was proposed [13], which nowadays is widely used in Anglo-Saxon countries. Type 3 lesion (wide injury of soft tissues as a consequence of a high-energy trauma) is subdivided into three groups according to the increasing severity of the damage to the soft tissues.

Tscherne and Gotzen's classification (the so-called Hannover classification) underlines the consequence of soft tissue injury on bone consolidation, subdividing into four grades of increasing severity of either closed or open fractures [14].

The "Seattle group" classification combines the Hannover classification into four grades of closed fracture with a modified version of Gustilo's classification into five grades of open fractures (quoted by Bonatz and Alonso [9]).

A more complete classification system (even if it is more difficult to apply) was proposed by the AO Group in 1980 [15]. It is based on three parameters: two types of fractures (closed and open), three categories of tissues (skin, muscles and tendons, neurovascular structures), and five grades of severity of the injury.

From this brief list it emerges that there are four parameters more difficult to detect [9]: description of the injury, indication for treatment, updating of the classification according to the mechanism of injury, and agreement on the classification.

In modern traumatology the concept of fracture is changing; in particular the distinction between closed and open fracture is less evident because a more relevant role is ascribed to soft tissue injury.

Prevention of Infection in Surgically Treated Fractures

If operative treatment is chosen, it is important to use an adequate program of infection prevention in the preoperative, operative, and postoperative phases [16].

Preoperative Phase

Investigations

All additional investigations should be carried out on an outpatient basis so as to avoid, if possible, having the patient wait for surgery in the hospital and thus to reduce the risks of infection from resistant germs. The routine preoperative blood tests requested by the anesthetist, should be completed with inflammatory indexes in order to detect a septic focus.

Patient on the Ward

The patient should be admitted to the ward the same day of surgery or at the earliest the day before; the patient should share a room with patients waiting for surgery, avoiding any contact with individuals who have suffered trauma or with a surgical wound at risk for infection.

Preparation Before Surgery

The site of the surgical incision must be managed prior to the arrival of the patient in the operating room [17]. A compress of antiseptic solution is applied to the area where surgery will take place; any shaving should be done immediately before surgery.

Transfer to the Operating Room

The patient should wear a sterile disposable skirt and be transferred to the operating area on a device used only for transporting patients inside the operating zone. If such a device is not available, the patient should be brought to the operating area lying on a dedicated stretcher, and a disinfectant carpet should be laid on the floor in the room outside the operating room.

Operative Phase

Surveillance of Instruments and Environment Sterility

The highest grade of sterility must be maintained in the operating room (Fig. 6).

Periodically the methods of sterilization should be checked and the effective sterility of the surgical instruments tested.

Pollution by air diffusion occurs when the environment contains corpusculated particles of 0.5–30 μm in the environment. These particles arise from two sources: from medical and nursing staff and from the air conditioning system.

Considering the first source, it should be remembered that it takes 16 h for particles of 1 μm to settle. The entrance of a staff member or a new patient or simply movement (transfer) inside the operating room or changing the position of a lamp or instruments is sufficient to resuspend the particles in a conventional operating room [18].

Considering the second source, the amount of corpusculated particles introduced with the air conditioning depends both on the quality of filters and on the velocity of flow, which, if irregular, can cause turbulence and keep the particles suspended. To address this problem, the laminar flow system was

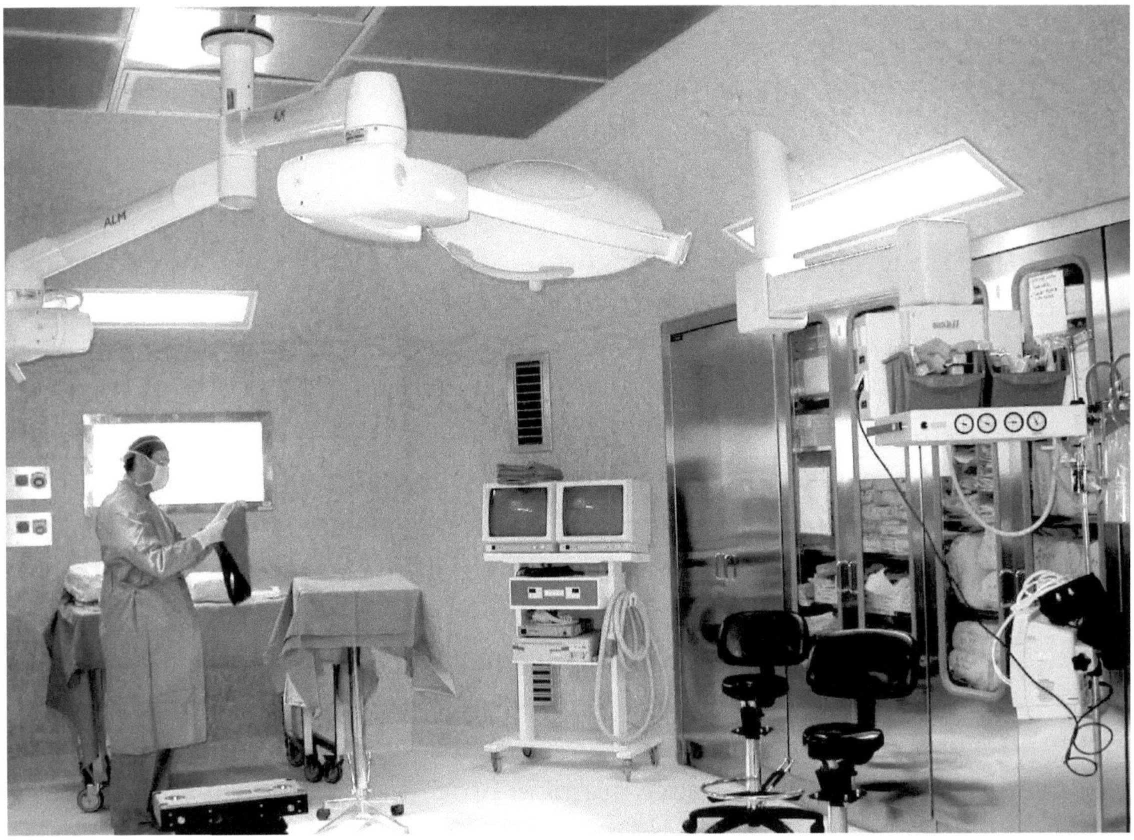

Fig. 6. A high grade of asepsis must be maintained in the operating room

developed in the 1960s, which consists in filtering the air to remove contaminants and then releasing the air at a speed moving it in a linear direction without turbulence [19]. The air flow direction can be horizontal or vertical. In general, vertical flow is more suitable for orthopaedic surgery; the advantage is that the anesthetist and his instruments are kept outside the area served by the flow, but it also requires particular attention to positioning of the surgical team.

The main requirements for a laminar flow are the quality of filters, the speed of flow (optimal is from 21 to 33 m/min), and proper maintenance [2]. It may be useful to check the quantity of corpusculated particles in the environment using specific devices that suck up a certain quantity of air and then to pour them on an Agar plate to verify the development of bacterial colonies.

Surveillance of the Behavior of the Operating Room Staff

Particles released from skin desquamation or air expiration from each member of the staff contribute to environmental pollution. The regular use of masks and head covers as well as suitable working clothes and shoes should be checked.

Surgeon's Preparation

The surgeon's preparation for surgery can be divided into three steps: preliminary clothing, scrubbing, and clothing for surgery.

Preliminary Clothing

Standard working clothes made of cotton allow the skin particles (coming from normal desquamation and carrying bacteria) to pass. The filter suits, "clean air suits", reduce the dispersion of skin particles in the air and then the risk of contamination of the surgical wound. This has been confirmed for orthopaedic surgery by Blomgren [20].

Surgical masks afford double protection for patients and surgical staff as well. The main properties of the masks are efficient bacterial filtration and splash resistance (that should be the highest possible) and the resistance to respiration (that should be the lowest).

Surgical caps should cover the head adequately and provide the highest and most effective bacterial filtration and splash resistance, like the surgical masks.

With regard to surgical masks and caps, two rules should be remembered: they need to be changed after each surgical procedure and always when wet.

Shoes and overshoes should be comfortable and never be put on to walk outside the operating room, to reduce the risk of contamination. They should have the same properties as surgical drapes.

Scrubbing

Scrubbing of hands and forearms is important because the skin of the surgeon, as the skin of the patient, contains germs. Cleaning with adequate liquid disinfectant soaps should be done meticulously, taking the necessary time; it is also useful to use a proper brush, which should not be too aggressive, however, in order to avoid skin microlesions.

Clothing for Surgery

Surgical gowns should have the same properties as the drapes: they should be disposable and impermeable. Cotton gowns cannot provide a safe barrier against "cross contamination" (transit of germs from the outside to the inside and vice versa). This is true for all the tissues that, like cotton, have interstices larger than 80 μm [21].

Very interesting are some of the special systems with complete isolation (such as "Freedom Aire", Stackhouse, USA), constituted by a helmet (with a miniaturized system of air conditioning, secured by a lumbar belt to the surgeon), headdress (with filter), and surgical gowns with total protection (with lens built in polycarbonate to protect the face) (Fig. 7).

Gloves are extremely important to prevent infections: the use of precau-

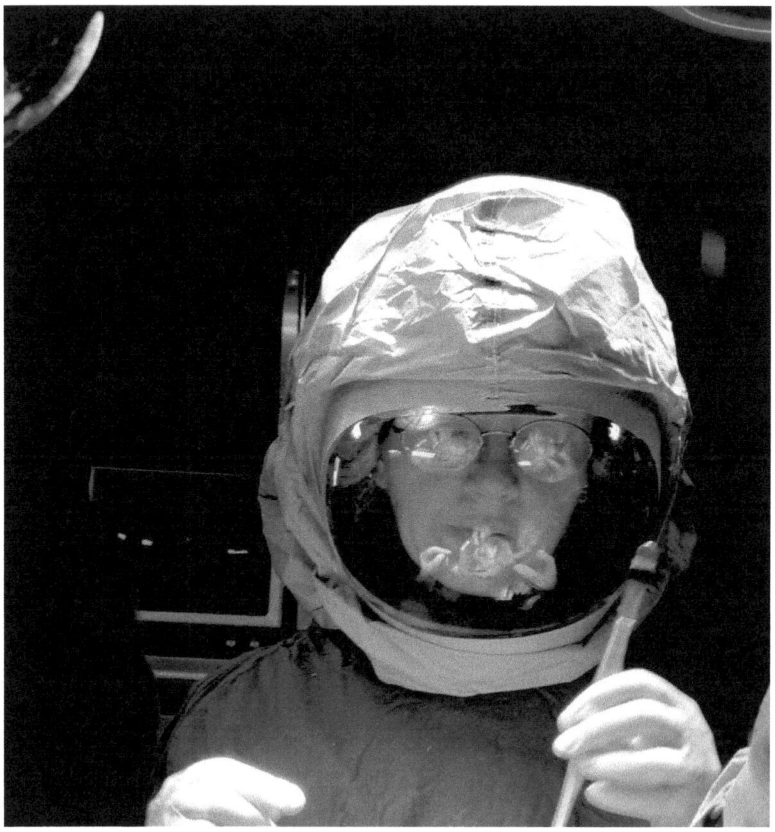

Fig. 7. "Total protection" of the surgeon by means of a complete isolation system

tions to reduce exposure to blood is crucial for the patient (and for the surgeon).

In single gloving, the frequency of glove perforation and resulting skin laceration in orthopaedic surgery is up to 58% [22], and 20% of these wounds cause blood leakage.

In double gloving (wearing two pairs of gloves), the integrity of the inner glove is maintained in up to 80% of cases in which the outer one is perforated [23]. Two layers of surgical gloves can reduce the number of breaks to the inner glove, which might allow cross-infection between the surgical team and the patient.

Double indicator gloves (as from Biogel, Regent, UK) represent a simple, effective, and more advanced system of protection that allows immediate identification of the perforation. If the outer glove is perforated, the entrance of organic fluids is made visible by the appearance of a colored spot [23, 24].

Preparation of the Surgical Field and Surgical Environment

"Draping is an important step in the surgical procedure and should not be assigned to an uninitiated assistant" [25]; considerable experience is required in placing the drapes, to avoid contamination of both the surgeons and the drapes.

The properties of surgical drapes are important as well: the use of disposable paper or fiber drapes remarkably reduces bacterial contamination of the environmental air compared to cotton drapes.

The use of impermeable drapes reduces the grade of contamination of the surgical wound by up to 92% due to the fact that the bacterial transit is higher when the tissue is wet [21, 27]. Finally, drapes with adhesive edges give a further barrier to the transit of germs because they adhere to the skin and improve the isolation of the surgical wound [27].

The surgeon-patient barrier should be under continuous control during the surgical procedure: for this reason, systems have been developed for monitoring the barrier: an interesting electronic monitoring system is ELPER Contact Detector (Selecta, Glasgow, UK), designed to detect glove holes, wet gowns, and glove permeability [28]. The ELPER system warns the surgeon immediately if his skin has come into direct contact with patient's blood [29]; any violation of the barrier is detected by the electronic system and at a predetermined threshold an alarm sounds.

Surgical Maneuvers

After accurate preparation of the surgical field and environment in order to create an effective surgeon-patient barrier, the rules of asepsis must be observed during the surgical procedure, eliminating unnecessary surgical steps and reducing "surgical trauma" (diminishing the invasivity, choosing the most appropriate type of implant and surgical technique, and reducing the length of time for the surgery) [19].

A case-by-case evaluation of the utility of aspirating drains should be carried out; the drain must exit through a separate stab wound and passive drains must be avoided [17]. The dressing applied should be occlusive enough to avoid the risk of secondary contamination [16].

Considering the implant, it should be chosen after careful evaluation in respect of: implant size, shape, and material [6].

The larger implants carry a higher infection risk, due to the wide surface the bacteria have for adherence. Similar evaluation should be made of the implant shape: experimental work in rabbit tibiae demonstrated that hollow intramedullary nails become infected more easily than solid nails.

Surgical grade stainless steel, known as 316-SL, is the orthopaedic alloy most prone to infection, according to many studies; chrome-cobalt (Co-Cr) alloys have an infection risk between those of stainless steel and titanium alloy, and titanium alloys have the lowest risk of infection. This seems due mainly to the presence of cytotoxic components in alloys. Stainless steel is composed of at least two cytotoxic components, nickel and cobalt; chrome-cobalt alloys are also composed of at least two cytotoxic components, cobalt and molybdenum. In titanium alloys only one component (Vanadium) is suspected of being toxic [6].

A recent study has shown, however, the presence of a marked inflammation and tissue reaction in the soft tissue covering stainless steel and titanium plates used for internal fixation of fractures of long bones independently of the material used [30].

Postoperative Phase

Prevention of infections during the first postoperative period consists in monitoring of patient's general condition (by clinical, instrumental, and laboratory examinations) and the control of local conditions, with constant surveillance of the surgical wound, providing the possibility of early diagnosis and early treatment if required.

References

1. Putti V (1942) Decalogo delle fratture. Chir Organi Mov 27:131–135
2. Dharan S, Pittet D (2002) Environmental controls in operating theatres. J Hosp Infect 51:79–84
3. Weitzel PP, Esterhai JL (1994) Delayed union, non-union and sinovial pseudoarthrosis. In: Brighton CT, Friedlander GE, Lane JM (eds) Bone formation and repair. AAOS, Rosemont, pp 505–527
4. Garg A, Court-Brown C (1999) Management of infection associated with tibial intramedullary nailing. Curr Med Lit (Orthopaedics) 12:7–9
5. Pascarella R, Gozzi E, Bertoldi E et al (2002) Il trattamento delle fratture esposte della tibia. Fissazione esterna e inchiodamento endomidollare differito paragonato ad inchiodamento endomidollare immediato. Giorn Ital Ortop Traumatol 28:227–232
6. Cordero J (2002) Influence of the implant to infection rate. Quad Infez Osteoartic 3:47–52
7. Lefèvre C, Le Nen D, Cabrol E et al (1993) Fractures diaphysaires de l'adulte. Encycl Méd Chir, App Locomoteur 14-031-A-60
8. Scott Levin L (1995) Personality of soft-tissue injury. Techn Orthop 10:65–72
9. Bonatz E, Alonso J (1995) Classification of soft-tissue injury. Techn Orthop 10:73–78
10. Cauchoix J, Duparc J, Boulez P (1957) Traitement des fractures ouvertes de jambe. Mem Acad Chir 83:811–822
11. Anderson LD (1984) Fractures. In: Tscherne H (ed) Fractures with soft-tissue injury. Springer, Berlin Heidelberg New York
12. Allgower M (1971) Weichteilprobleme und Infektionsrisiko der Osteosynthese. Langenbecks Arch Chir 329:1126–1136
13. Gustilo RB, Anderson JT (1976) Prevention of infection in the treatment of 1025 open fractures of long bones. J Bone Joint Surg Am 58:453–458
14. Tscherne H, Gotzen L (1984) Fractures with soft tissue injuries. Springer, Berlin Heidelberg New York

15. Muller M, Allgower M, Schneider R (1991) Manual of internal fixation. Springer, Berlin Heidelberg New York
16. Salvi V (2003) Il ruolo del chirurgo ortopedico nella prevenzione delle infezioni operatorie. Quad Infez Osteoartic 4:39–47
17. Fry DE (2003) Surgical site infection: pathogenesis and prevention. Medscape.com/viewprogram:1–17
18. Vielpeau C, Locker B, Van Nedervelde T et al (1989) Le risque infectieux en chirurgie orthopédique. Encycl Méd Chir, Techniques Chirurgicales Orthopédie–44–005, pp 1–18, Elsevier, Paris
19. Ritter MA (1999) Operating room environment. Clin Orthop Relat Res 369:103–109
20. Blomgren J, Hoborn J, Nystrom B (1990) Reduction of contamination at total hip replacement by special working clothes. J Bone Joint Surg Br 72:985–987
21. Hoborn J (2003) Controllo delle infezioni e norme tecniche per camici chirurgici, teli e set chirurgici per la copertura del paziente. Intern Meeting: La sicurezza nelle sale operatorie italiane e i nuovi standard europei. Milan
22. Sanders R, Fortin P, Ross E et al (1990) Outer gloves in orthopaedic procedures. J Bone Joint Surg Am 72:914–917
23. Wigmore SJ, Rainey JB (1994) Use of coloured undergloves to detect glove puncture. Br J Surg 81:1480
24. Laine T, Aarnio P (2004) Glove perforation in orthopaedic and trauma surgery. J Bone Joint Surg Br 86:898–900
25. Crenshaw AH (1987) Surgical techniques. In: Crenshaw AH (ed) Campbell's operative orthopaedics, 7th edn. Mosby, St. Louis, Vol 1, pp 3–22
26. Hoborn J (1990) Wet strike-through and transfer of bacteria through operating barrier materials. Hyg Med 15:15–20
27. Werner HP, Hoborn J, Schon K et al (1991) Influence of drape permeability on wound contamination during mastectomy. Eur J Surg 157:379–383
28. McIntyre IM, Currie JS, Smith DN et al (1994) Reducing the risk of viral transmission at operation by electronic monitoring of the surgeon-patient barrier. Br J Surg 81:1076–1078
29. Perugia L, Traina GC (1994) AIDS and surgery. Intern Orthop 18:397–399
30. Voggenreiter G, Leiting S, Brauer H et al (2003) Immuno-inflammatory tissue reaction to stainless-steel and titanium plates used for internal fixation of long bones. Biomaterials 24:247–254

Nonunions: Treatment Objectives and Options

Redento Mora, Gabriella Tuvo, Stefano Gili, Milena Miceli

Treatment Objectives

The main objective in the management of nonunions is fracture healing; the second objective is restoration of the limb function, either by correcting any shortening or angular, rotational, translational deformity or by eliminating the stiffness of the adjacent joints. Joint stiffness can be treated by using the most appropriate nonoperative techniques (physiotherapy, CPM, or hinged braces) or operative methods (arthrotomy, arthrolysis, or myolysis).

In the particular case of infected nonunions, the treatment aim is nonunion healing and eradication of infection and to gain a functional limb. To accomplish these objectives, considerable time is needed and multiple operative procedures are often required. In selected patients in whom many previous procedures have failed and who have extensive bone and soft tissue loss and neurovascular damage, amputation can be considered.

Treatment Options

Nonsurgical Methods

Pharmacological Therapy

The positive influence of medical treatment with calcium and vitamin D3 on the fracture healing process has been demonstrated in animal experiments [1] and also in humans [2], where these drugs seem to act over the first 6 weeks after fracture.

Several studies were also performed in order to determine whether bisphosphonates can have favorable effects on fracture repair, but the results are still unclear. It remains to be investigated whether the effect of calcium and vitamin D supplementation could be extended to some types of nonunions.

Mechanical Stimulation

Even if in particular cases (mainly in the upper limbs) nonunion can be left untreated (so-called benign neglect [3]), in general, mechanical stimulation with functional weight-bearing (through axial movement and micromotion enhancement) can promote bone healing in delayed unions or nonunions. In specific types of nonunions, keeping the fracture stable or improving the fracture stability, with casting or bracing, can promote progressive bone callus formation and bone healing. In most cases, however, these treatments are insufficient and a more complex approach is required.

Biophysical Stimulation

Electrical Stimulation

Electrical stimulation is effective in hypertrophic nonunions, but it cannot be used to correct a deformity or shortening and is ineffective in the presence of a gap [4]. Three forms of electrical stimulation are available for treatment of nonunions: direct current (DC), inductive coupling (IC), and capacitive coupling (CC). The biologic principle is based on the observation that mechanically stimulated bone cells produce an electrical field, which mediates bone cell proliferation by mimicking the electrical stimulus of mechanical stress [3].

Ultrasound Stimulation

Low intensity pulsed ultrasound may accelerate healing of fresh fractures and nonunions, positively influencing the phases of fracture repair [5–7]. Ultrasound influences cell activity, affecting ionic permeability of the cell membrane and second messenger activity. Ryaby reported that low intensity ultrasound increases calcium incorporation in both cartilage and bone cells [8]. Furthermore, ultrasound may increase blood flow through the dilation of capillaries and the enhancement of angiogenesis, thus optimizing the environment that is conductive to nonunion healing [9].

Extracorporeal Shock Waves

High-energy extracorporeal shock wave therapy (obtained by means of electrohydraulic, or electromagnetic, devices) has been shown to be effective in the treatment of nonunions. Shock waves act through several processes [10–12]: vascular (inducing microfissures and hematoma), increasing local blood flow and oxygen, breaking the linkage between molecules of tricalcium phosphate and giving rise to microcrystals of hydroxyapatite and the cavitation effect with high energy liberation.

Surgical Methods

In noninfected nonunions, treatment is specific for hypertrophic, normotrophic, and atrophic types. For the hypertrophic type, treatment is based upon a stable immobilization; in the other two types a biologic stimulation is required as well.

Several surgical procedures have been used in order to treat long bone nonunions: osteosynthesis by means of internal fixation or external fixation, bone marrow injection, bone grafting, use of bone substitutes, and use of growth factors.

Osteosynthesis

Internal Fixation

Intramedullary locked nailing is commonly used in treating noninfected long bone nonunions. Canal reaming destroys the endosteal blood supply, but blood flow is fully restored in 12 weeks [13]. Intramedullary nailing provides stable immobilization and also allows early partial weightbearing. In many cases the use of adjuvant bone grafting is indicated [3].

Many nonunions can be treated with compression plates [14, 15]. Conventional plating provides only the environment stability for bone healing, but does not provide the osteogenic stimulus; therefore, bone grafting is often associated with plating. Because conventional plating presents some problems, such as damage to periosteal blood flow and creation of osteoporotic areas beneath the plate, a special kind of plate has been developed in recent years in order to overcome these problems: LC-DCP (limited contact - dynamic compression plates) [16] and LCP (locking compression plates) [17].

External Fixation

Axial external fixation is often employed in cases of noninfected and infected nonunions [18, 19]. In these cases, it has some important advantages (rigid immobilization of bone fragments, absence of implanted hardware, and respect of the blood flow) and some disadvantages (minimal axial loading, risk of pin tract infection and, most importantly, nonunion cannot be treated “dynamically”).

In treating long bone hypertrophic nonunions, circular external fixation has made significant progress, mainly considering that bone nonunion is often associated with other problems (in particular: shortening deformity) that can be treated at the same time using this method [20].

In normotrophic nonunions, in which the biologic reaction of the bone is reduced but not absent, the use of compression-distraction techniques improves the reaction capacity by activating the osteogenic potential.

In atrophic nonunion, the bone gap contains tissue without any biologic reaction capability. In these cases transosseous osteosynthesis acts at the nonunion site (after resection of the atrophic zone) and at the metaphysis (by means of corticotomy and bone transport). The vascularization of the whole segment is increased, with a high stimulation on different tissues [21].

In infected nonunions, treatment is similar to that for noninfected nonunions but it should be associated with *débridement* and antibiotic therapy. In particular, in infected nonunions with bone loss, which represent the main indication for these techniques, infected bone and soft tissues can be completely removed and the structure of the bone segment completely restored without previous sterilization of the infection, soft tissue closure, or use of a bone graft [22].

Bone Grafting

Bone grafting has been the basic technique used for the treatment of long bone nonunions for many years, in the form of bone autografts or allografts [7]. Bone autografts can be nonvascularized or vascularized.

Nonvascularized autogenous bone grafting can be used as an isolated bone grafting or associated with internal or external fixation (adjunctive bone grafting) or in the form of nonvascularized fibula.

The indications for bone grafting as an isolated procedure are currently rare, but include intertibiofibular grafting for tibial nonunions in cases of bone loss or soft tissue damage at the anterior aspect of the leg [23].

Bone grafting associated with internal or external osteosynthesis employs cancellous bone chips or structural corticocancellous grafting. A segment of nonvascularized fibula is sometimes used to fill a large bone defect. The transplanted fibula can hypertrophize, especially in children, to a significant degree.

The use of vascularized grafts (from ribs, ipsilateral or contralateral fibula, or iliac crest) is based on microvascular surgery. In particular cases, composite osteocutaneous or osteomyocutaneous vascularized grafts may be employed.

Bone allografts, harvested from cadavers and usually stored by freezing or irradiation methods, are generally distributed through tissue banks [24–27]. This material is employed mainly for reconstruction of nonunions with bone defects. The advantages of bone allografts include ready availability and no donor-site morbidity; possible disadvantages include the risk of transmission of infectious agents and the risk of fracture due to bone fragility.

Bone Marrow Injection

Harvesting autologous bone grafts can be associated with considerable morbidity [28]. Because bone marrow incorporates the osteoinductive properties of bone grafting (0.01% of marrow cells are osteogenic stromal stem cells), experimental studies have provided evidence that local autologous bone marrow injections can stimulate nonunions to heal [3, 29]. The technique is simple: marrow is obtained from the iliac wing and directly injected into the nonunion site, which should be stabilized by cast bracing or by osteosynthesis.

Bone Graft Substitutes

The ideal bone graft substitutes are biocompatible and resorbable, structurally similar to bone, cost effective, and have the properties of osteoconduction and osteoinduction. Many kinds of "bone alternatives" are commercially available: they are osteoconductive but minimally osteoinductive, and offer a low structural integrity [27].

Today ceramics made of calcium phosphate are generally used: hydroxyapatite (HA), tricalcium phosphate (TCP), and biphasic ceramics (a combination of HA and TCP). Favorable results were achieved in the management of nonunions by Meyrueis et al. [30].

Growth Factors (or Bone Growth-Promoting Factors)

Healing can be biologically stimulated by locally implanting growth factors that have osteoinductive properties. Growth factors alone induce local bone formation only to a very limited degree; a biodegradable delivery system is needed in order to obtain a gradual release of growth factors over time [31]. Osteoinductive growth factors can be obtained today by means of recombinant synthesis, but they have some disadvantages: their application is expensive and they are not autologous.

Considering that some growth factors are stored in platelet alpha granules, it has been suggested that autologous activated platelets be used as a source of growth factors in order to improve osteointegration. By means of autologous growth factor (AGF) technology, an AGF gel can be prepared and employed in order to stimulate osteogenesis in long bone nonunions [32].

References

1. Delgado-Martinez AD, Martinez ME, Carrascal MT et al (1998) Effect of 25-OH-vitamin D on fracture healing in elderly rats. J Orthop Res 16:650–653
2. Doetsch AM, Faber J, Lynnerup N (2004) The effect of calcium and vitamin D3 supplementation on the healing of the proximal humerus fracture: a randomised placebo-controlled study. Calcif Tissue Int 75:183–188

3. Weitzel PP, Esterhai JL (1994) Delayed union, non-union and synovial pseudoarthrosis. In: Brighton CT, Friedlander GE, Lane JM (eds) Bone formation and repair. AAOS, Rosemont (Illinois), pp 505–527
4. Bray TJ (1994) A prospective, double-bind trial of electrical capacitive coupling in the treatment of nonunions of long bones. J Bone Joint Surg Am 76:820–826
5. Heckman JD, Ryaby JP, McCabe J et al (1994) Acceleration of tibial fracture healing by non-invasive, low intensity pulsed ultrasound. J Bone Joint Surg Am 76:26–34
6. Hadjiargyrou M, McLeod K, Ryaby JP et al (1998) Enhancement of fracture healing by low intensity ultrasound. Clin Orthop Relat Res 355[Suppl]:216–229
7. Rodriguez-Merchan EC, Forriol F (2004) Nonunion: general principles and experimental data. Clin Orthop Relat Res 419:4–12
8. Ryaby JT, Bachner EJ, Bendo JA et al (1989) Low intensity pulsed ultrasound increases calcium incorporation in both differentiating cartilage and bone cell cultures. Proceedings ORS 35th Annual Meeting, Las Vegas
9. Rubin C, Bolander M, Ryaby JP et al (2001) The use of low-intensity ultrasound to accelerate the healing of fractures. J Bone Joint Surg Am 83:259–270
10. Corrado EM, Russo S, Gigliotti S (1996) Le onde d'urto ad alta energia nel trattamento delle pseudoartrosi. Giorn Ital Ortop Traumatol 22[Suppl. 2]:485–490
11. Russo S, Marlinghaus E, Amelio E et al (2000) The shock waves in treatment of bone pseudoarthrosis: clinical and experimental evaluation of osteo-angiogenetic response. Giorn Ital Ortop Traumatol 26[Suppl. 1]:6–12
12. Russo S, Amelio E, Galasso O et al (2001) La litotrissia extracorporea nel trattamento delle pseudoartrosi ossee. Min Ortop Traumatol 52:261–267
13. Rhinelander FW (1974) Tibial blood supply in relation to fracture healing. Clin Orthop Relat Res 105:34–81
14. Siebert CH, Lehrbass Sokeland KP, Rinke F et al (1997) Compression plating of tibial fractures following primary external fixation. Arch Orthop Trauma Surg 116:390–395
15. Zinghi GF, Rollo G, Trono M (eds) (2004) La pseudoartrosi delle ossa lunghe. Timeo, Bologna
16. Perren SM (1991) The concept of biological plating using the limited contact-dynamic compression plate (LC-DCP): scientific background, design and application. Injury 22[Suppl. 1]:1–41
17. Frigg R (2003) Development of the locking compression plate. Injury 34[Suppl. 2]:6–10
18. Green SA, Moore TA, Spohn PJ (1988) Nonunion of the tibial shaft. Orthopaedics 11: 1149–1157
19. Lortat-Jacob A (1997) Principes de traitement chirurgical de l'infection osseuse. Infection sur os non solide. Encycl Méd Chir, Techniques Chirurgicales–Orthopédie 44–082, Elsevier, Paris
20. Mora R (2000) Tecniche di compressione-distrazione. Indicazioni e limiti. Amplimedical, Milano
21. Paley D (1990) Treatment of tibial nonunion and bone loss with the Ilizarov technique. Instr Course Lect 39:185–197
22. Umiarov GA (1986) Classification of nonunions of the long bones complicated by infection, and principles of treatment. Sborn Trud CITO 30:5–9
23. Reckling PW, Waters CH (1980) Treatment of nonunions of fractures of the tibial diaphysis by posterolateral cortico cancellous bone grafting. J Bone Joint Surg Am 62:936–941

24. Volkov M, Bizer V (eds) (1972) Homotransplantation du tissu osseux en orthopédie infantile. Éditions de Moscou, Moscow
25. Imamaliev AS (ed) (1978) Homoplasty of the articular ends of bones. Mir, Moscow
26. Perry CR (1999) Bone repair techniques, bone graft and bone graft substitutes. Clin Orthop Relat Res 360:71–86
27. Greenwald AS, Boden SD, Goldberg VM et al (2002) Bone graft substitutes: facts, fictions and applications. Proceedings AAOS 69th Annual Meeting, Dallas
28. Roesgen M (1990) The regenerative ability of the iliac crest following spongiosa removal in man. Induction by phosphate ceramics? Unfallchirurg 16:258–265
29. Connolly J, Guse R, Lippiello L et al (1989) Development of an osteogenic bone-marrow preparation. J Bone Joint Surg Am 71:684–691
30. Meyrueis JP, Cazenave A, Le Saint B et al (1998) Utilisation d'une céramique macroporeuse biphasée en traumatologie. À propos de 108 cas. Rev Chir Orthop 84[Suppl. 2]:59–64
31. Ripamonti U, Pipino F (2003) Le Bone Morphogenetic Proteins (BMPs). Dalla ricerca alla clinica. Giorn Ital Ortop Traumatol 29:124–140
32. Hood AG, Biggi F (2003) The use of autologous growth factors to stimulate osteogenesis. Aggiorn Club Ital Osteosint 9:47–52

Compression-Distraction Systems

Redento Mora, Barbara Bertani, Gabriella Tuvo, Giovanni Battista Galli

Introduction

There are a few basic elements of circular external fixation systems, as underlined by Kalnberz [1]. They can be summed up as: bone fixation elements, rings which encircle the bone segment, rods connecting the rings, connecting elements between rods and rings, and connecting elements between rings and bone fixation elements. Many other elements can be added (Fig. 1). However, they differ in importance and number from system to system, and their effectiveness is often questionable.

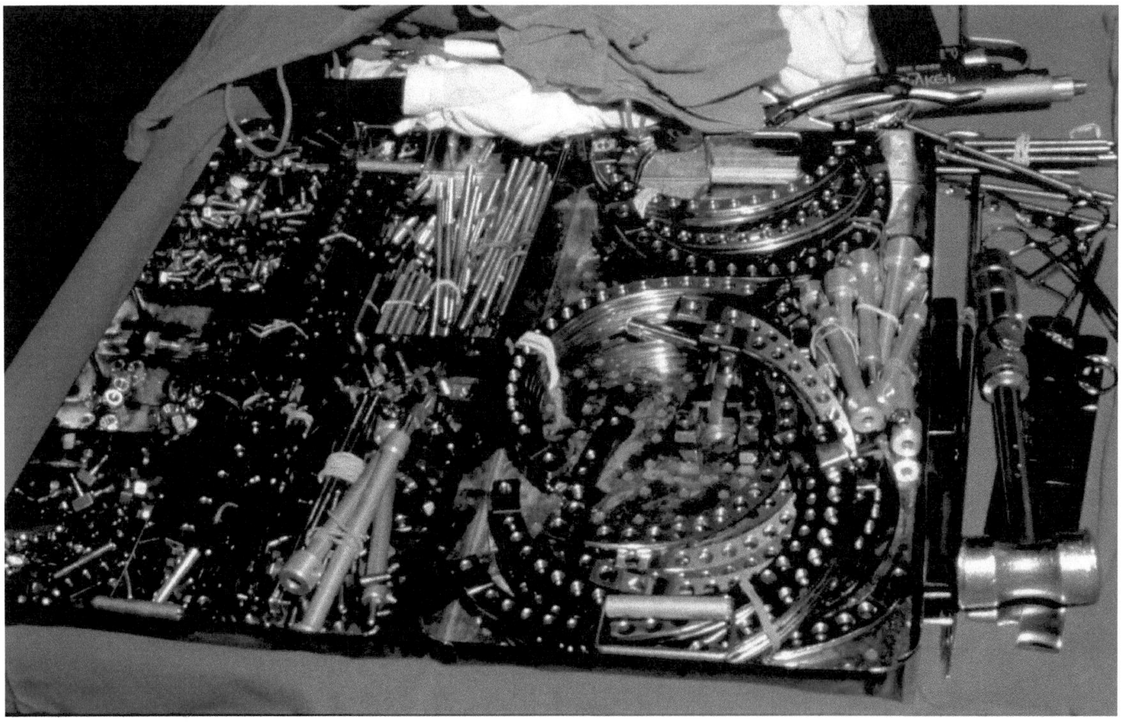

Fig. 1. The components of the original Ilizarov compression-distraction system

In the last few decades many different circular external fixation systems have been proposed, but only some of them have been successful and gained widespread recognition (thanks to their particular features and versatility), mainly, but not only, in Eastern Europe.

A particularly detailed description of these systems goes beyond the scope of this chapter, but some aspects, particularly featuring a limited number of systems developed in the Soviet Union and in Western countries, will be discussed. Each of them shows interesting features, even though their success has been very different.

Ilizarov System

The most well known system is certainly that of Ilizarov, developed at the Kurgan KNIIEKOT Institute [2] (Fig. 2).

The original device, made with steel, fundamentally consists of flat half-rings, which are connected in pairs and compose the apparatus rings. On the surface of the rings, longitudinally threaded rods (fixed by nuts and used to connect the rings) can be passed through holes displaced by 10°.

The bone fixation elements, in the original apparatus, are thin metallic wires (1.5 or 1.8 mm in diameter) fixed to the rings by dedicated buckles or special cannulated or slotted bolts and put under tension with a specific tensioner.

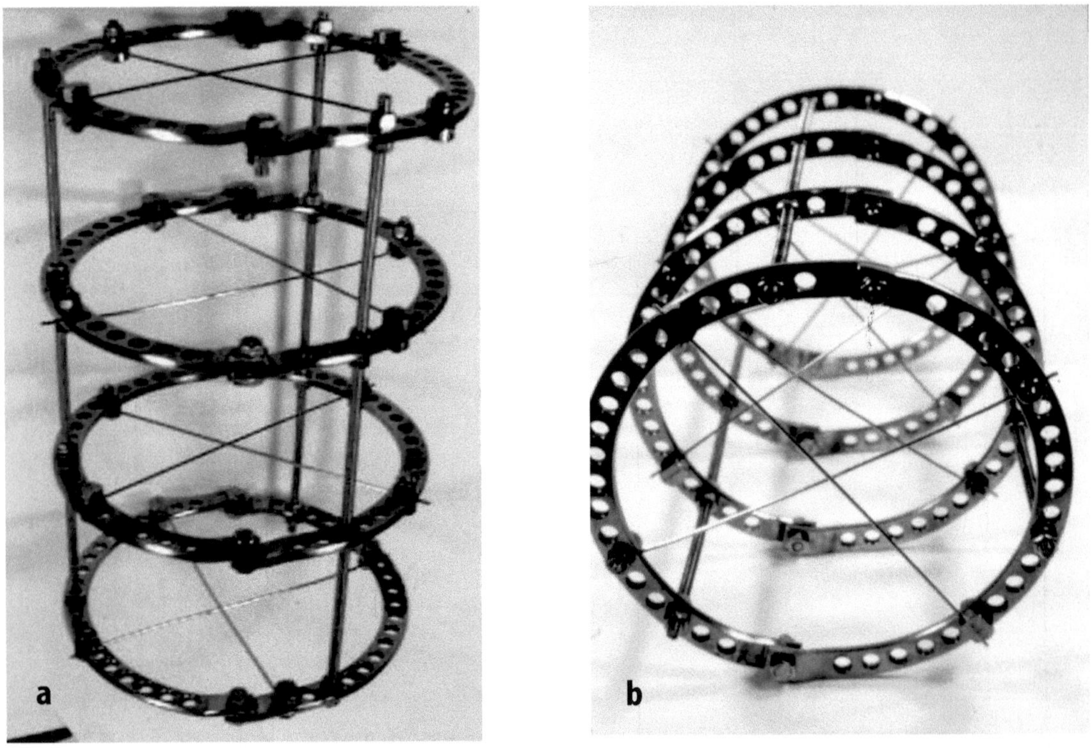

Fig. 2a, b. The Ilizarov apparatus, developed at the KNIIEKOT Institute of Kurgan

In this system the wide range of equipment with optional elements enhances the creation of many configurations, more or less complex, and is suitable for any kind of treatment. This feature offers a wider edge of control and always allows the best position to be achieved between the fragments.

The original system, planned by Ilizarov, progressively evolved after it became known in Western countries, and even benefited by the increasing knowledge of the other kinds of compression-distraction systems, mainly used in Eastern Europe.

Concerning the essential components of the Ilizarov system, the initial focus was primarily on transosseous wires. Actually they represented an obstacle to patient tolerability, most of all at the limb root level, because they required an excessively bulky and complex assembly.

A good initial compromise, mainly used in the 1980s at the Orthopaedic Department of the University of Pavia, involved connecting some Hoffmann System components to the Ilizarov apparatus in the proximal humerus and proximal femur assembly.

Since 1986 a special fixation system developed by Catagni and Cattaneo has been used for the proximal portion of humerus and femur. This device consists of 90° and 120° arches, half-pins (4 to 6 mm in diameter), pin fixation bolts, and special oblique supports to connect arches to rings [3].

Then other elements were developed: lighter and radiotransparent composite half-rings as alternatives to the classic steel half-ring at one or more assembly levels, and graduated telescopic rods, to promote the execution and the control of compression or distraction through the simple rotation of the head of the rod (mainly used for limb lengthening).

During the following years, Green suggested an increasingly wider use of half-pins fixed to the rings through special buckles called "Rancho Cubes" not only at the limb root level but at any level of fixation instead of wires, in order to improve patient compliance and reduce the risk of inflammation and infection [4]. This is the "Rancho mounting technique", named from the Californian Orthopaedic Centre "Rancho Los Amigos Hospital", where this technique was developed.

Moreover, in a systematization proposed by Catagni et al. [3], the different types of assemblies developed by mixed use of wires and screws were named "hybrid assemblies" and divided into hybrid traditional (HT) and hybrid advanced (HA), according to the prevalence of wires or screws used for assembling it.

We believe, however, that it is more useful to call the assemblies made by combined use of wires and screws "mixed" and reserve the term "hybrid" for those assemblies using external axial fixation components connected to external circular fixation components.

Then, a new Ilizarov system (the "Acute Trauma Ilizarov") was proposed some years ago in the United States. In this system, even more extensive modifications have been added to the original idea, the intention being to make the assembly even faster in trauma applications (by means of "Quick connect" rods, adjustable pin clamps for both rods and rings) [5].

The risk of this series of modifications and changes to the basic elements is related to the creation of a sort of confusion among orthopaedic surgeons approaching these techniques as a result ot the extreme schematization or too detailed description of the assembly.

The secondary parts for the system have also progressively evolved and can be employed for particular assemblies.

The most interesting and useful among them are described in Chapters 10–14.

Volkov-Oganesian System

The Volkov-Oganesian system [6], developed at the CITO (Central Institute of Traumatology and Orthopaedics) of Moscow, is made up of four titanium rings connected to each other by longitudinally threaded rods and characterized by the presence, between the two central rings, of an orthogonal screw system. With this system angular, transverse, and rotational dislocations of bone fragments can be carefully corrected (Fig. 3).

Transosseous wires, 2 mm in diameter, are fixed to the rings at pre-established sites and are then tightened by a grooved screw. The use of this apparatus is quite difficult, because the wires must be inserted in an established direction and angulation. In a model of the device developed by Umiarov (personal communication) [7] pins or half-pins 4 mm in diameter can be employed instead of wires.

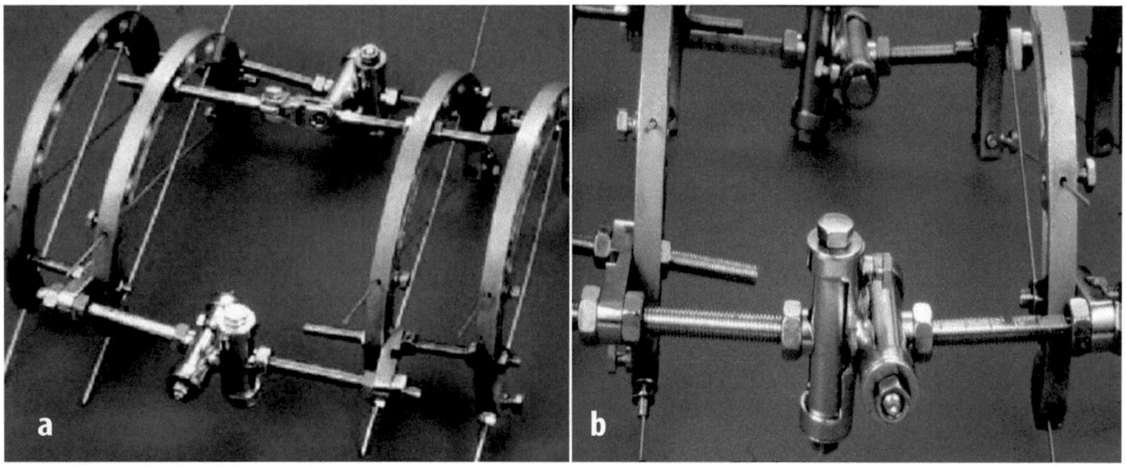

Fig. 3a, b. The Volkov-Oganesian device, developed at the CITO Institute of Moscow

Kalnberz System

The Kalnberz apparatus [1] was developed at the LNIITO Institute of Riga (Latvia) and shows some interesting features. First of all, it is distinguished by the ring composition, which is not metallic but plastic (made of fiberglass), and by the section (flat or octagonal). Moreover, even in the first version of the apparatus, pins or half-pins 4 mm in diameter could be used instead of crossed wires. These features allow a wide range of solutions in the application of the bone fixation elements and a stable bone fragment fixation.

Metallic, threaded rods (rigid or elastic) or, alternatively, fiberglass rods, connect the rings to each other. Their internal surface is gripped by clamps, which allow all the required movements to be made rapidly.

According to the rods employed, the assemblies are classified into three different groups: "rigid universal system" (rigid titanium rods), "stress system" (elastic titanium rods), and "rigid simplex system" (fiberglass rods).

The use of plastic elements decreases the apparatus weight, assuring complete radiotransparency.

Moreover, it is often useful to shape the rings, cutting segments of different length on demand.

Made up of exclusively five kinds of elements (wires or pins, rings, rods, clamps, and nuts), this system couples the facility of management with wide flexibility (Figs. 4, 5).

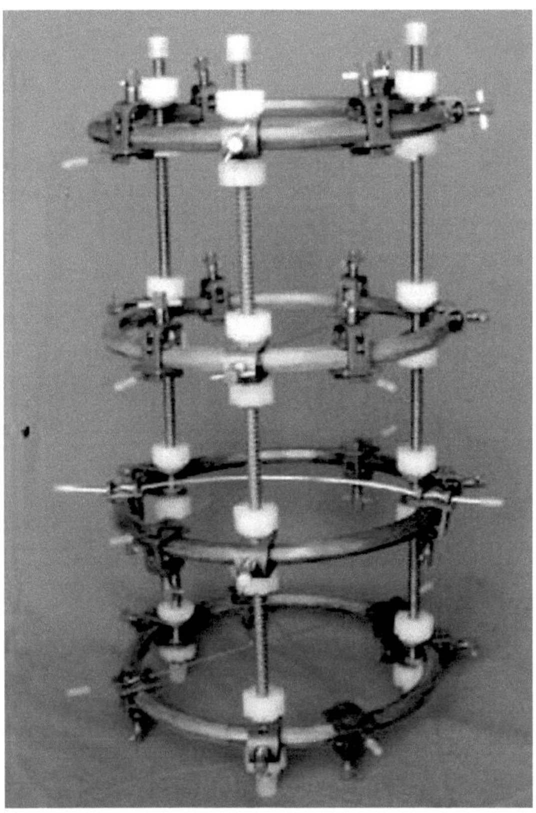

Fig. 4. The Kalnberz "Rigid Universal" apparatus, developed at the LNIITO Institute of Riga

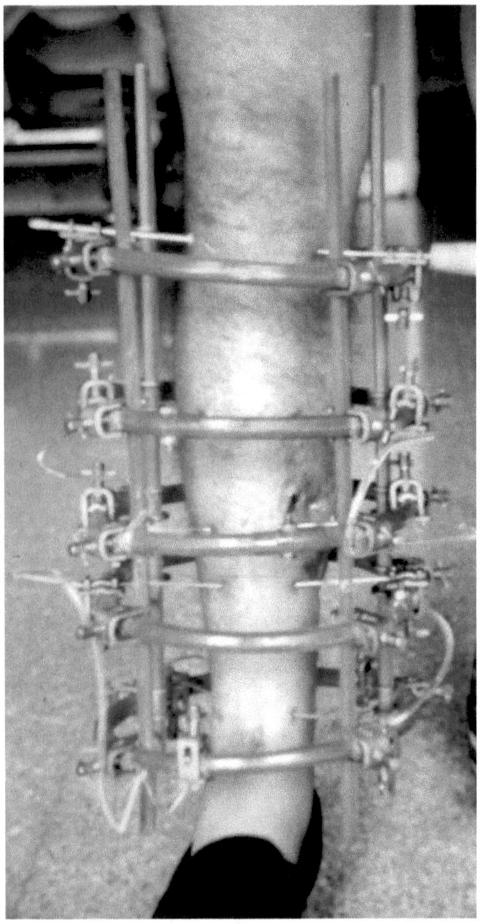

Fig. 5. Treatment of a tibial nonunion with the Kalnberz "Rigid Simplex" apparatus

Fischer System

Another system was planned by Fischer at the Department of Orthopaedic Surgery of Minnesota State University in Minneapolis [8]. It is based on a very flexible apparatus, made up of aluminium or titanium rings, connected to each other by special rods that allow movements in each individual plane and that are connected to the bone by steel or titanium pins. These pins are 5 mm in diameter and can be inserted in every spatial plane. Transosseous wires can be used even in this system instead of the screws (Figs. 6, 7).

Taylor Spatial Frame

The Taylor Spatial Frame is a multiplanar circular external fixator [9]. It combines ease of application and computer accuracy in reducing fractures or nonunions and in correcting deformities. The basic unit consists of two full rings that are connected by six diagonally oriented, adjustable struts. The struts are connected to each ring by universal joints. Fixation to the bone is

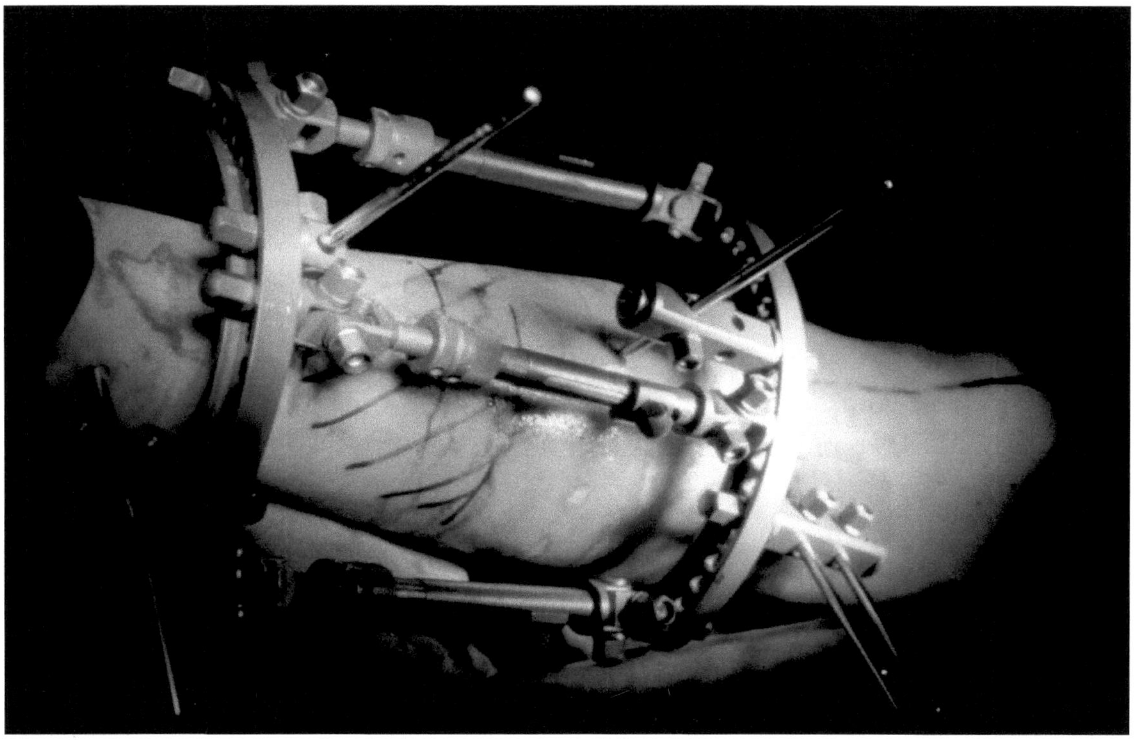

Fig. 6. Management of a tibial nonunion by means of the Fischer device, developed at Minnesota State University

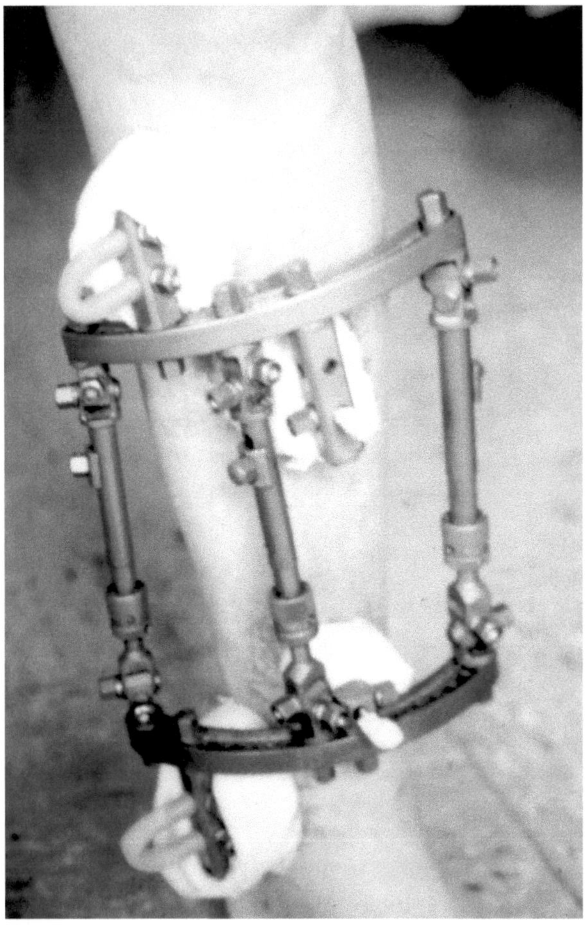

Fig. 7. Fischer apparatus applied to a leg with a tibial delayed union

achieved with transosseous wires, half-pins, or a combination of the two. Additional stability can be achieved by adding a second ring above or below the site of the lesion.

The device is modular and offers the possibility of using full rings, half-rings, or 2/3 rings of various diameters, and different strut lengths are available (Fig. 8).

The accuracy of displacement or deformity correction by this device is dependent on analysis of the radiograms. Thirteen parameters describing the fixator, displacement or deformity, and position of the fixator to the bone are entered into a computer, and a computer program provides the proper adjustments of the six modular struts needed to obtain reduction or correction.

Adjusting the struts changes the orientation of one ring to the other, and this results in a spatial change of one bone fragment to the other one. Adjustments during the postoperative period are also possible by changing the strut length and can be done by the patient, according to a special schedule, which is also generated by the software [10, 11].

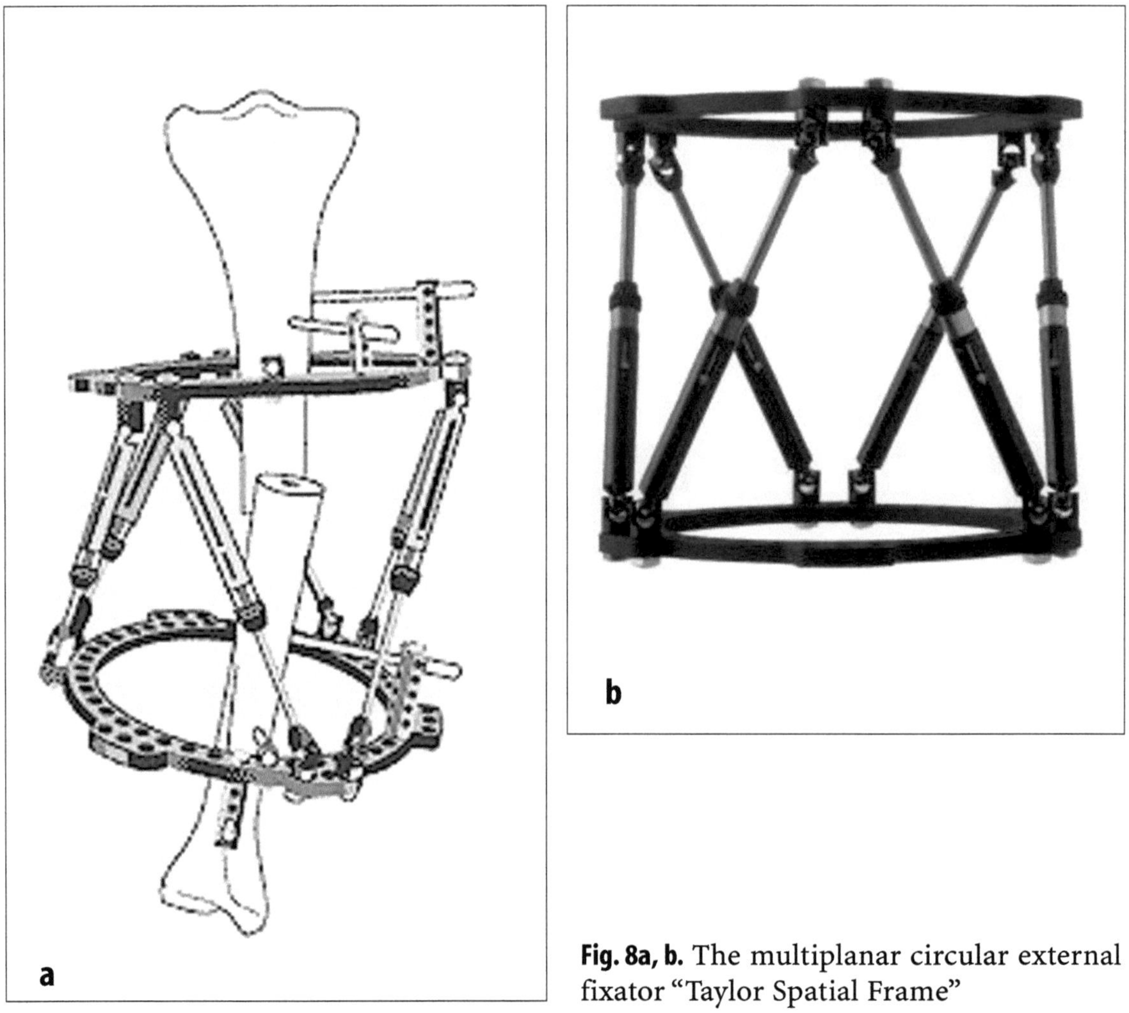

Fig. 8a, b. The multiplanar circular external fixator "Taylor Spatial Frame"

Hybrid Ring Fixator

The "hybrid" ring fixator is designed for fixation of proximal and distal tibial fractures, particularly those involving the joints [12–15]. The device is composed of one ring (of various diameters) fixed to the proximal or distal tibial metaphysis by wires and connected by clamps to one or more rods or to an axial external fixator, coupled to the tibial diaphysis by pins (Figs. 9, 10).

If rods are employed, the use of more than one rod gives additional stability to the frame.

To restore a good articular surface, a preliminary open reduction and stabilization with cannulated screws (in combination with bone grafting if required) can be performed.

Conclusion

This short introduction to compression-distraction systems shows some important features of circular external fixation. The use of screws instead of

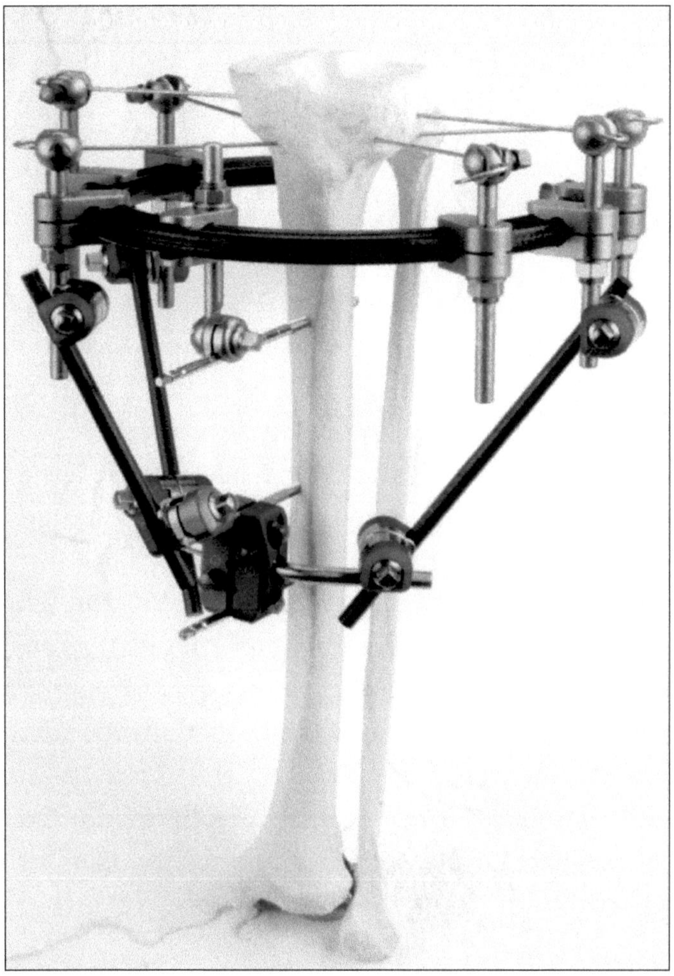

Fig. 9. Hybrid frame "Tenxor"

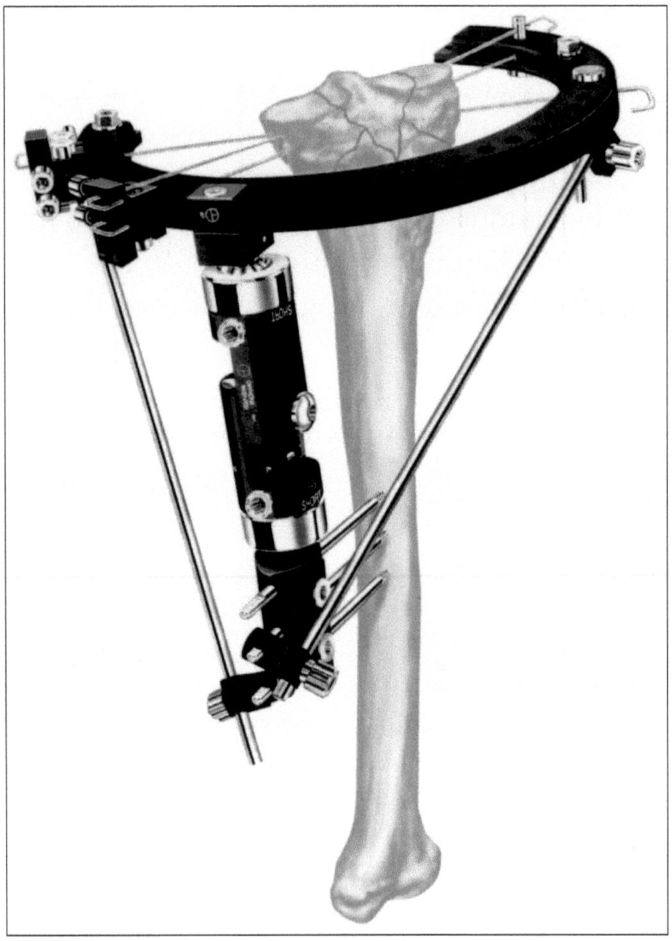

Fig. 10. Hybrid fixation system "Orthofix"

or in addition to Kirschner wires, already in use even in the early versions of many of the systems described, was further improved in the Ilizarov system. This system is now the most widely used system in Western countries due to the more or less important (and more or less useful) modifications suggested by many authors both in Europe and United States (the so-called "hybrid assemblies", which more properly should be called "mixed assemblies").

Moreover, some of the axial external fixation systems still used in Western countries and elements or systems of circular external fixation (so-called hybrid systems) have been created to be compatible with each other [14].

The aim, al least in theory, should be to combine the advantages of the two fixation systems, decreasing some assembly problems at specific sites, improving stability, and enhancing tolerability.

The success of the systems presented here are different in orthopaedic surgery and traumatology, and some of them are still not well known in Western countries. In any case, indications for their use should be evaluated according to the following parameters: assembly stability, flexibility, ease of application and management, kind of pathology to treat and the resulting better or worse possibility of reducing interfragmentary movement in traumatology or correcting deformities in orthopaedic surgery, and the frequency of adjustments needed during the treatment [16].

Ultimately, an overall evaluation of the characteristics of these systems favors the versatility of the Ilizarov system, both regarding the original idea and its further development, which seems to be higher than in the other systems and suggests that it should be employed in the most complex cases.

References

1. Kalnberz VK (1981) Compression-distraction apparatus. Stress and rigid system. LNIITO, Riga
2. Ilizarov GA, Green SA (1992) Transosseous osteosynthesis. Springer, Berlin Heidelberg New York
3. Catagni MA, Malzev V, Kirienko A (eds) (1994) Advances in Ilizarov apparatus assembly. Medicalplastic, Milan
4. Green SA, Harris NL, Ishkanian J, Marinow H (1992) The Rancho mounting technique for the Ilizarov method: a preliminary report. Clin Orthop Relat Res 280:104–116
5. Smith & Nephew Orthopaedics (1996) Acute trauma Ilizarov. Smith and Nephew Richards, Memphis
6. Volkov MV, Oganesian O (1987) External fixation: joint deformities and bone fractures. International University Press, Madison
7. Umiarov GA (1988) Personal communication
8. Fischer DA (1983) Skeletal stabilization with a multiplane external fixation device. Clin Orthop Relat Res 180:50–62
9. Binski JC (2002) Taylor spatial frame in acute fracture care. Techn Orthop 17:173–184
10. Binski JC (2003) Treatment of the fractures with the Taylor spatial frame. Proceedings 8th Italian Congress ASAMI, Lecco
11. Morandi M (2003) Taylor spatial frame. Minerva Ortop 54:54–56
12. Helfet DL, Koval K, Pappas J et al (1994) intraarticular pilon fracture of the tibia. Clin Orthop Relat Res 298:221–228
13. Barbieri R, Schenk R, Koval K et al (1996) Hybrid external fixation in the treatment of tibial plafond fractures. Clin Orthop Relat Res 332:16–22
14. Saleh M, Yang L, Nayagam S (1997) Can a hybrid fixator perform as well as the Ilizarov fixator? J Bone Joint Surg Br 79 [Suppl. 4]:462
15. Anglen JA (1999) Early outcome of hybrid external fixation for fracture of the distal tibia J Orthop Trauma 13:92–97
16. Aronson J, Harp JH (1984) Factors influencing the choice of external fixation for distraction osteogenesis. AAOS Instr Course Lect 39:175–183

Compression-Distraction Methods

Redento Mora, Barbara Bertani, Luisella Pedrotti, Gabriella Tuvo, Stefano Gili

Preoperative Planning

The preoperative planning should include both clinical and instrumental investigations, evaluation of the patient's psychological conditions, planning of the device assembly, and choice of the correct surgical technique.

Clinical and Instrumental Investigations

The clinical investigations should include an accurate anamnesis and a careful general and local physical examination (Fig. 1).

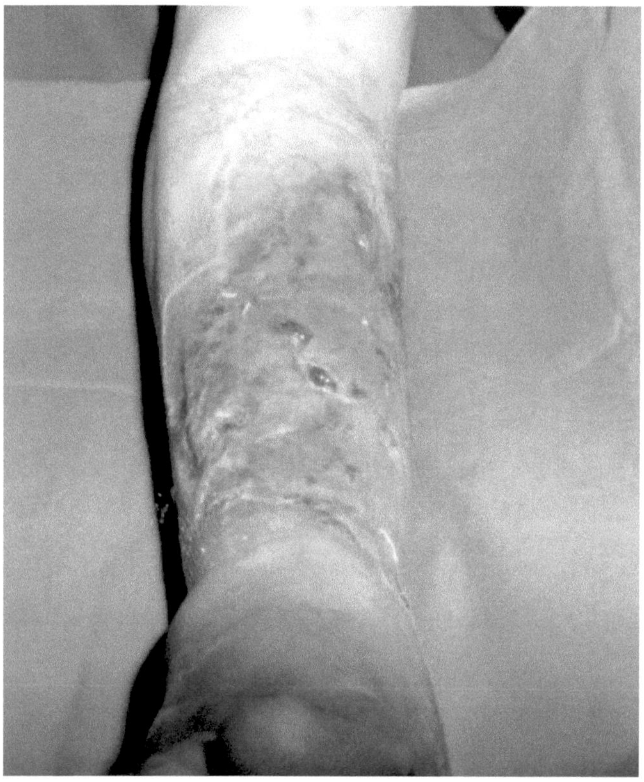

Fig. 1. Patient with tibial nonunion: the skin and the soft tissues are in very poor conditions

Special attention should be given to the state of the skin and soft tissues in the areas in which transosseous wires and screws will be applied, considering that they will affect the patient's tolerability and the general stability of the device.

Instrumental assessments include radiographic examinations and other examinations, such as bone scan, computed tomography, and MRI. It is also useful to image the extremity that needs to be treated, especially for simple or complex defomities.

Patient Preparation

Psychological Preparation

During the meeting with the patient (and his or her family) it is advisable to explain the aspects of the device and the details of the operation, the possible problems and their solutions, as well as the expectable level of tolerability.

Rehabilitation Preparation

The measures that can be taken aim mainly to make elastic, by means of muscle stretching techniques, the site of interest, and to increase the control of muscular contraction and relaxation [1].

Planning the Device Assembly

The configuration and all possible modifications during treatment must be preliminarily defined (especially when using the Ilizarov system, in which new rings cannot be added except with great difficulty and loss of time because the connection rods must pass through the holes of the rings).

It is necessary to foresee any possible maneuvers of displacement reduction or correction of the deformities, and it is necessary to decide whether to preassemble the device or to gradually assemble it during the operation.

Finally, the proper surgical technique must be chosen for each patient individually.

Operative Planning

Anesthesia

The anesthesiologic problems connected with the use of compression-distraction techniques are related to: age of the patient, kind of orthopaedic pathology or trauma, length of the operation, postoperative pain, and risk of vascular and neurological damage (with subsequent need for immediate or early modification of the mounting) [2]. Thus, in this particular type of surgery, the anesthesia must block the transmission and the integration of the nociceptive stimulus at the level of the reticular system, thalamus, cortex (general anesthesia) or at the peripheral or medullary level (regional anesthesia), but also allow an early evaluation of possible motor disorders that occurred during the operation.

The type of anesthesia must obviously be adapted to these particular needs, choosing among several possibilities: general anesthesia, regional anesthesia, or combined general and regional anesthesia [3].

General anesthesia has the advantage of allowing an immediate control (as soon as the patient wakes up) for neurological problems. Postoperative pain, which is often intense, is not well controlled with the use of major and minor analgesic drugs, because the experience of surgery can represent quite a shock for the patient.

Regional anesthesia for operations on the lower limbs has improved in recent years. It uses central blocks (continuous lumbar epidural anesthesia and selective spinal anesthesia) and peripheral blocks (troncular anesthesia), which all have advantages and disadvantages.

Continuous lumbar epidural anesthesia has the advantage of producing a sensitive block of good quality without motor block (with low-dose, local anesthetic drugs) and allows complete control of postoperative pain (by means of local anesthetics and/or morphine administered in bolus or by infusion).

Selective spinal anesthesia produces a sensitive block of good quality but also a motoric block; the control of postoperative pain is good (if modest amounts of morphine are added); finally there is a limit of time of the block of about 3 h.

Among the most commonly used blocks is the so-called "bi-block" (block of the sciatic and femoral nerves), applied by using an electroneurostimulator [4, 5]. This technique is less invasive and only involves a low rate of complications compared to the other methods of regional anesthesia. It also can obtain an effective sensitive and motor block of the leg and the distal third of the thigh (therefore, the lower limb is not completely anesthetized). The control of postoperative pain is good; the time limit for the block is about 3 h.

For regional anesthesia in operations of the upper limbs peripheral blocks are used. The qualities include those of a good sensitive block, often combined with a motor block.

In interscalenic blocks, the risk of complications must not be underestimated; finally, for this kind of surgery the length of the anesthesia is excessive.

Combined general and regional anesthesia is employed in selected cases. In particular, when using the "bi-block" technique, regional anesthesia must often be complemented by hypnotic and opiate drugs.

Surgery

From the time the patient arrives until he or she leaves the operating room at the end of the surgery, the stages of preparation and execution of the operation should follow precise rules, governed by experience.

Putting the Patient on the Operating Table

Several types of supports for surgically treated limbs have been described and introduced in the past few decades, but, as underlined by Kalnberz [6], the majority of these solutions are not very practical. However, the use of some simple tricks after the patient has been put on the operating table in supine position is more than enough in most cases (Fig. 2): a folded cloth can be placed under the buttock and, after preparation of the operating field, the lower limb can be slightly elevated by means of some folded cloths.

Concerning the upper limbs, the forearm does not require particular supports and only a table is needed for hand surgery. For the humerus, too, support on the table for hand surgery in cases of nonunion is sufficient.

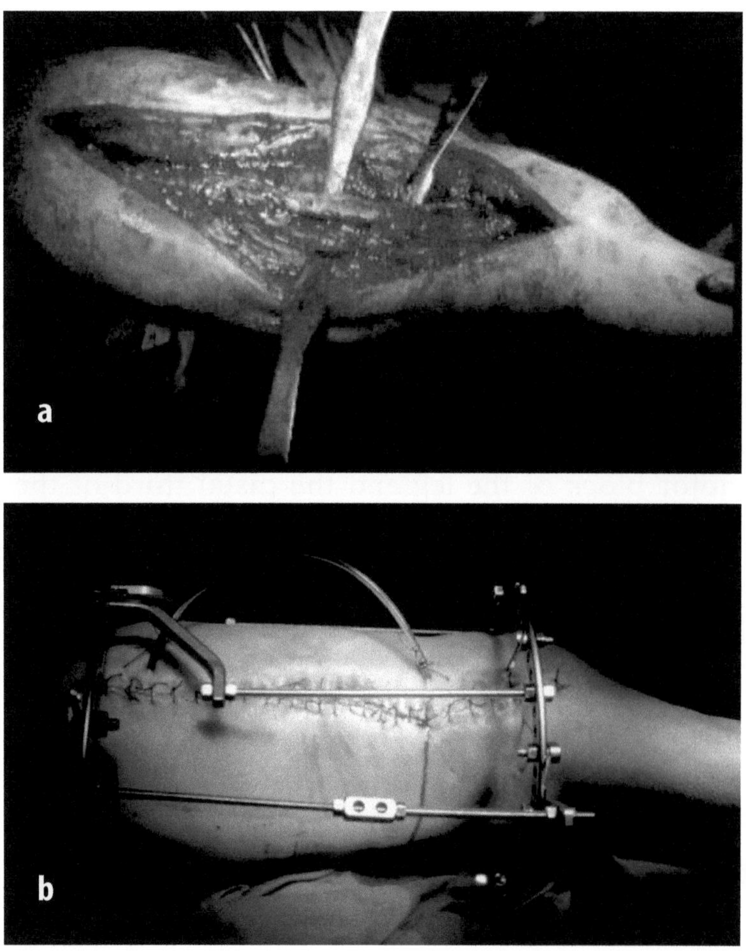

Fig. 2a, b. Operative treatment of an infected nonunion of the femur without any kind of support of the lower limb

Application of a Tourniquet

Considerable doubts exist regarding the use of this device. Generally, a tourniquet should not be applied when transosseous osteosynthesis is employed, especially in trauma surgery, to avoid the risk of not recognizing vascular lesions caused by the passage of wires and screws, even if this means the operation time is longer. In the simplest cases, for which operative technique is completely standardized, application of a tourniquet makes the operation faster and easier, without adding complications.

Preparation of the Surgeons

Preparation of the surgeons must obviously be as accurate as for any other operation, with extra care regarding the potential danger of the use of transosseous wires: two pairs of gloves must be worn and changed every 25 min in order to avoid accidental injuries to the hands and contamination during application of the external fixation device [7, 8].

Surgical Field

The preparation of the operating field must meet two critical requirements: the operating field must be wide and completely cover the upper or the lower limb, in order to have the limb axis in sight at all times. Secondly, the field must also be prepared as simply and practically as possible: in fact the surgeon must frequently move around the patient during the various stages of the operation, for reasons of both safety and ease (Fig. 3).

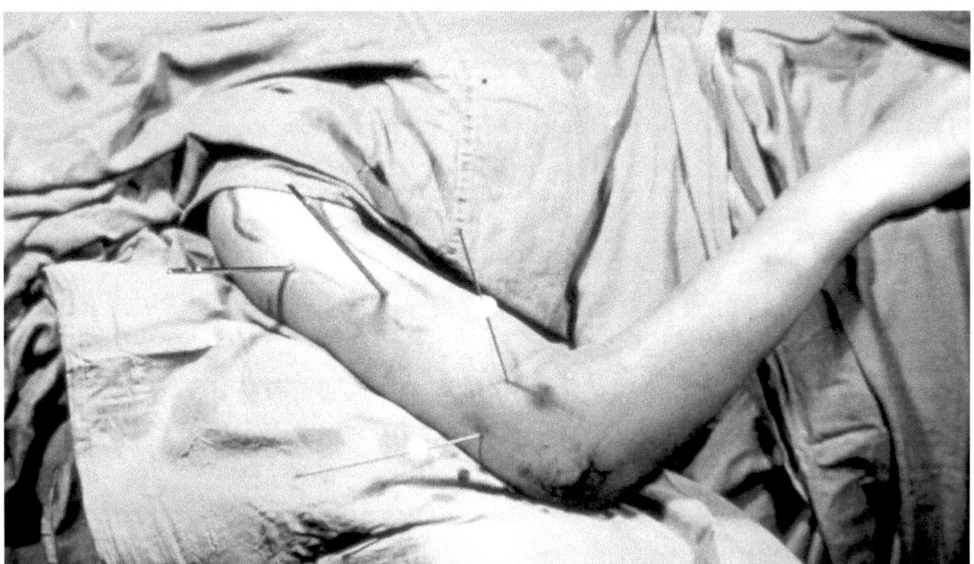

Fig. 3. Wide operating field for the upper limb

Preoperative Landmarks

The points and lines, drawn with a dermographic pencil before the beginning of the operation, are actually very useful as this drastically reduces the exposure to the image intensifier during the operation.

It is always advisable to trace these points and lines after the surgical field has been prepared to ensure that the levels of the proximal and distal joints and the level of nonunion are precisely indicated.

Surgical Procedure

Surgery must be the "natural consequence" of the preoperative planning and of the stages of preparation described above. Depending on the type and severity of the nonunion, different types of devices and mounting must be chosen, deciding on the possible use of radiotransparent elements and/or the use of wires or screws.

It is important to remember that the mounting that requires the smallest number of wires or screws is the best: particular attention must be given to stability because if it is insufficient the patient will experience pain and the entire treatment may fail.

The need for radioscopic controls can be reduced to minimum if the preparation has been accurate and the surgeon is well experienced. In fact, the use of x-rays can often be limited to the final control after the surgery.

Some interesting observations, based on anatomical research and instrumental investigations, have recently been presented about the use of bone fixation elements at the leg in the proximity of the knee and ankle joints [9, 10]. According to these studies, bone fixation elements should not be applied at distances less than 15 mm from the knee joint or less than 12 mm from the ankle joint in order to obtain safe and extracapsular application.

External fixators are effective for managing bone, but problems may arise with soft tissues. We are not referring to vessels and nerves, which must obviously be respected, but rather the skin, subcutaneous tissue, fasciae, muscles and tendons, because problems may develop such that the number of clinical control examinations required may markedly rise. In particular, tension of soft tissues, caused by the bone fixation elements in both longitudinal and transverse directions, must be avoided (Fig. 4).

First of all, apart from the pain during both rest and movement, inflammation or necrosis (that adds problems for the patient) may develop. Secondly (basically when wires are used, and when no particular care is taken to avoid bending and torsion when connecting the wires on the rings), other issues are added, such as the alteration of the normal venous and lymphatic flow, with resulting edema and local inflammation.

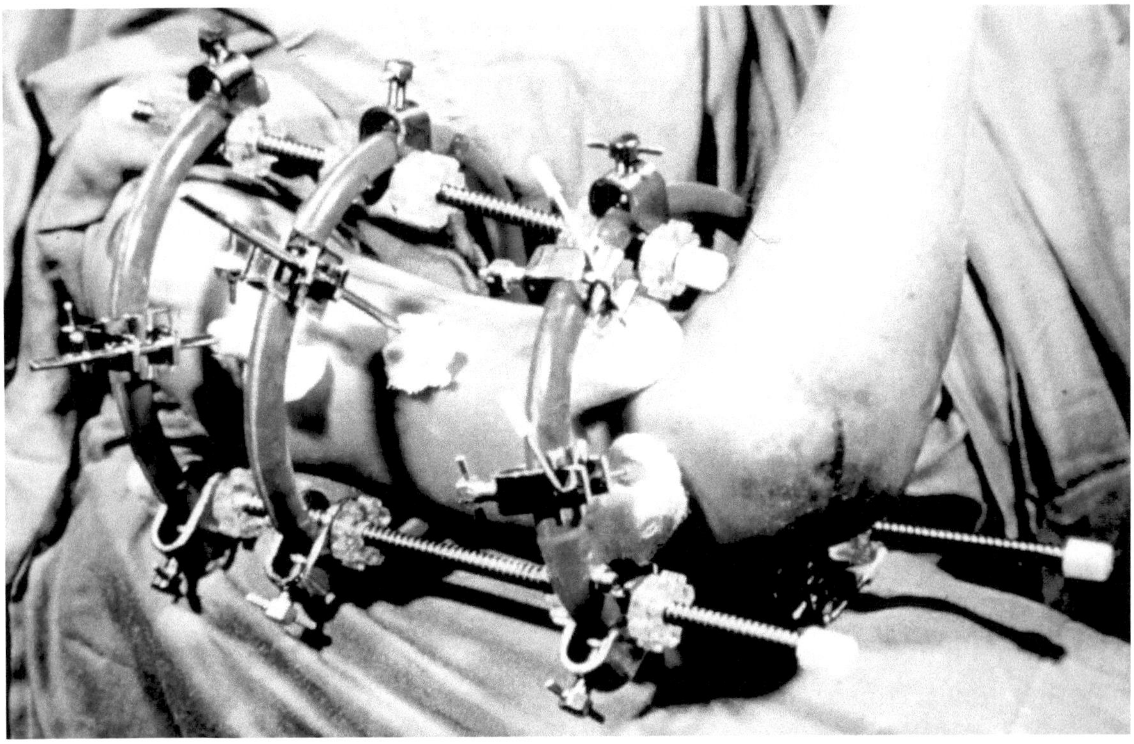

Fig. 4. Mounting of the Kalnberz device on the humerus, avoiding tension of the soft tissues

Another particularly important aspect is the prevention of postoperative joint stiffness. This can occur in all joints, but particularly in the knee in the case of femoral mountings [11]. The main rule to follow for the prevention of joint stiffness is maintaining the correct position of the joint while inserting the bone fixation elements in proximity of the joint. In fact, it is necessary that they be inserted through the flexor muscles with the joint extended and through the extensor muscles with the joint flexed.

During the surgical procedure the previously planned general program must be strictly adhered to, also in relation to possible future adjustments. The external circular fixation systems are different from one another, especially with regard to the difficulty of inserting new rings to the initial structure. With the Kalnberz system, for example, in which the fiberglass rings are applied externally to the rods, it is easy to insert new rings, but in the Ilizarov system, where the rods must go through holes in the rings, the need for insertion of a new ring may involve a great loss of time. Thus, it is very important that the rings that will be used in the future are inserted in the original structure (for example, in the case of bifocal compression-distraction osteosynthesis).

Site of Application of the Device

The site of application of the compression-distraction device is surely one of the most important considerations. Particular care must be given to the mounting stability, which is provided not only by the use of an adequate number of rings and wires or screws, but also by applying them at the appropriate levels and correct angles.

The importance of the soft tissues must always be kept in mind. The size of the soft tissues of the thigh, in particular, often represents an obstacle to applying a circular external fixator, due to matters of space.

Generally speaking, the more the mounting involves the root of the limb, the worse it is to use a circular external fixator. For this reason, when treating the humerus or the femur, it is advisable to take all precautions that will improve the tolerability, without reducing the stability of the structure.

Finally, it is very important from a psychological point of view to maintain at least partial mobility of the proximal and distal joints during treatment. On the other hand, considering that the first goal is healing and that this strictly depends on the device stability, it is sometimes necessary to postpone joint motion maintenance for a short period of time and use an assembly to bridge a joint.

Humerus

The use of external fixation with good results in the management of humeral shaft fractures was described by Burny et al. [12] and De Bastiani et al. [13]. The methods of axial or circular external fixation, indeed, can be advantageously employed in humeral trauma and represent a valid alternative to internal fixation techniques, owing to ease of use, simple reduction and stabilization, and good tolerability [14, 15].

With regard to the differences between axial and circular external fixation in humeral trauma surgery, axial fixators are believed to be better tolerated, less cumbersome, and less of a risk for the vessels and nerves [16]. Circular systems, however, offer the advantages of a more stable fixation and a better adaptability to the different kinds of injuries.

The mounting is based on three or four levels of fixation, depending on the exact position of the fracture (Fig. 5). If wires are used, the smallest size is recommended (1.5 mm in the Ilizarov system) [17–19].

Proximally, the lateral half-ring connected to two wires in anterior-posterior and posterior-anterior direction, as originally used in Ilizarov technique, has been now replaced in all systems by a lateral arch connected to two screws, as in the original Kalnberz system. Distally, the use of a posterior half-ring (or a 5/8 ring) connected to two wires allows a wider range of motion of the elbow. If more stability is needed, a complete ring may be used (that tem-

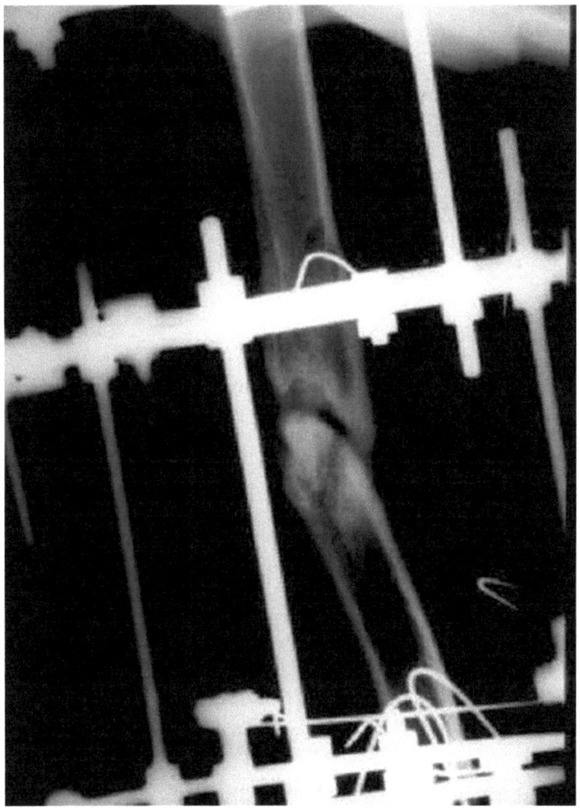

Fig. 5. Humeral nonunion treated with an Ilizarov compression-distraction device

porarily limits the flexion). Alternatively to the wires, two screws (lateral and medial) with oblique anterior-posterior direction can be used.

At the intermediate level, a tendency has been observed in the past few years to use screws instead of wires or mixed mountings for bone fixation. This does not really provide any advantage to the patient, however, in terms of stability or tolerability.

Forearm

At the forearm, indications for treatment with external fixators are more limited [20]. Here, maintaining the length, reduction of angular and rotational displacements, and conservation of the interosseous space must always be under control. These objectives are reached by means of internal osteosynthesis, but in cases of infection external fixation is indicated as a temporary or definitive means of fixation [21–23].

When treating nonunions of the forearm with a circular external fixator, the construction is based on the use of three or four rings, depending on the level and on the kind of the injury (mono-osseous or bi-osseous; *see* Fig. 6).

Small wires are used (1.5 mm). An important rule is to connect the distal wires to the rings only after eliminating the rotatory displacement of the fragments; otherwise, the reduction would be impossible [24–26]. As an alternative to the wires, screws can be used, performing mixed mountings.

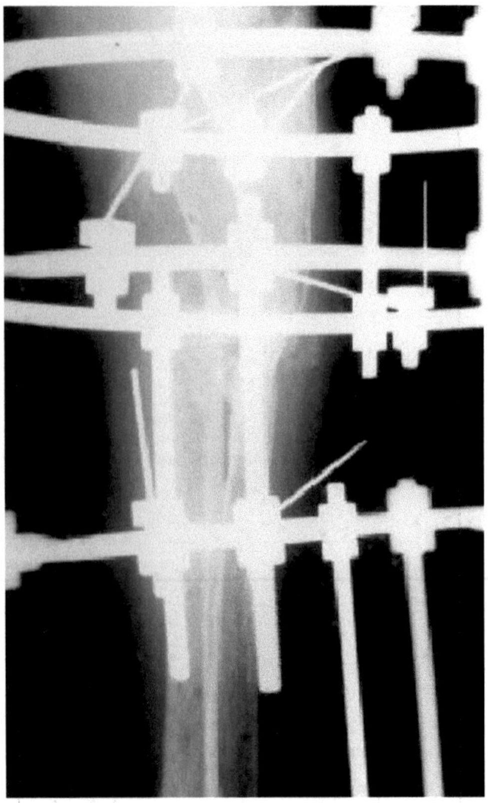

Fig. 6. Treatment of a forearm nonunion with an Ilizarov compression-distraction apparatus

Femur

In the lower limbs, the versatility and stability of compression-distraction systems have improved their diffusion, especially for use at the tibial level. For the femur, the indication is more limited because of the low tolerability and the difficulty of obtaining (with standard mountings) effective reduction, correction, and stability and because of the frequent occurrence of knee joint stiffness.

Patient compliance, in fact, can be reduced for numerous reasons: thickness of the soft tissues of the thigh (often increased by edema in a standing position); size of the device; high level of traction delivered by the powerful muscles of this area that often require complex mountings; and frequent incidence of so-called "minor" problems, such as serous secretion and superficial inflammation at the level of the holes of wires or screws.

Circular external fixation methods are indicated in the treatment of femoral injuries mainly when internal synthesis or axial external synthesis does not ensure adequate stabilization [27].

Considering the theoretical advantages of circular external fixation, especially in cases of infected nonunions that develop as a result of "high energy" open diaphyseal femoral fractures, non-"standard" configurations can be employed using special tricks aimed to reposition the fragments and thus avoid the risk of injuries to vessels and nerves and at the same time provide good stability of the synthesis and reduce pain for the patient. These special tricks consist basically of partial or total use of screws instead of wires, changes of the distal part of the mounting, combination with internal osteosynthesis, Novikov reduction nails, and double-threaded screws.

Standard mountings for femoral trauma surgery are based on three or four levels of fixation, depending on the fracture site (Fig. 7). When using wires as bone fixation elements, they must always be of the largest diameter (1.8 mm in the Ilizarov system).

The current tendency to replace crossed wires with nontransfixing screws in the mounting (Fig. 8) [28, 29] certainly does not represent anything new considering that the circular systems developed in the former Soviet Union and largely used in the Eastern countries involve the use of wires, screws, and wires and screws at the same time (Volkov-Oganesian system in the evolution proposed by Umiarov; Kalnberz system) [6, 30].

The widespread use of screws instead of transfixing wires, connected to 90° or 120° arches at the proximal level of the mounting improves patient compliance, while maintaining a good level of stability of the device. With this solution the use of transfixing wires close to the sagittal plane, which causes pain and trouble for the patient, can be successfully replaced. It is important that one of the two screws fixed to the arch is inserted anteriorly through a

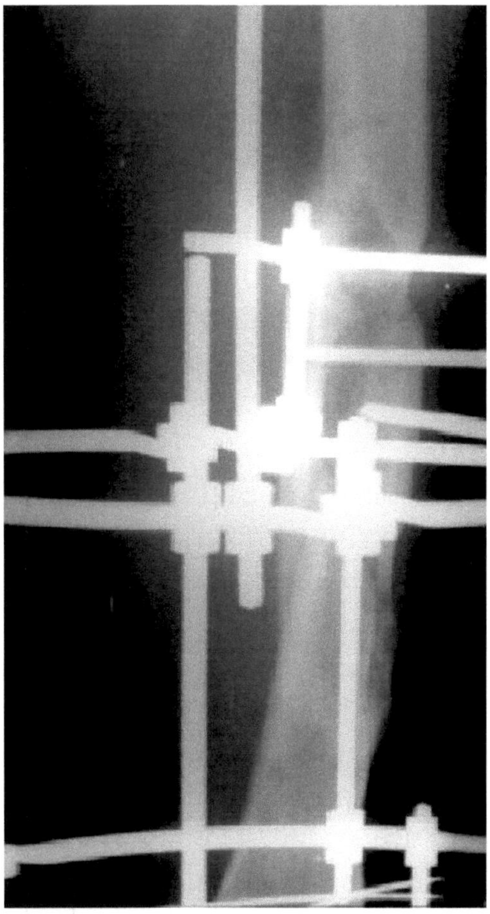

Fig. 7. Femoral nonunion treated with an Ilizarov compression-distraction device

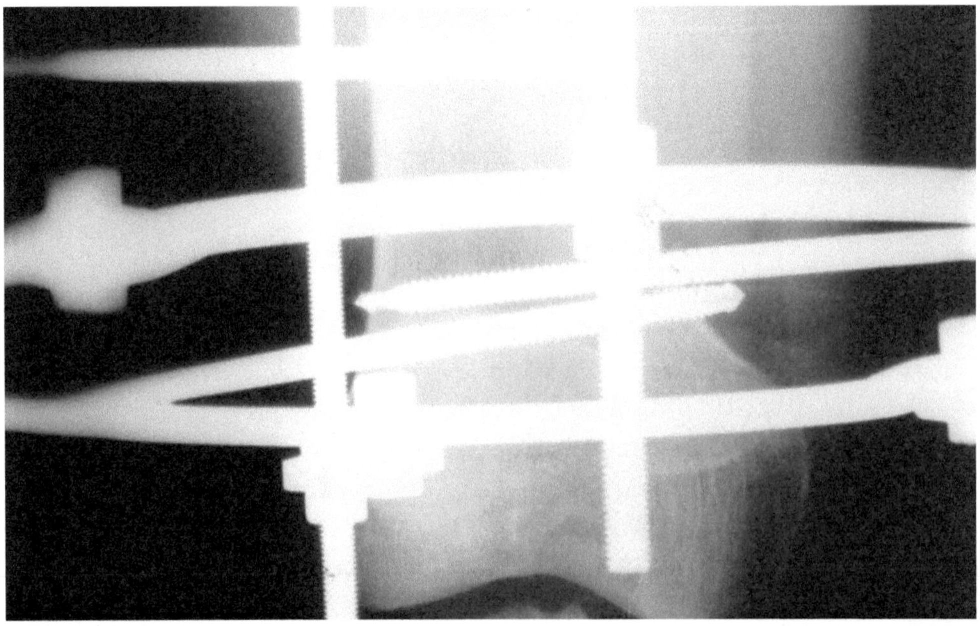

Fig. 8. Femoral nonunion in which wires are replaced by screws at the distal part of the femur

sagittal plane and the other laterally through a coronal plane (with an angulation of 90° between them; *see* Fig. 9): this prevents the arch from leaning backwards and makes things easier for the patient, especially in supine position.

At the intermediate level, it may be useful to use mixed mountings, which do not reduce the stability of the device, to reduce the number of transfixing elements. This can be combined with internal osteosynthesis, intended both as synthesis with Kirschner wires or screws to fix small fragments and as intramedullary synthesis (generally with elastic nails of small diameter) to maintain a certain alignment of the fragments, and can be used successfully in some cases to simplify the external assembly (reducing bulk and improving tolerability) [31].

The Novikov nails (developed at the Latvian Orthopaedic Institute of Riga) (Fig. 10) represent a simple and intelligent tool to obtain, in certain cases, reduction and stabilization of small fragments almost atraumatically. These consist essentially of a Steinmann nail with a blunted end, connected with a micrometric movement system that is easily fixed on one of the rings.

The blunted end is inserted through the soft tissue in contact with the bone; then the nail is gradually inserted until a complete reduction and stabilization of the fragment is obtained [6].

The double-threaded screws, developed by our department in collaboration with the Latvian Orthopaedic Institute of Riga (Fig. 11), are a great improvement when treating fractures with compression-distraction systems.

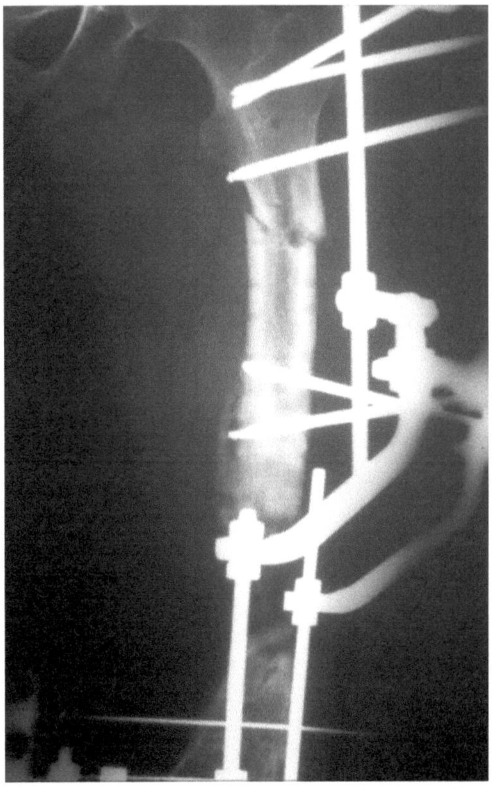

Fig. 9. One of the screws fixed to the proximal arch of the apparatus is inserted anteriorly and the other laterally

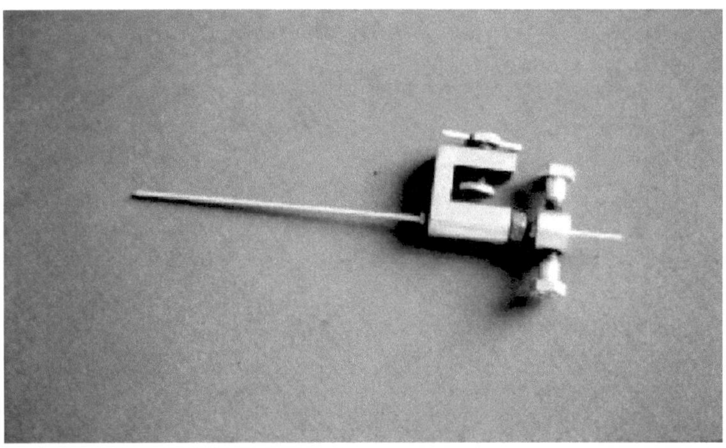

Fig. 10. Novikov nail

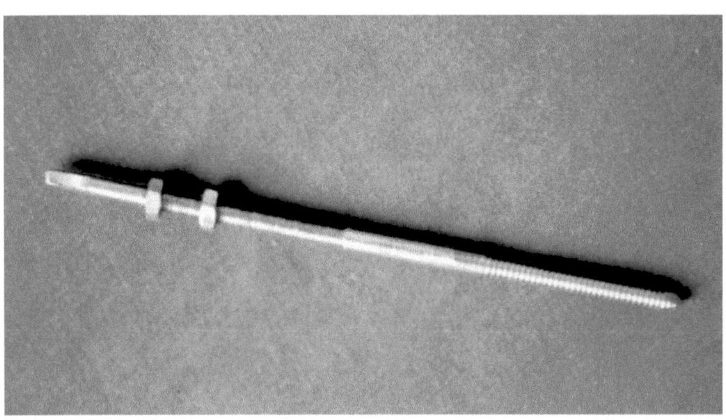

Fig. 11. Double-threaded screw

These screws, which have one thread in their apical part to firmly fix the fragment in which they are inserted and a second thread in their basal part connected to one of the rings, can provide a micrometric correction of the displacements [27].

For the intraoperative prevention of the knee joint stiffness, particular kinds of fixation on the distal part of the assembly have been created. The main rule to follow for the prevention of joint stiffness is to maintain the correct position of the joint while inserting the bone fixation elements (especially transosseous wires). Next to the joint itself, in fact, it is necessary that they be inserted through the flexor muscles with the joint extended and through the extensor muscles with the joint flexed.

Moreover, special kinds of fixation have also been proposed as an alternative to the classic fixation with crossed wires on the transverse plane to reduce the transfixion of the tendinous-fascial-muscular and capsular-ligamental structures:

- Fixation with a transfixing screw in the coronal plane [6, 32];
- Fixation with crossed wires in the coronal plane [33];
- Fixation with two nontransfixing screws in the transverse plane with an oblique posterior-lateral and posterior-medial direction [29, 34].

When completing the femoral assembly, wires or screws must be applied, if possible, in proximity of the coronal plane of the limb, avoiding angles of over 60° in relation to the poor movement of the soft tissues on the medial and lateral surface of the thigh [32].

Tibia

The leg is considered the most simple and least dangerous application site for a compression-distraction apparatus in traumatology, even if that probably is not true. As regards the differences between axial and circular external fixation in tibial traumatology, they follow those previously presented for humeral traumatology.

Mountings that have been proposed for the tibia are very different: the use of screws as an alternative or in addition to small wires at this level may sometimes be useful. Therefore there is a wide range of possible configurations (Fig. 12). Even at the tibial level the combination of external and internal osteosynthesis can be used in certain cases to reduce the bulk of the external assembly [31].

Assembly Types

The priorities for treating a pathological condition are often the opposite of those for patient tolerability. For this reason, the characteristics of the various

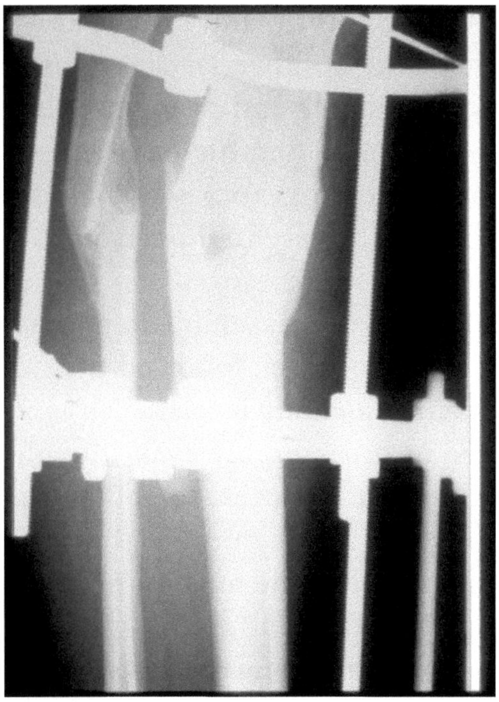

Fig. 12. Tibial nonunion treated with an Ilizarov compression-distraction apparatus

models of circular external fixators must be known in detail and the configurations that meet the standards given in Table 1 must be chosen.

Table 1. Types of Assembly

Feature to be considered	"Modern" mountings	"Classic" mountings
Mounting assembly	Preassembly[1]	Intraoperative assembly
Bone fixation elements	Screws[2]	Wires
Levels of fixation	Less levels[3]	More levels
Extension	Limited (far from the joints)[4]	Wide (close to the joints)
Radiotransparency	Radiotransparent elements[5]	Radio-opaque elements

[1]The preassembly is simpler yet less versatile and less adaptive
[2]The assembly with screws is more rigid and (maybe) better tolerated
[3]The assembly with fewer levels of fixation is better tolerated but less stable
[4]The assembly far from the joints is also better tolerated but less stable
[5]The assembly with radiotransparent rings can be controlled better radiographically but is more (sometimes too) elastic

Execution of the Assembly

The preassembly has gained favor in the last few years because it supports the notion of constructing a personalized apparatus for a given pathology. Here, the treatment is based on multistage planning [35]:

- Stage of designing of the structure (based on the clinical and radiographic examinations), with a precise calculation of the number, level, and distribution of the external elements and of the number and orientation of the bone fixation elements. Then a scheme of the apparatus on a transparency of the bone segment, obtained from the radiograph, is prepared.
- Stage of preassembly, generally assembling only the essential parts of the apparatus. Then the device is sterilized.
- Surgical assembly stage, with initial fixation of the preassembled apparatus to the bone segment at the proximal and distal level, followed by the application of the bone fixation elements at intermediate levels.

Our experience suggests not using any type of preassembly even though there could be (theoretically) some advantage. In fact, the preassembly must be virtual; in other words, the scheme must be clear in the mind of the surgeon and based on extremely accurate planning (which is the most important stage of the treatment). Therefore the best is when the real assembly takes place at the moment of surgery, step by step, to obtain from the system the highest versatility and maximum patient tolerability with the only disadvantage of a minimally longer-lasting operation [36].

Bone Fixation Elements

Since they first appeared, some compression-distraction systems, such as the Kalnberz system [6] and the Fischer system [37] have provided the possibility to use more than one kind of bone fixation element (screws, small wires). In the most commonly used system (Ilizarov system) the trend to use a mixed assembly has gradually asserted itself, especially after it became established in Western Europe and the USA.

Using screws has the disadvantage that the assembly is less elastic (probably reducing the capacity of adaptation to functional requests of the bone during the treatment, typical of the assemblies using small wires) and the advantage of an improved tolerability by the patient, thanks to the reduction of soft tissue transfixion.

Levels of Fixation

Another technique has recently become popular: using mountings with a lower number of levels of fixation, for the usual reason of improving tolerability. This solution has been forwarded by the introduction of improvements in the structure of the external elements and the bone fixation elements, by the creation of new accessory elements, and by the improvement of modern methods of treatment, which in certain cases has allowed the mounting to be simplified without significantly reducing the stability.

The rule to always follow is: the reduction in the number of levels of fixation must never reduce the stability of the mounting, which is the most important factor of the treatment.

Extension

Stable fixation of a bone segment requires mounting with levels of fixation close to the nonunion site or to the area of corticotomy, and levels of fixation close to the proximal or distal epiphysis of the long bone. These represent the cause of major tolerability problems, and one recently established solution is to use mountings that "move away" from the joints. This possibility must be used within careful limits because even here the main rule is to maintain the stability of the device. This must never be reduced by oversimplified constructions.

Radiotransparency

The rings of carbon fiber of the Ilizarov system (introduced in recent years) and rings and rods of fiberglass of the Kalnberz system "Rigid Simplex" show the important advantage of radiotransparency. This is particularly useful in the most complex mountings when x-ray examination cannot demonstrate important details because they are covered by metallic elements of the device (Fig. 13).

In particular, in the Ilizarov system the radiotransparent components may be used to partially or totally replace the radio-opaque metallic components.

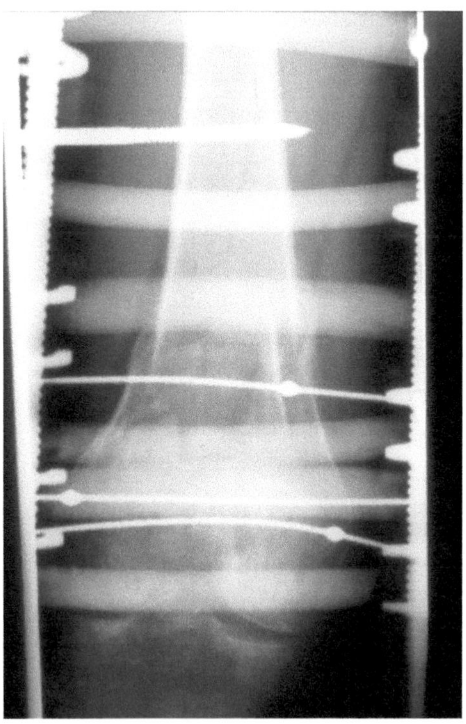

Fig. 13. Radiotransparent fiberglass rings of the Kalnberz "Rigid Simplex" system

Complications

The potential intraoperative complications (that basically consist in injuries to vessels and nerves) [38] must be immediately recognized to be treated successfully. For the prevention of these complications, full knowledge is required of the anatomy of the limbs. Numerous anatomic-topographic tables are available that follow the lead of the classic Eycleshymer and Schoemaker atlas [39]. They are useful for the surgeon when wires and screws need to be inserted. Among these atlases, the most useful are surely those that also indicate the direction in which the bone fixation elements are going to be applied [6] (Fig. 14).

Suprisingly, an important and "critical" aspect represented by the postoperative complications, has been underestimated by most Authors. Actually, only Green [38, 40, 41] and Paley [42] have addressed this complex problem. In particular Paley [42] proposed an interesting classification of three kinds of complications that can appear during a limb lengthening, distinguishing between "difficulties" (divided into "problems" and "obstacles") and true complications. This classification can even be extended to complications observed during the treatment of nonunions of the long bones.

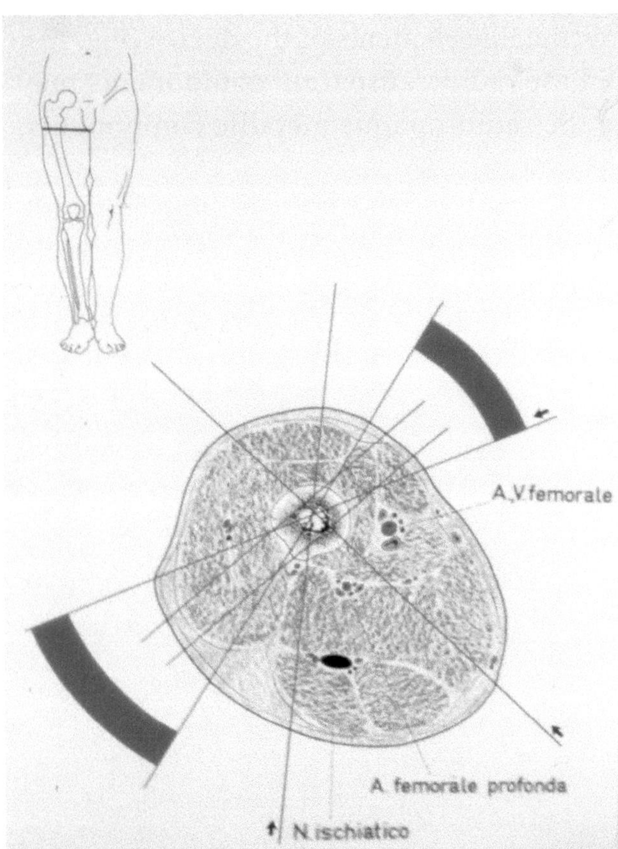

Fig. 14. Anatomic topographic table with the indications for the safe and correct insertion of wires and screws

- The "problems" appear during the treatment and can be solved before it is over, with nonsurgical techniques.
- The "obstacles" also appear during the treatment and can be solved before it is over, but with surgical methods.
- The "true complications" appear during the treatment and remain unsolved at the end of the treatment. These are divided into "minor" and "major" (solvable with nonsurgical or surgical techniques, respectively) and permanent (nonsolvable even after the end of the treatment).

A bleeding during or immediately after inserting a wire can be generally stopped by removing the wire and compression. A vascular lesion after inserting a screw is normally more dangerous and requires removal of the screw and an arteriographic control to actually see what damage has been done and possibly how to treat it.

A nervous lesion caused by a rotating wire that tears a nerve may be difficult to treat; therefore, especially in endangered areas, wires should be inserted through the soft tissues by gradually pushing them or by gentle traction, whereas rotation must be used only when the wire is inserted through the bone.

Clearly, maximum care must always be taken, and thus one should never hesitate to carry out any investigation that may help to locate the exact position of the principal vessels and nerves of the area of interest (arteriographic study, examination by means of electroneurostimulation).

Radiographic Control

A final radiographic control at the end of the operation, but with the patient still on the operating table and under anesthesia and in a sterile environment, is always advisable as any kind of correction could still be performed under ideal conditions.

Dressing

Before moving the patient from the operating table, a simple dressing must be applied. This dressing must fulfill two basic requirements [36]:

1. No dressing should be applied at the points of insertion of screws and wires (Fig. 15) (such as gauzes, bandages and more or less complex devices to keep them stable (caps from antibiotic bottles, sponges). In this case the dressing would probably promote local maceration and inflammation.
2. Dressing of the wounds with a light bandage. Only in cases in which compression is considered useful should a compressive bandage be employed, not a circular one but rather connected to some elements of the mounting (generally connecting rods).

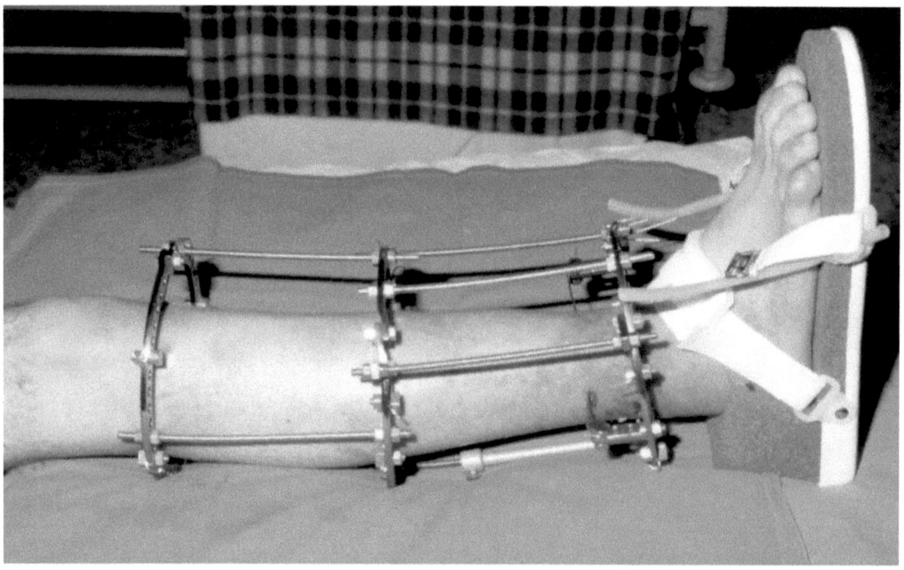

Fig. 15. No kind of dressing is applied to the leg

Completing the Medical Records

In the medical record of the operation it is advisable to be very precise, especially when dealing with complex mountings, as it is easy to forget in the following weeks which components have been used. It is surprising to see how difficult it can be, after some time, to remember the location and the direction of the wires, and even with the assistance of x-rays it can sometimes be difficult to solve the problem.

Therefore it is very useful to have a schematic drawing to refer to when the components have to be removed.

Postoperative Planning

Putting the Patient on the Bed

The postoperative regimen actually begins by putting the patient on the bed, and the rules to follow are simple:

- The patient must be placed on the bed in the most comfortable yet functional way possible.
- For both legs and arms it is advisable to use soft cushions that can be easily modeled in order to keep the limb slightly higher and to protect other parts of the body with which the external fixation device must not come in contact.
- Using properly modeled cushions, or with simple braces, a comfortable support can easily be created for the sole, with the aim of avoiding equinus deformity, which develops rapidly and is difficult to correct.

Rehabilitation

Rehabilitation treatment begins very soon. It is mainly based on active and passive joint mobilization, isometric contractions to reactivate the muscles of the operated limb, early functional loading for the upper limb, and weight bearing and walking for the lower limb (Fig. 16).

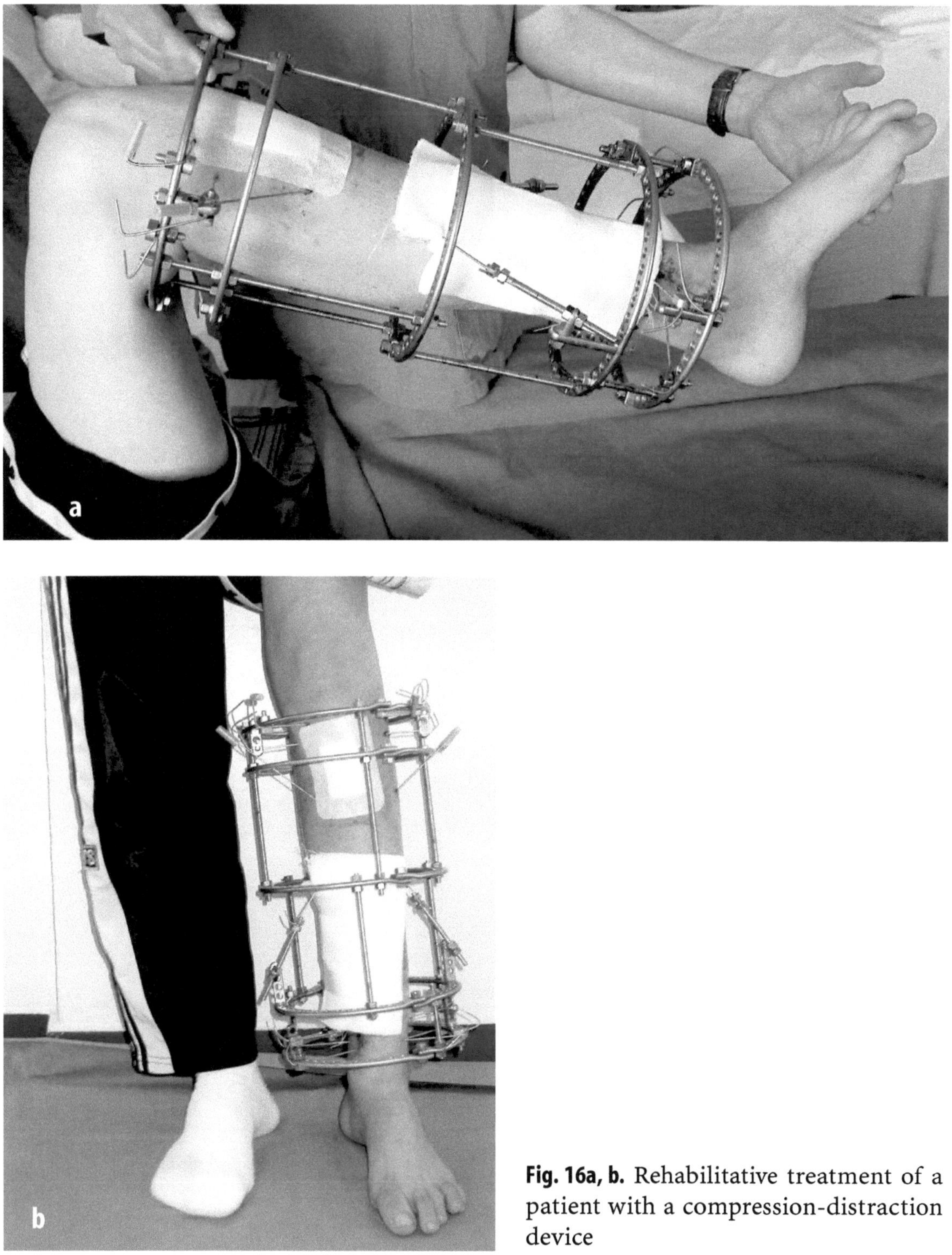

Fig. 16a, b. Rehabilitative treatment of a patient with a compression-distraction device

Useful add-ons to the rehabilitation treatment are massage (used for its pain-relieving effect) and vascular exercise, which improves venous return [1].

The CPM devices and the "Dynasplint" braces are important tools to gradually correct joint stiffness in flexion or in extension [43].

Postoperative Problems

Particular care must be given to treating both immediate or late postoperative problems, without forgetting the importance of prevention in planning and performing the surgical treatment.

There are four types of postoperative problems: injuries to vessels or nerves, inflammatory or infectious conditions (superficial and deep), bad scars or defacing, or joint stiffness.

Bleeding may start even weeks or months after application of the fixator, generally due to the erosion of the wall of a vessel caused by a bone fixation element. After removing the wire or the screw, an arteriogram will help to see what kind of damage has occurred and what kind of treatment to use. In treatments based on distraction, vascular or nervous injury can appear because of the distraction of the soft tissues. In these cases, interruption of the distraction or even proceeding to temporary compression treatment is generally enough to solve the problem.

Inflammatory and infectious conditions at the site of insertion of wires or screws represent the most common problems (Fig. 17). The reason is simple and has been well explained by Green [44]: "The transfixion of a limb with a wire or a screw violates the principal barrier against the bacterial invasion".

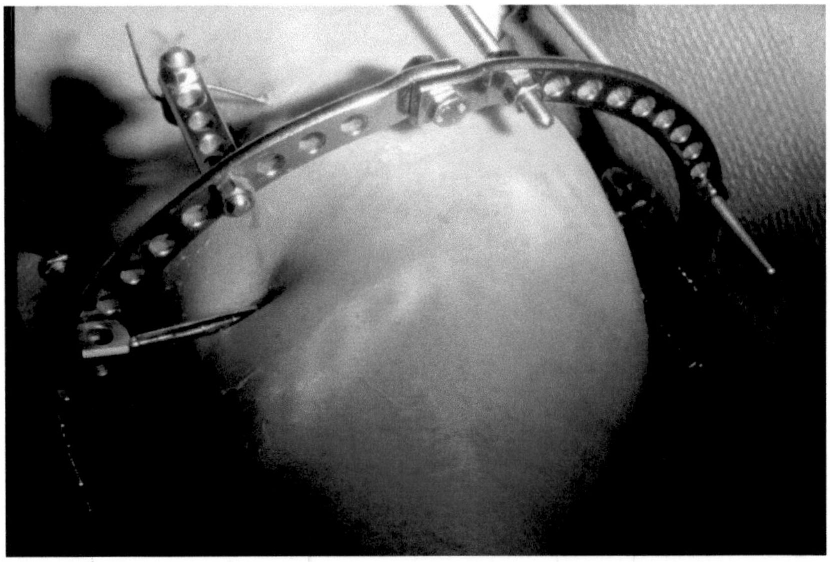

Fig. 17. Signs of inflammation at the pin tracts

Basically these are superficial problems that can be solved with an adequate treatment (local medications, general antibiotic therapy) and only rarely require more radical solutions (removal of the bone fixation element and replacing it at a different site and with a different direction).

Deep infections are rare and appear on x-rays as an osteolysis or as a sequestrum (Fig. 18). They require antibiotic therapy, removal of the bone fixation element, and surgical cleansing with *débridement* or in some cases with marginal resection of the infected bone, using the same treatment as for chronic osteomyelitis.

As always, the best treatment is prevention, which must be based on two rules:

1. Avoid necrosis of the tissues, which can be caused during the insertion of wires and screws by wrapping of the tissues or by overproduction of heat and, after insertion of the bone fixation element, by excessive tension of the soft tissues (this is generally a consequence of a wrong technique of insertion or of an incorrect connection to the external device, followed by straining in flexion of the wire or the screw).
2. Avoid excessive movement of the tissues around the bone fixation element, produced by an unstable mounting.

Particular solutions have been studied in an attempt to reduce the rate of infections of those areas in which screws and wires are present:

- Titanium screws [43] that do not interfere with the bactericidal action of the white blood cells (while standard iron screws do).
- Screws covered by hydroxyapatite [45] that allow a more stable fixation of the bone, reducing micro-movements and the risk of infection.
- Silver plated screws [46]. The antibacterial properties of silver create a layer that works as a barrier against infection.

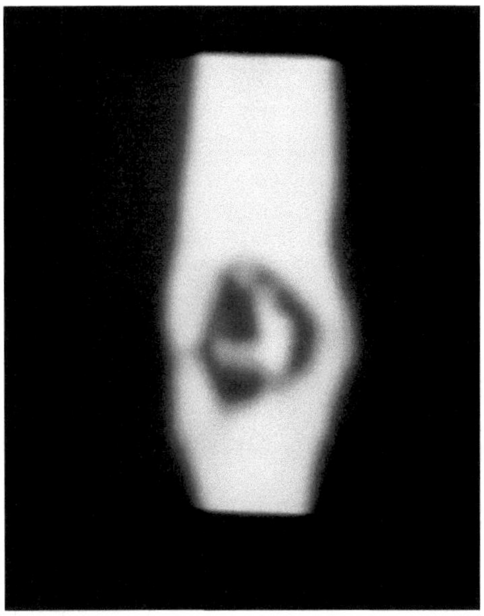

Fig.18. Deep infection after wire insertion

- Screws covered with sleeves of PMMA (polymethylmethacrylate) soaked in antibiotic (tobramycin) to prevent local infections [47].

The scars at the site of previous points of passage of wires or screws (Fig. 19) are an almost unavoidable inconvenience when dealing with axial or circular external fixation. These can be (within certain limits) avoided by a precise preoperative planning and by correctly performing the operation (insertion of the bone fixation elements avoiding tension of the soft tissues when no important modifications of the configuration in the postoperative phase are planned, and on the contrary, applying wires or screws by creating a "reserve" of soft tissues in cases of internal or external lengthening of the limb or correction of serious deformities, so an overload of tension of the soft tissues during the gradual correction period can be avoided).

Knee stiffness is often observed when using a circular external fixation device at the level of the femur; this is rare in other joints (Fig. 20).

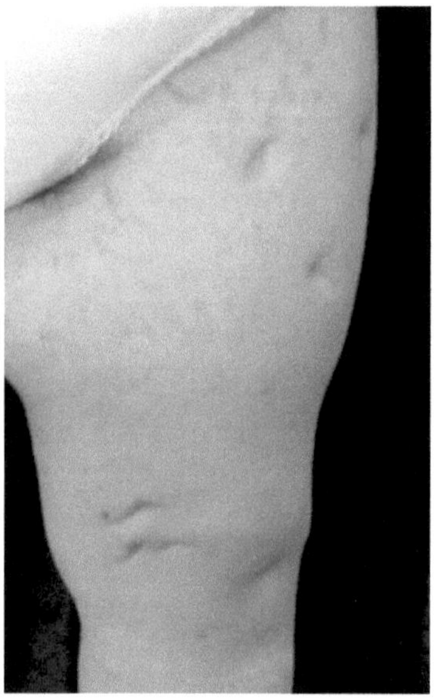

Fig. 19. Scars at the site of previous passage of wires

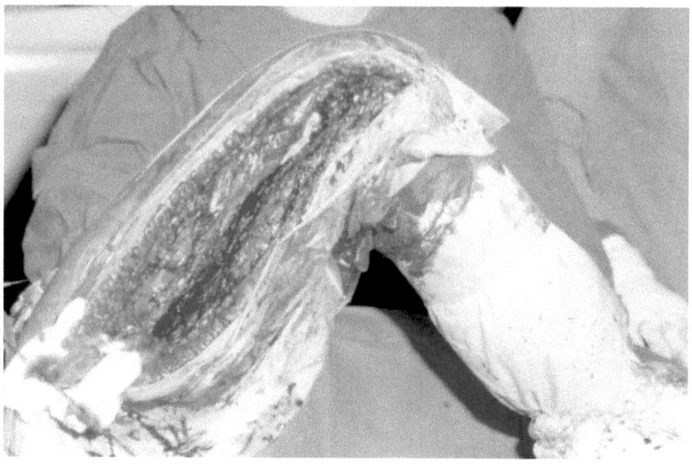

Fig. 20. Operative treatment according to Judet for a persistant knee stiffness after removal of a femoral Ilizarov device

As underlined above, knee stiffness can be avoided or reduced in two ways: correct position of the knee when inserting wires or screws (generally, bone fixation elements should go through the flexor muscles with the knee extended and through the extensor muscles with the knee flexed) and using particular techniques in order to reduce soft tissue transfixion.

The postoperative treatment is based on kinesitherapy, focusing on flexion and extension exercises for the knee, both active and passive (using CPM devices if needed), and using particular braces such as "Dynasplint".

Periodical Controls

Programming the periodical controls represents another key part of the treatment. In contrast to internal synthesis and axial external fixation techniques, the methods of circular external fixation, which allow the gradual correction of complex deformities, require frequent controls of the patient because of the high number of bone fixation elements used (with the resulting risk of inflammation, which must be quickly treated).

These methods are often dynamic methods and require modifications during treatment, and clinical controls must be added to the instrumental controls for the correct evaluation of the formation of callus or regenerated bone and the position of the bone fragments. It is therefore advisable to schedule clinical controls every 15 days and instrumental controls every month.

The instrumental examinations that have proven to be most useful are x-rays and sonographic and extensimetric studies.

Standard x-rays remain the most important examination as they are simple and provide consistent information about the callus or the regenerated bone. A delayed union may take place because of the late formation of bone trabeculae or a disorientation of the fibers in the interfragmentary space. In nonunions, bone trabeculae are absent, and fibers projecting from one fragment to another cannot be seen. The x-ray control of the formation of regenerating bone shows the first signs of ossification in the first month after the operation. These consist in a slight opacity of the area of interest, which presents as a normally cylindric shape. This opacity extends regularly inside the gap. Within weeks, the opacity intensifies and the lines begin to get bigger and blend together. After about 4 months a thin cortical shell appears and gets stronger in the fifth and sixth months after surgery. In case of faulty ossification, the regeneration resembles an "hourglass".

Sonographic evaluation of bone callus formation and bone regeneration has the double advantage of reducing the total number of radiographic examinations during treatment and of showing the early phases of bone callus and regeneration during the first 4 weeks, in which the radiographic examination still does not give useful information.

Aspects similar to those of developmental morphology of the bone callus (previously described) can be observed during the study of the stages of progressive formation of regenerating bone in cases of correction of simple or complex deformities of the long bones, reconstruction of bone defects, and distraction osteosynthesis of hypertrophic nonunions.

The extensimetric examination calculates the mechanical properties of the bone callus or regenerating bone by measuring the deformations of the fixator-bone system in the progressive stages of consolidation.

A useful and simple to use extensimetric device for the Ilizarov system has been developed and tested in some Italian orthopaedic centers: the Orthopaedic Department of the University of Pavia has actively taken part in creating this [48]. This extensimetric device is a transducer for biomedical measures with which the deformations of the external fixator are quantified by the repeated movements during the treatment.

The equipment consists of an extensimetric rod that can be easily fixed to the rings of the circular fixator (in the most anterior position and on the rings that are proximally located to the involved area) and in a system of analog-digital conversion connected to a computer.

Flexion-extension, walking and "bending" tests can be performed. These examinations, regularly repeated (every 15–20 days) during the treatment, give important information about the solidity of the mounting and on the evolving stages of the stiffness of the bone callus and regenerating bone. Analysis of the charts of maximum deformation helps identify some different stages and to create a "deformation curve" during the treatment.

For the entire treatment period a rehabilitation program must be created. It must be as useful as possible and not follow a predetermined scheme, but rather must be adaptable to the type of pathology, to the type of treatment, and to its aim.

Three main rules to follow during the rehabilitation of patients with a circular external fixator must never be forgotten:

- Active and passive joint mobilization, allowing an early functional load, maintaining the correct position of the joints proximal and distal to the interested bone segment.
- Clinical and instrumental information, and all the modifications made to the system, are registered with care on the medical record of the patient.
- All clinical and instrumental controls and all the decisions made during the treatment must be programmed, when possible, right from the beginning of the postoperative period.

References

1. Iorio L, Forte R, Spinelli R (1990) Problemi di riabilitazione. Giorn Ital Ortop Traumatol 16[Suppl. 1]:222–228
2. Mazzarello F, Puncuh F, Lampugnani E et al (1997) Limb external devices application: anesthetic procedures comparison. Gaslini 29:55–60
3. Chiaranda M, Minoja G (1997) Anestesia. In: Dionigi R (ed) Chirurgia. Masson, Milano
4. Fanelli G, Nobili F, Agostoni M et al (1991) Il blocco femoro-ischiatico con l'utilizzo di un elettroneurostimolatore per l'anestesia locoregionale del ginocchio. Minerva Anestesiol 9:514–515
5. Pagani I, Paparella F, Preseglio I et al (1996) Anestesia locoregionale nella chirurgia ortopedico-traumatologica dell'arto inferiore con fissatori esterni. Minerva Ortop Traumatol 47:551–554
6. Kalnberz VK (1981) Compression-distraction apparatus. Stress and rigid system. LNIITO, Riga
7. Traina GC (1993) AIDS e chirurgia. Chirurgia 6:1–7
8. Perugia L, Traina GC (1994) AIDS and surgery. Int Orthop 18:397–399
9. De Coster TA, Crawford MK, Kraut MA (1999) Safe extracapsular placement of proximal tibia transfixation pins. J Orthop Trauma 13:236–240
10. Vora AM, Haddad S, Kadakia A et al (2004) Extracapsular placement of distal tibial transfixation wires. J Bone Joint Surg Am 86:988–993
11. Ceciliani L, Mora R, Di Castri U et al (1995) Fissazione esterna in traumatologia e rigidità. Giorn Ital Ortop Traumatol 2[Suppl. 1]:215–221
12. Burny F, Hinsenkamp L, Donkerwolcke M (1979) External fixation of the fractures of the humerus. In: Vidal J (ed) Hoffmann external fixator. Université de Montpellier, Montpellier
13. De Bastiani G, Aldegheri R, Renzi Brivio L (1984) The treatment of fractures with a dynamic axial fixator. J Bone Joint Surg Br 66:538–543
14. Mora R, Pedrotti L, Benazzo F et al (1999) Indicazioni e limiti della fissazione esterna monoassiale e circolare nell'arto superiore. Giorn Ital Ortop Traumatol 25[Suppl. 1]: 215–218
15. Mollica Q, Mora R, Falzarano G et al (2000) L'uso della fissazione esterna nel trattamento delle fratture diafisarie di omero. Atti del 10° Congresso CIOD, Sesto di Pusteria
16. De la Caffinière JY (1990) Le fixateur externe circulaire en traumatologie. Springer, Paris
17. Andreev D, Mishev P (1980) Anatomical study aimed at the determination of the optimal zones and directions of passing external fixation pins through the humerus. Ortop Travm (Sofia) 17:10–16
18. Ilizarov GA, Golikov VD, Sherd SI et al (1982) Transosseous osteosynthesis with the Ilizarov apparatus in the fractures of the humerus. KNIIEKOT, Kurgan
19. Benedetti GB, Argnani F (1991) Fractures of the humerus. In: Bianchi Maiocchi A, Aronson J (eds) Operative principles of Ilizarov. Williams and Wilkins, Baltimore
20. Mc Auliffe JA (1997) Forearm fixation. Hand Clin 13:689–701
21. Mears D (1983) Skeletal external fixation. Williams and Wilkins, Baltimore
22. Jupiter JB (1990) External fixation in the upper extremity. AAOS Instr Course Lect 39:209–218

23. Been JN, Seligson D, Ashby Howard P (1996) Temporary circular external fixation for forearm fractures in complex circumstances. Tech Orthop 11:196–200
24. Ilizarov GA, Devjatov AA, Safonov VA et al (1977) Transosseous osteosynthesis of diaphyseal fractures of the forearm by means of the Ilizarov apparatus. KNIIEKOT, Kurgan
25. Kalnberz VK, Klesis V (1985) Management of diaphyseal fractures of the forearm and their complications by meams of the Kalnberz external fixator. LNIITO, Riga
26. ASAMI Group (1991) Fractures of the forearm. In: Bianchi Maiocchi A, Aronson J (eds) Operative principles of Ilizarov. Williams and Wilkins, Baltimore, pp 160–169
27. Mora R, Ceciliani L (1992) Classification and methods of treatment of nonunions using compression-distraction systems. Proceedings 14th International Hoffmann External Fixation Conference, Granada
28. Catagni MA, Malzev V, Kirienko A (1984) Advances in Ilizarov apparatus assembly. Medicalplastic, Milan
29. Catagni MA, Mendlick RM (1996) Femoral fractures. Tech Orthop 11:160–173
30. Volkov MV, Oganesian OV (1978) Treatment of lesions of the bones and joints by the devices of Authors. Meditsina, Tashkent
31. Feraboli F, Manenti R, Bellini C et al (1991) Fissazione esterna ed inchiodamento endomidollare elastico. Minerva Ortop Traumatol 42:249–260
32. Volkov M, Oganesian O (1987) External fixation: joint deformities and bone fractures. International University Press, Madison
33. Pavolini B (1986) X-crossing wires in the distal tibia. Tech Orthop 11:208–209
34. Herzenberg JE, Scheufele LL, Paley D et al (1994) Knee range of motion in isolated femoral lengthening. Clin Orthop Relat Res 301:49–54
35. Marini MM (1997) Preassemblies in complex fractures. Utopia or reality? Gaslini 29:24–29
36. Mora R (2000) Tecniche di compressione-distrazione. Amplimedical, Milano
37. Fischer DA (1983) Skeletal stabilization with a multiplane external fixation device. Clin Orthop Relat Res 180:50–62
38. Green SA (1990) Complications of pin and wire external fixation. AAOS Instr Course Lect 39:219–228
39. Eycleshymer A, Schoemaker D (1911) A cross-section anatomy. Appleton-Century, New York
40. Green SA (1983) Complications of external skeletal fixation. Clin Orthop Relat Res 180:109–116
41. Green SA (1984) Complications of external fixation. AAOS Instr Course Lect 33: 138–143
42. Paley D (1991) Problems, obstacles and complications of limb lengthening. In: Bianchi Maiocchi A, Aronson J (eds) Operative principles of Ilizarov. Williams and Wilkins, Baltimore, pp 352–366
43. Paley D, Chaudray M, Pirone AM et al (1990) Treatment of malunions and malnonunions of the femur and tibia by detailed preoperative planning and the Ilizarov techniques. Orthop Clin North Am 21:667–691
44. Green SA (1996) External fixation mounting for difficult locations. Tech Orthop 11:115–124
45. Caja VL, Moroni A (1996) Hydroxyapatite coated external fixation pins. An experimental study. Clin Orthop Relat Res 325:269–275

46. Trace R (1997) Antimicrobial silver coating reduces external fixation pin-tract infections. Orthop Today 17:1–2
47. Voos K, Rosenberg B, Faghri M et al (1998) Use of tobramycin-impregnated polymethylmethacrylate pin sleeve for the prevention of pin-tract infection in goats. J Orthop Trauma 13:98–101
48. Ceffa R, Bombelli M, Boero S et al (1997) Extensimetric monitoring of healing in the treatment with the lizarov apparatus. Bull Hosp Joint Dis 56:41–45

Treatment of Noninfected Nonunions: Techniques Other Than Compression-Distraction Methods

LUISELLA PEDROTTI, REDENTO MORA, BARBARA BERTANI

Introduction

Bone consolidation is the result of a complex cellular recruitment and differentiation process. A number of methods have been developed to modulate this cellular process in nonunions. Besides compression-distraction techniques, both nonsurgical (biophysical stimulation methods) and surgical treatments (including various techniques of osteosynthesis and methods for biological stimulation) can be attempted. Moreover, physical and biological mechanisms can often be combined.

Biophysical stimulation methods include electrical stimulation, low intensity ultrasound, and shock wave therapy. Biological stimulation methods include bone grafting, bone substitutes, and growth factors (GFs). The osteosynthesis techniques include stabilization with internal fixation or axial external fixation.

Biophysical Stimulation Methods

These methods have shown to be effective in some types of nonunions. Moreover, it should be emphasized that deformities or shortening cannot be corrected with this kind of stimulation nor has it been effective in the presence of a gap [1].

Electrical Stimulation

Electrical and electromagnetic devices have been shown to be effective in the management of delayed unions and nonunions [2]. The development of these treatment methods is based on the discovery that dry bone [3] and hydrated bone [4] have electrical properties. In brief, mechanically stimulated bone cells produce an electrical field, which mediates cell proliferation [5]. In the past few years, some studies gave further information about the action of the electrical fields on signal transduction pathways and on GFs [2, 6].

Three modalities of electrical stimulation of bone growth are presently available for nonunion treatment:

- Direct current (DC) stimulation employing percutaneously implanted electrodes (invasive method). With this method a constant current of about 20 μA and 1 V is generated between two electrodes inserted in the nonunion site. This technique has quite a high rate of good results (78%–86%), according to some Authors [7, 8] (Fig. 1).
- Electromagnetic stimulation by inductive coupling (IC) uses magnetic fields (noninvasive method). This technique, developed by Bassett et al. [9], is based on the action of pulsed electromagnetic fields produced by external devices that generate a current of 20 mV and about 10 μA/cm^2 in the tissues. Bassett et al. [9] reported a success rate of 87% in the management of nonunions.
- Capacitive coupling (CC) stimulation employs electrodes placed on the skin (noninvasive method). Disk-shaped electrodes to which transducer gel has been applied are placed on the skin and transmit a uniform electric current (3–6 V, 5–10 mA) at the nonunion site. A success rate of 82% has been reported [10].

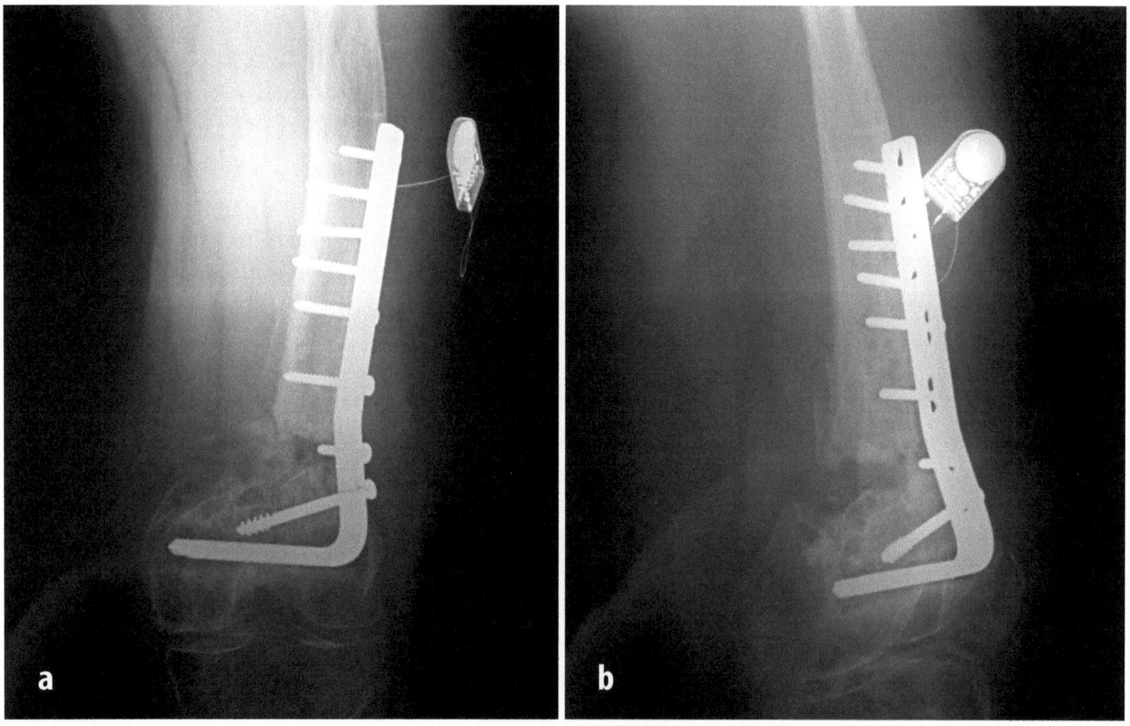

Fig. 1a, b. Atrophic nonunion of the distal metaphysis of the left femur in a 26-year-old man treated with plating, autologous bone grafting, and electric stimulation

Double-blind studies to test the efficacy of electrical stimulation on long bone nonunions were performed and gave statistical evidence of these good results [11, 12]. In conclusion, this treatment has proven to be effective, particularly in hypertrophic nonunions.

Ultrasound Stimulation

Ultrasound is a form of mechanical noninvasive energy transmitted through the skin. High-intensity ultrasound (500 mW–3 W/cm^2) induces an intense warming of tissues and is employed in physical therapy to reduce pain and muscular contracture.

The use of ultrasound to stimulate fracture healing was initiated in Germany in the 1960s [13, 14], employing a continuous wave signal of relatively high intensity (of about 500 mW/cm^2), but these treatments carried the risk of bone necrosis. Low-intensity ultrasound (1–50 mW/cm^2) releases a relatively low amount of warmth and has insignificant thermal effects; echographic techniques have been developed according to these principles. Therefore, starting in the 1970s, this idea was developed. These researchers used pulsed low-intensity ultrasound of about 30 mW/cm^2, producing only little increase in temperature. This kind of treatment can be left in place for long periods of time [15, 16].

More recently, pulsed low-intensity ultrasound has proved to be efficacious in the management of both noninfected nonunions [17, 18] and infected nonunions [19]. Large series have been published by Duarte [15] (success rate: 85%), Mayr et al. [20] (success rate: 86%), and Rubin et al. [21] (success rate: 91%), confirming the clinical efficacy of this kind of treatment in delayed unions and nonunions.

The mechanism of action of low-intensity ultrasound is still not completely clarified, but a variety of mechanisms are involved (some biological and some physical) influencing cell activity, affecting ionic permeability of the cell membrane and second messenger activity. Moreover, low-intensity ultrasound may increase calcium uptake in bone and local blood flow, enhancing angiogenesis [21].

Extracorporeal Shock Wave Therapy

Extracorporeal shock wave lithotripsy has been employed with success for many years in the management of kidney stones and bile-stones. Starting from these applications and considering that the acoustic impedance of some of the crystals in kidney stones and in bone hydroxyapatite (HA) are similar, this technique has also been applied in orthopaedics and traumatology to treat delayed unions and nonunions.

The first papers on this topic were published at the end of the 1980s, but the first reports of a clinical series appeared in 1991, by Valchanov and Michailov, who treated a group of patients at the Bulgarian Military Academy in Sofia [22]. Since then, numerous studies, both clinical and experimental, have been published, proving the favorable effects of the high energy shock waves on reparative osteogenesis [23–28].

High energy extracorporeal shock wave therapy (ESWT) is given by means of electrohydraulic or electromagnetic devices. A location instrument is generally employed, such as a surgical x-ray C-arm or an ultrasound device, to direct precisely the pressure field. Treatment protocols differ in number of applications, number of shots, power of single trains of shock waves, and target of shock waves. The power of trains of shock waves must be adjusted to the size of the skeletal segment: for large bones the power is 2 kV using electrohydraulic devices, 0.6–1 mJ/mm^2 using electromagnetic devices.

In conclusion, the mechanism of action of this method has not been completely clarified yet, but it seems that shock waves act through several processes: induction of microfissures and hematoma, increase in local blood flow, interruption of linkage between molecules of calcium phosphate, and a cavitation effect with liberation of energy [27, 28].

Surgical Methods

Techniques of Osteosynthesis

Plating Osteosynthesis

Plating osteosynthesis can be defined as a kind of "static fixation" because its rigidity is constant from the beginning to the end of treatment. Classical plating techniques provide environmental stability but cannot provide osteogenic stimulation, mainly in cases of atrophic nonunions: in these cases bone grafting should be associated with the treatment [29–31].

These techniques have some advantages in the management of nonunions [30]: accurate correction of a malalignment combined with nonunion; easy application of bone grafts or bone substitutes at the nonunion site, if required; good management of periarticular and intrarticular nonunions. However, they also have some important drawbacks: weight-bearing must be delayed; dissection of soft tissues and periosteal destruction may increase the risk of infection and persistence of nonunion; creation of osteoporotic zones may facilitate delayed unions and refractures (Figs. 2, 3).

The disadvantages have been partially resolved by the development of new kinds of plates in recent years: limited contact-dynamic compression plates (LC-DCP) [32] and more recently locking compression plates (LCP) [33] and

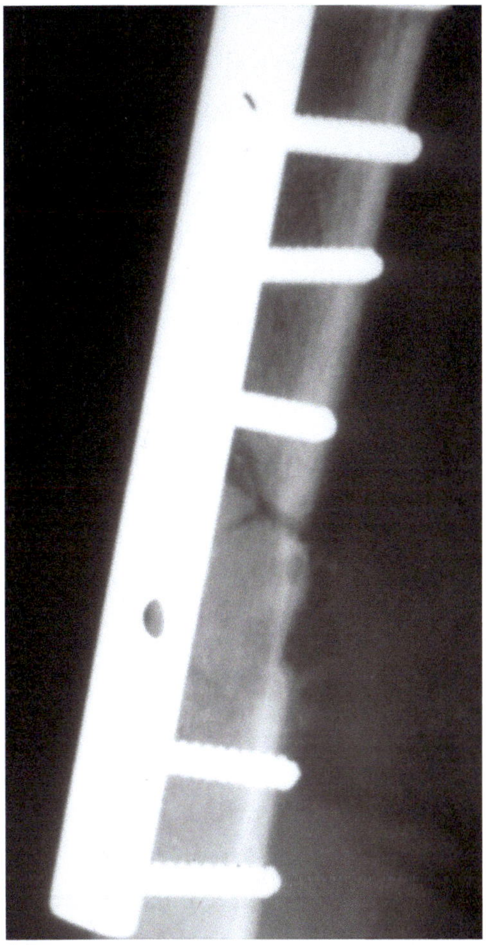

Fig. 2. Nonunion of the right humerus in a 56-year-old woman treated with plating

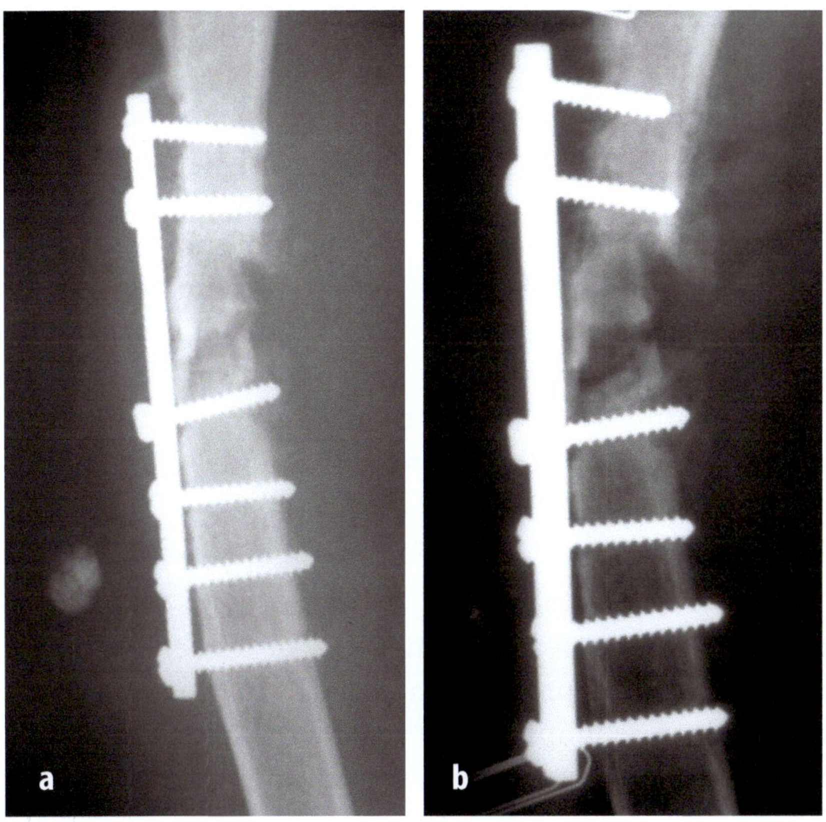

Fig. 3a, b. Same case as in Fig. 2. **a** Infection with failure of the internal fixation 4 months after osteosynthesis. **b** Worsening of the infection and hardware mobilization 6 months after osteosynthesis

less invasive stabilization systems (LISS) [34]. LCP plates have both the advantages of standard plates and screws and locked internal fixators (LIF) thanks to a combined hole which allows fixation with standard screws, auto locking screws, and a mixed fixation with both types of screws. LISS plates are an internal fixation device: they can be used at the distal femur and at the proximal lateral tibia. The premolded plate can be applied under the muscles using an adapted instrumentation, and it is left in proximity of the bone but not in contact with it. Screws can be applied percutaneously and can be locked to the plate through the threaded connection screw-internal fixator.

Series reported by Helfet et al. [35], Wiss et al. [36], and Zinghi et al. [31] show satisfactory results obtained by means of the "static fixation" by plating in noninfected nonunions.

Intramedullary Nailing

Intramedullary nailing, in the current "locked" version, can be defined as a kind of "dynamic fixation" because, as for external fixation, its stiffness can be adjusted during the treatment. By removing the proximal or distal screws (called dynamization), the callus formation is stimulated.

Intramedullary nailing, distinguished in two categories (nails applied with or without reaming), has some advantages [30]: it allows early weight bearing thanks to its stability; and the nail can be inserted in most cases without opening the fracture site, minimizing the soft tissue damage and increasing the consolidation rate compared to plating. In particular, in treating long bone nonunions, the debris produced by the reaming procedure, with their osteoinductive and osteoconductive elements, seems to be very effective in reinitiating the healing cascade. In some cases, nevertheless, adjuvant bone grafting is required [5].

Disadvantages of this technique are: limitations of indications (nonunions with bone loss or periarticular nonunions are contraindications for the use of intramedullary nails); complications are difficult to treat (postoperative infections can infect the whole diaphysis); and it is often difficult or impossible to remove a broken nail (Figs. 4–6).

In the series reported by Galpin et al. [37] and by Wiss and Stetson [38] satisfactory results are reported in the management of noninfected nonunions.

Axial External Fixation

Axial external fixation is achieved by means of unilateral or bilateral frames, depending on whether half-pins or full-pins are employed. If all pins are coplanar, the external device is defined as uniplanar. In biplanar frames, pins enter the bone at an angle to one another, to provide increased stability [30, 39].

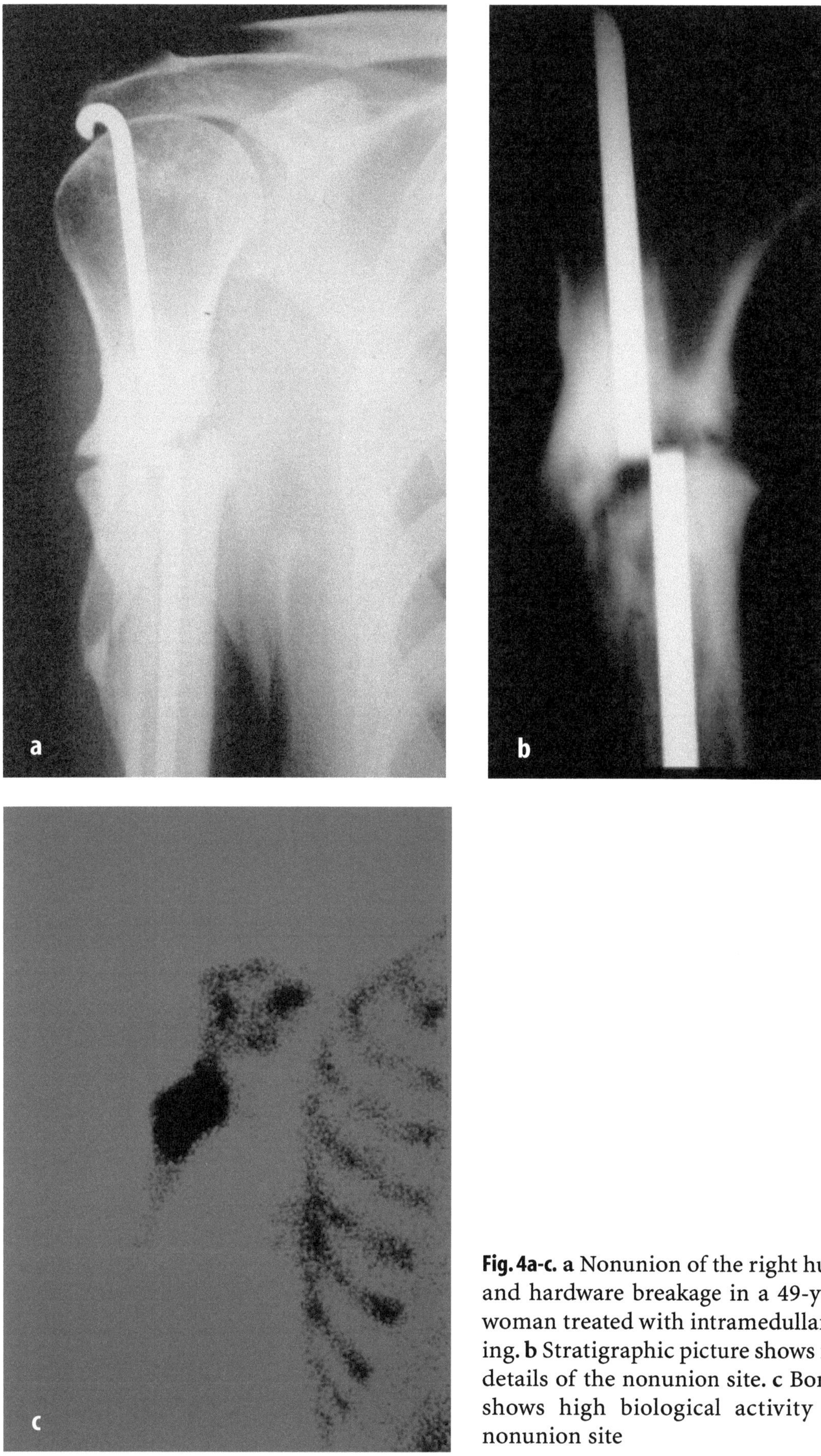

Fig. 4a-c. **a** Nonunion of the right humerus and hardware breakage in a 49-year-old woman treated with intramedullary nailing. **b** Stratigraphic picture shows further details of the nonunion site. **c** Bone scan shows high biological activity at the nonunion site

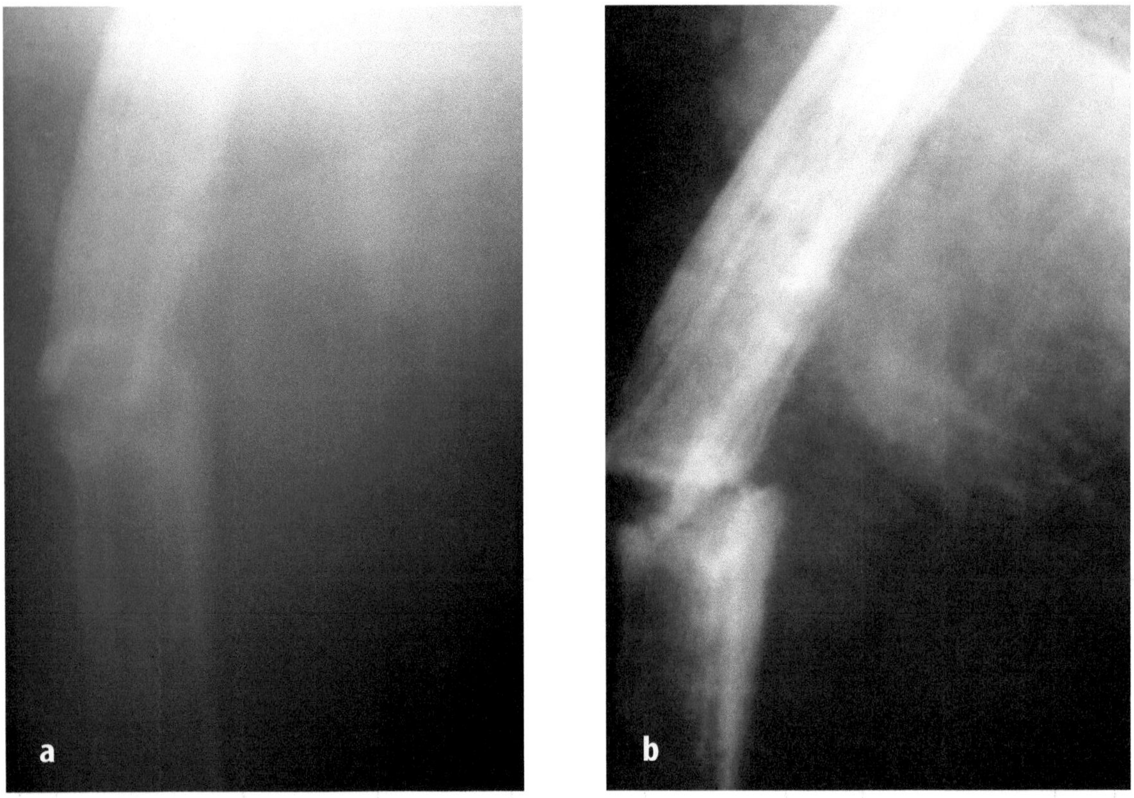

Fig. 5a, b. Nonunion of the right femur in a 59-year-old woman after previous treatment with axial external fixation

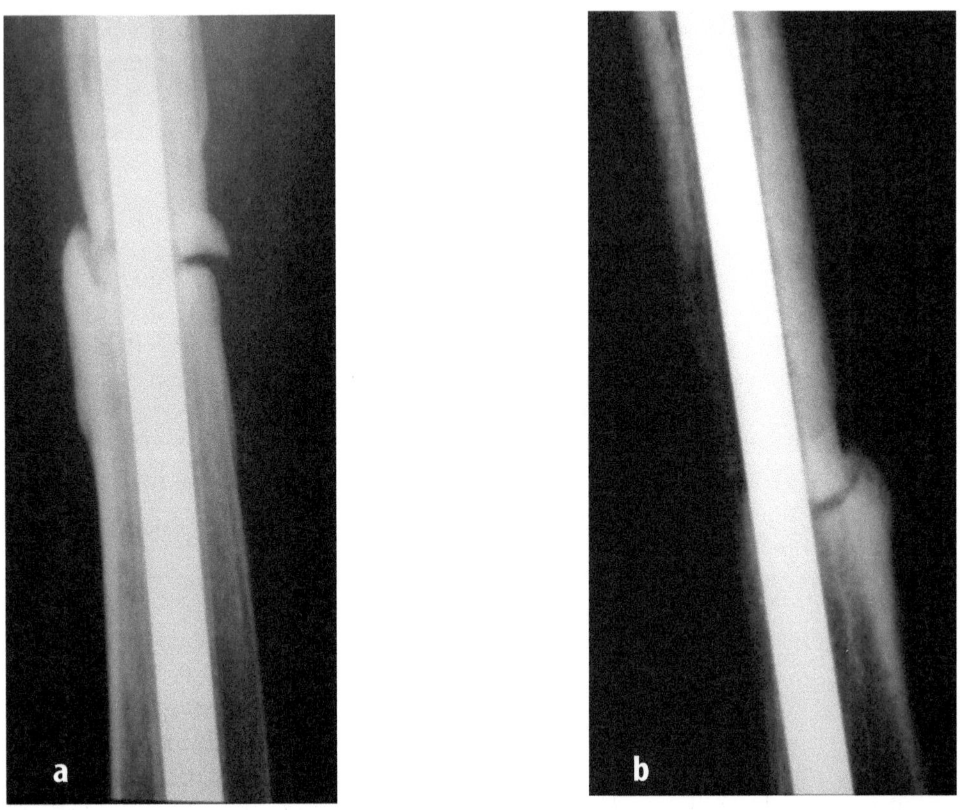

Fig. 6a, b. Same case as in Fig. 5. Persistence of nonunion 9 months after intramedullary nailing

This kind of osteosynthesis (which can be defined "dynamic fixation" such as intramedullary nailing) has many advantages: good stabilization of fragments, no implanted hardware, and respect of blood circulation. It has also many important disadvantages: difficulty of good reduction of displacements or correction of deformities; minimal axial loading; risk of pin tract infection; and difficulty of really "dynamic" treatment (Fig. 7).

Good results obtained with this technique have been reported in the literature [40].

Biological Stimulation Methods

Osteoconductive biomaterials act as a support for the growing bone tissue when put in contact with the bone fragments. Such materials are useful to fill the gap left from loosened bone. They need to be biocompatible, resorbable (if possible), and porous, with holes of a diameter between 100 and 500 μm.

Osteoinductive biomaterials induce bone regeneration by stimulating the progenitor cells to differentiate and proliferate as bone cells. There are biochemical osteoinductive factors and GFs (these will be treated in a separate section).

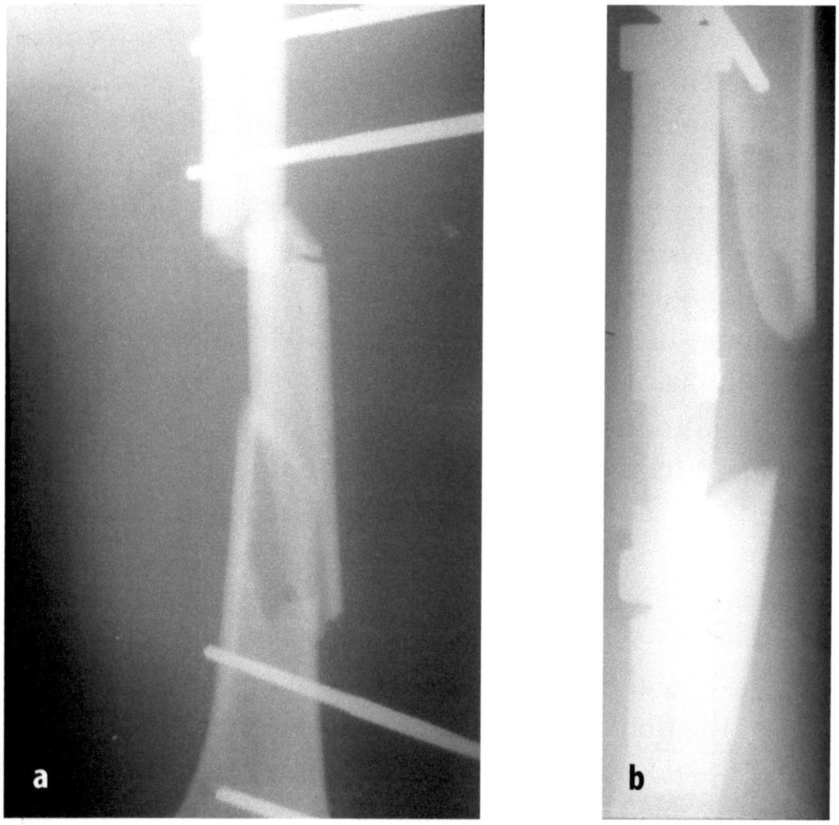

Fig. 7a, b. Poor reduction with axial external fixation of a femoral nonunion after a bifocal fracture in a 20-year-old man

Osteogenic biomaterials, unlike osteoinductive biomaterials, also give progenitor cells, which are associated with support. Bone grafts and bone marrow can be considered part of this group (and are treated in an appropriate section).

Bone Grafting

Bone grafting was the basic technique employed for many years in the management of nonunions [18]. Various types of bone grafts (autografts, allografts, and xenografts) have been characterized and used in the past, but autologous bone grafts, in the nonvascularized and vascularized forms, are certainly the most effective. Therefore, an autologous graft is still the best material for application at the nonunion site and the results obtained using other techniques should always be compared with the success rate obtained using autologous bone grafts.

Autologous bone grafts have three primary characteristics: they have an excellent osteoconductive framework (derived from collagen and HA); they contain osteoinductive factors (including bone morphogenetic proteins, BMPs, that induce or modulate bone formation), and they contain cells with osteogenic potential. These qualities are derived mainly from cancellous bone grafts, whereas cortical bone grafts give perfect support but have a low osteoinductive action and can only be incorporated very slowly.

Nonvascularized autologous bone grafts can be used alone or combined with another form of internal or external osteosynthesis, or in the form of nonvascularized fibula. Currently, the only indication for using autologous bone grafts alone in nonunions is as an intertibiofibular graft for tibial nonunion in cases of bone loss or soft tissue damage on the anterior aspect of the leg [41]. Combined autologous bone grafts are employed both in the form of cancellous bone chips or as structural corticocancellous grafts: this is the most frequent type of autologous transplantation.

Nonvascularized fibula may be used to fill large bone defects. It can hypertrophy with time, but this bone, despite hypertrophy, is often mechanically inadequate and a further fracture may occur.

The use of vascularized grafts requires microvascular surgery. The difference between vascularized and nonvascularized grafts is that vascularized grafts are transferred from a living tissue and therefore (at least theoretically) their healing potential is definitely higher.

Vascularized bone transfer techniques involve the ribs and, more frequently, ipsilateral or contralateral fibula (Figs. 8-11) or iliac crest. The indications for local transfer of the fibula are limited, however (bone defects with a short proximal or distal tibial segment are difficult to manage), and there are many disadvantages (prolonged immobilization is needed in order to protect the fibula while it heals) [30].

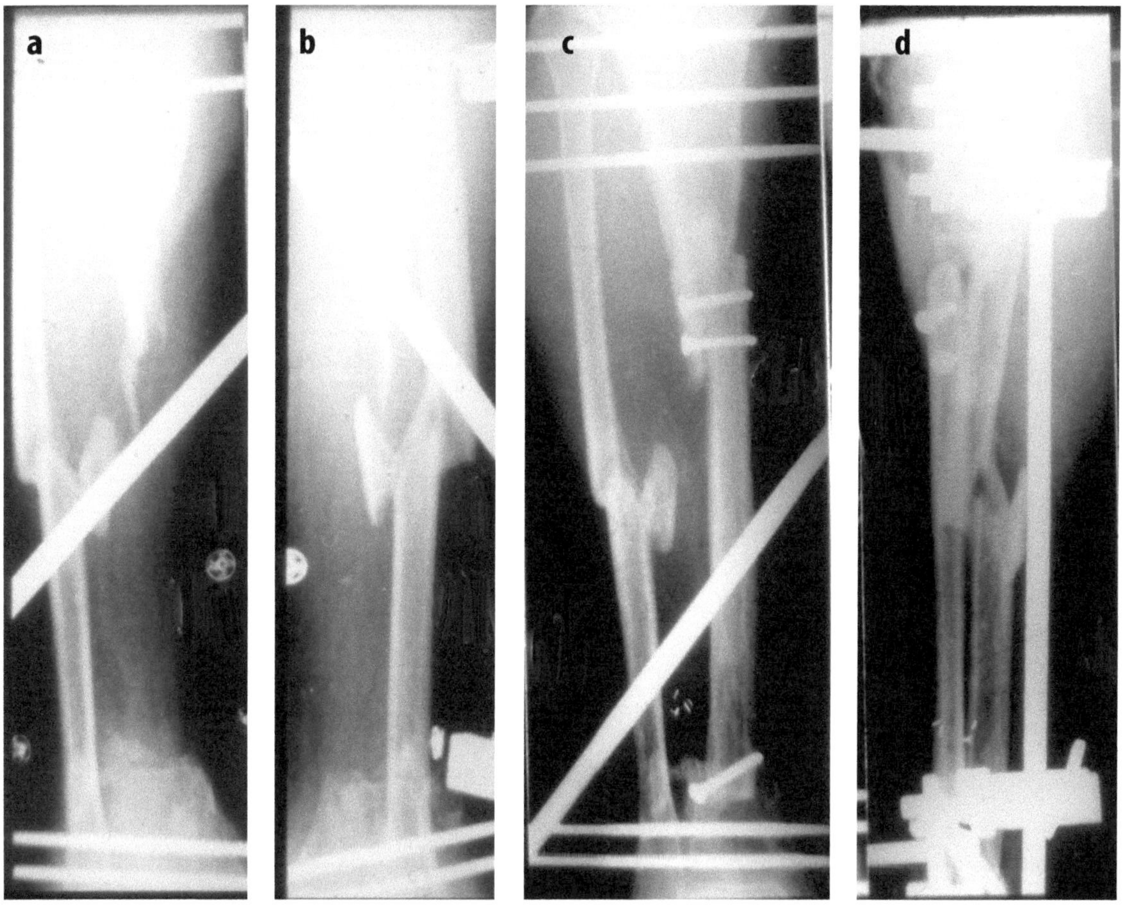

Fig. 8a-d. a, b Diaphyseal nonunion of the right tibia with bone loss in a 28-year-old man treated with a Hoffman axial external fixator. **c, d** Treatment with vascularized bone graft (contralateral fibula) fixed by means of proximal and distal screws

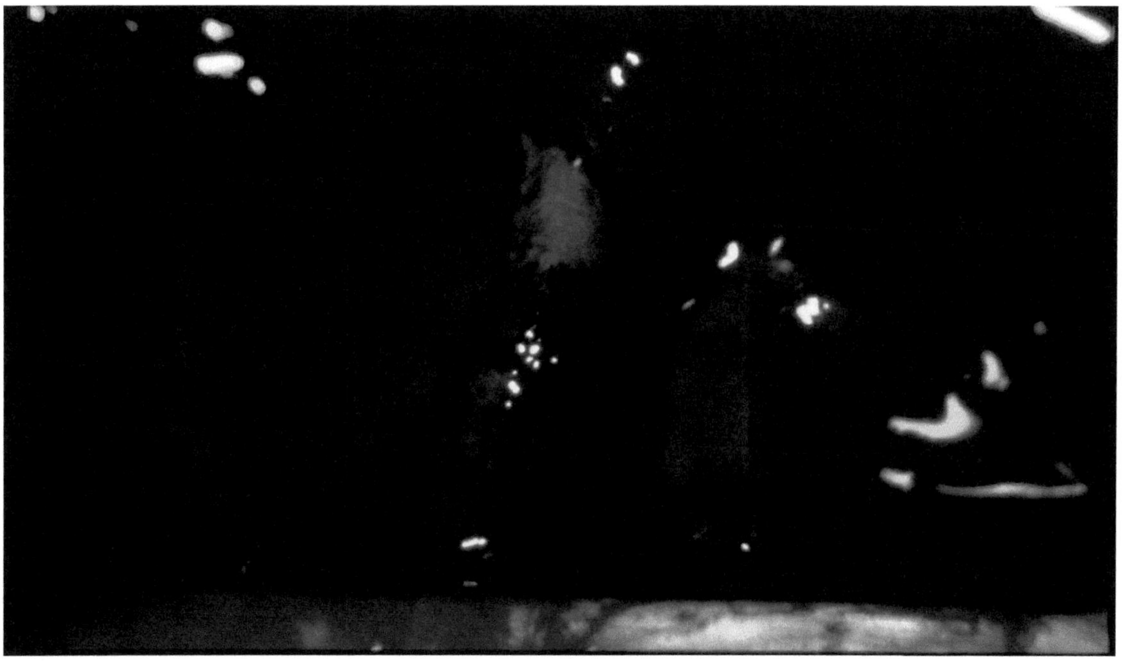

Fig. 9. Same case as in Fig. 8. Microvascular anastomosis during the operative procedure

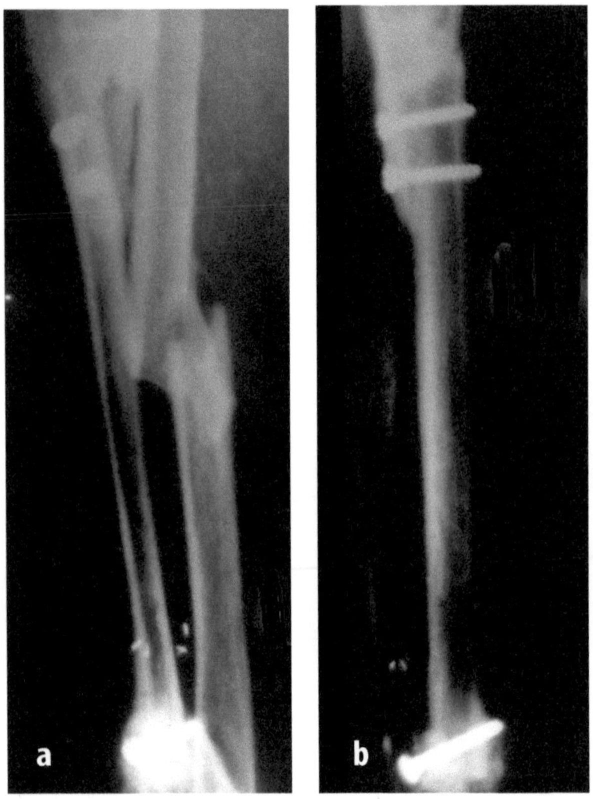

Fig. 10a, b. Same case as in Fig. 8. X-rays 3 months after bone grafting show good formation of bone callus

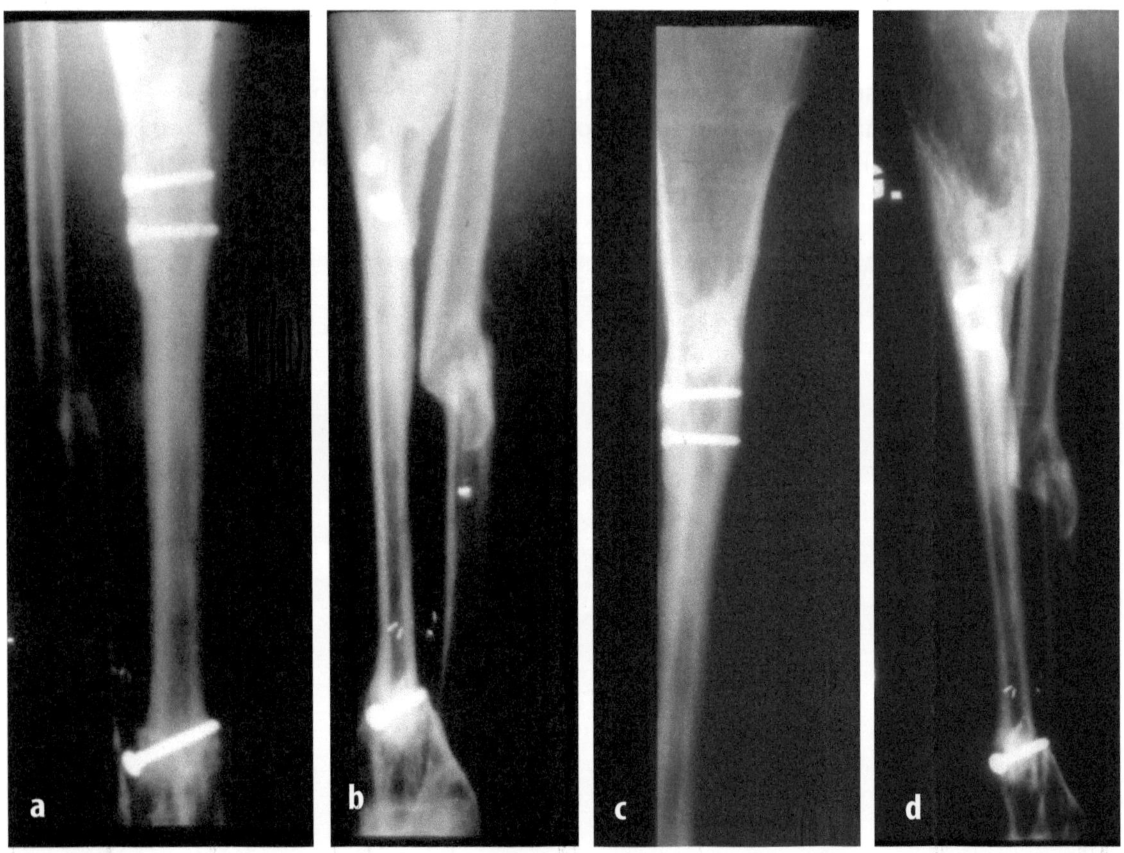

Fig. 11a-d. Same case as in Fig. 8. **a, b** X-rays at the removal of the external fixator (6 months after bone grafting) show complete consolidation. **c, d** X-rays after 5 years show considerable hypertrophy of the bone graft

In the free vascularized bone transfer technique the bone can be transferred alone or with overlying soft tissues (composite osteocutaneous or osteomyocutaneous vascularized grafts). This surgical procedure is technically demanding and donor site morbidity can be a major consequence.

Bone allografts must be harvested by a sterile procedure, and the sterile preparations in various shapes and sizes should be preserved by freezing, irradiation, or lyophilization [30, 42–45].

Allografts are stored in special tissue banks and are employed mainly for reconstruction of bone defects. Advantages include ready availability and no donor site morbidity; possible disadvantages include risks of infection, fracture, and transmission of infectious agents.

In traumatology today, the use of bone xenografts is extremely rare.

Bone Substitutes

An "ideal" bone alternative should be biocompatible, resorbable, structurally similar to bone, easy to use, osteoconductive, osteoinductive, and cost effective [45]. Commercially available bone substitutes differ in composition and mechanism of action. Moreover, they are osteoconductive but have limited osteoinduction, and generally offer minimal structural integrity [45].

Ceramics made of calcium phosphate are the bone substitutes most frequently used today. Polycrystalline ceramic structures are designed to reproduce synthetically calcium phosphate as found in the extracellular matrix of normal bone, giving an osteoconductive substrate for the bone regeneration. Materials more frequently employed to prepare polycrystalline ceramics are hydroscyopatite (HA) and tricalcium phosphate (TCP). The composition of HA closely approximates the mineral component of the bone with a Ca/P rate of 1.7, while TCP has a Ca/P rate of 1.5. The Ca/P rate correlates with its solubility; therefore, TCP ceramics can be resorbed 12 times more quickly than HA ceramics.

By combining HA and TCP in various ratios, it is possible to produce biphasic ceramics (or biceramic phosphates) with specific characteristics. For example, a structure composed of 75% HA and 25% TCP has the best equilibrium between mechanical strength and reasorption time. [46]. In clinical application, favorable results were observed in the management of a series of long bone nonunions [47]. The clinical introduction of these materials can avoid, ultimately, having to harvest an autologous bone graft.

In cases of wide bone loss, or when a more osteoinductive activity is required, additional materials with osteoinductive action can be included [for example: mixture with autologous bone graft, and a combination with demineralized bone matrix (DBM)].

Finally, in order to evaluate the results obtained with these "bone alternatives", it is important to remember that the variety of the commercially available materials makes it difficult to compare results, that the levels of difficulty in forming new bone vary in different healing environments, and that the behavior of a bone substitute in one site cannot be used to predict its performance in another site [45].

Growth Factors

Biologic stimulation of healing in nonunions can be obtained by means of locally implanted GFs with osteoinductive properties. In particular, the bone morphogenetic proteins (BMPs), members of the TGF superfamily, have proven to be capable of initiating the bone healing cascade through recruitment and interaction with mesenchymal cells [48, 49], which are stimulated towards differentiation to an osteochondroblastic lineage.

The first studies on the use of BMPs in nonunions were performed using purified human BMP (hBMP) [50], but later the ability to produce BMPs by means of recombinant gene technology (rhBMPs) made it possible to widely extend experimental and human studies [51]. Recently, two kinds of rhBMPs were approved by the US Food and Drug Administration for trauma: BMP-7 for use in recalcitrant nonunions (nonunions that have failed to respond to other treatment modalities) and BMP-2 for acute open tibial fractures.

Since these GFs alone induce very limited bone formation, the recombinant BMPs require a carrier or delivery system in order to exert the maximum biological activity by means of a gradual release over time [52, 53]. A number of carriers and delivery systems (including type I collagen, synthetic polymers, and hyaluronic acid gels) have been used in experimental and clinical models. Autologous bone grafts and some bone graft substitutes, including DBM and calcium phosphate containing preparations (HA, TCP, Bioglass), are also potential carriers.

Today it is unclear which carrier is best for transporting these molecules to receptors. Some preliminary clinical studies, published by Giltaji [54] on the association BMP – collagen carries and Cherubino et al. [55] on the assocation BMP – autologous bone graft showed favorable results.

These same properties of RhBMPs, however, impose caution in their application: Current formulations of BMP require an open procedure. Large amounts of recombinant protein are required to produce a clinically evident effect. They are expensive. They are not autologous. There is the risk of ectopic bone formation and compression on the soft tissues. Moreover, BMPs have been found in high concentration in some malignant tumors, and the consequences of a systemic diffusion of BMP are still not completely clarified [56–59].

Considering that in the white blood cells and especially in platelets alpha granules contain high concentrations of several GFs that are released with the platelet degranulation, it has been suggested that autologous GFs be used in combination with bone grafts in order to improve osseointegration in nonunions.

An autologous growth factor (AGF) gel can be obtained by isolating and concentrating platelets and white cells to levels sevenfold of circulating levels in patients. Then, 1 ml of thrombin is mixed with 10 ml AGF extract and applied to the graft material to obtain a malleable and plastic composite. The graft-gel composite can be implanted in order to stimulate osteogenesis in long bone nonunions [60].

Another technology is based on concentrating platelets by gradient density centrifugation in order to obtain the so-called platelet-rich plasma (PRP), which contains GFs capable of stimulating the proliferation of mesenchymal cells [61].

The published data about the use of the AGF and PRP procedures in the management of nonunions include a limited number of cases but the preliminary results appear to be favorable.

References

1. Bray TJ (1994) A prospective, double-blind trial of electrical capacitive coupling in the treatment of nonunions of long bones. J Bone Joint Surg Am 76:820–826
2. Ryaby JT (1998) Clinical effects of electromagnetic and electric fields on fracture healing. Clin Orthop Relat Res 335[Suppl]:205–215
3. Fukuda F, Yasuda I (1957) On the piezoelectric effect in bone. J Physiol Soc Jpn 12:1158–1162
4. Friedenberg ZB, Brighton CT (1966) Bioelectric potentials in bone. J Bone Joint Surg Am 48:915–923
5. Weitzel PP, Esterhai JL (1994) Delayed union, non-union and synovial pseudoarthrosis. In: Brighton CT, Friedlander GE, Lane JM (eds) Bone formation and repair. AAOS, Rosemont (Illinois), pp 505–527
6. Fitzsimmons RJ, Ryaby JT, Mohan S et al (1995) Combined magnetic fields increase IGF-II secretion in osteoblast cultures. Endocrinology 136:3100–3106
7. Brighton CT, Pollack SR, Windsor RE (1981) Acceleration of fracture healing in the rabbit fibula by a capacitively coupled electric field. Trans Bioelect Repair Growth Soc 1:36
8. Patterson D (1984) Treatment of non-union with a constant direct current. A totally implantable system. Orthop Clin North Am 15:47–59
9. Basset CA, Mitchell SN, Gaston SR (1981) Treatment of ununited tibial diaphyseal fractures with pulsing electromagnetic fields. J Bone Joint Surg Am 63:511–523
10. Benazzo F, Mosconi M, Todesca A et al (1996) L'induzione dell'osteogenesi riparativa con campi elettrici. Minerva Ortop Traumatol 47:291–295
11. Sharrard W (1990) A double-blind trial of electromagnetic field for delayed union of tibial fractures. J Bone Joint Surg Br 72:347–355
12. Scott G, King JB (1994) A prospective double-blind trial of electrical capacitive coupling in the treatment of non-union of long bones. J Bone Joint Surg Am 76:820–826

13. Knoch HG (1967) Konservative Behandlungsmöglichkeiten durch Ultraschall bei verzögerter Kallusbildung. Beitr Orthop 14:720–723
14. Klug W, Knoch HG (1987) Aktivierung der Knochenbruchheilung durch Ultraschall. Z Physioter 39:91–98
15. Duarte LR (1983) The stimulation of bone growth by ultrasound. Arch Orthop Trauma Surg 101:153–159
16. Heckman JD, Ryaby JP, McCabe J et al (1994) Acceleration of tibial fracture healing by non-invasive, low intensity pulsed ultrasound. J Bone Joint Surg Am 76:26–34
17. Duarte L, Choffie M (1994) Review of nonunions treated by pulsed, low-intensity ultrasound. Proceedings of the Orthopaedic Health Conference, São Paulo
18. Rodriguez-Merchan EC, Forriol F (2004) Nonunion: general principles and experimental data. Clin Orthop Relat Res 419:4–12
19. Meani E, Romanò CL, Messina JC et al (2000) Ultrasuoni pulsati a bassa intensità nel trattamento delle pseudoartrosi settiche. Giorn Ital Ortop Traumatol 26[Suppl. 1]:21–26
20. Mayr E, Frankel V, Ruter A (2000) Ultrasound. An alternative healing method for nonunions? Arch Orthop Trauma Surg 120:1–8
21. Rubin C, Bolander M, Ryabi JP et al (2001) The use of low intensity ultrasound to accelerate the healing of fractures. J Bone Joint Surg Am 83:259–270
22. Valchanov VD, Michailov P (1991) High energy shock waves in the treatment of delayed and nonunion fractures. Int Orthop 15:181–184
23. Schlaberger R, Senge T (1992) Non invasive treatment of long bone pseudoarthrosis by shock waves. Arch Orthop Trauma Surg 111:224–227
24. Sukul DM, Johannes EJ, Pierik EG et al (1993) The effect of high energy shock waves focused on cortical bone: an in vitro study. J Surg Res 54:46–51
25. Haupt G (1997) Use of E.S.W. in treatment of pseudoarthrosis, tendinopathy and other orthopaedic diseases. J Urol 158:4–11
26. Ghisellini F, Ceffa R, Gandini G et al (2000) La litotripsia extracorporea a onde d'urto nella terapia della pseudoartrosi. Giorn Ital Ortop Traumatol 26[Suppl. 1]:17–20
27. Corrado EM. Russo S, Gigliotti S (1996) Le onde d'urto ad alta energia nel trattamento delle pseudoartrosi. Giorn Ital Ortop Traumatol 22[Suppl. 2]:485–490
28. Russo S, Amelio E, Galasso O et al (2001) La litotrissia extracorporea nel trattamento delle pseudoartrosi ossee. Minerva Ortop Traumatol 52:261–267
29. Siebert CH, Lehrbass Sokeland KP, Rinke F et al (1997) Compression plating of tibial fractures following primary external fixation. Arch Orthop Trauma Surg 116:390–395
30. Perry CR (1999) Bone repair techniques, bone graft and bone graft substitutes. Clin Orthop Relat Res 360:71–86
31. Zinghi GF, Rollo G, Trono M (2004) La pseudoartrosi delle ossa lunghe. Timeo, Bologna
32. Perren SM (1991) The concept of biological plating using the limited contact-dynamic compression plate (LC–DCP): scientific background, design and application. Injury 22[Suppl. 1]:1–41
33. Frigg R (2003) Development of the locking compression plate. Injury 34[Suppl. 2]:6–10
34. Schandelmaier P (1999) Stabilization of distal femoral fractures using the LISS. Techn Orthop 14:230–246
35. Helfet DL, Jupiter JB, Gasser S (1992) Indirect reduction and tension band plating of tibial nonunion with deformity. J Bone Joint Surg Am 74:1286–1297

36. Wiss D, Johnson DL, Miao M (1992) Compression plating for non-union after failed external fixation of open tibial fractures. J Bone Joint Surg Am 74:1279–1285
37. Galpin RD, Veith RG, Hansen ST (1986) Treatment of failures after plating of tibial fractures. J Bone Joint Surg Am 68:1231–1236
38. Wiss D, Stetson WB (1994) Non-union of the tibia treated with a reamed intramedullary nail. J Orthop Trauma 8:189–194
39. Solomin L (2005) Principles of external fixation with the Ilizarov apparatus. Morsar, St. Petersburg
40. De Bastiani G, Aldegheri R, Renzi Brivio L (1984) The treatment of fractures with a dynamic axial fixator. J Bone Joint Surg Br 66:538–545
41. Reckling PW, Waters CH (1980) Treatment of nonunions of fractures of the tibial diaphysis by posterolateral corticocancellous bone grafting. J Bone Joint Surg Am 62:936–941
42. Volkov M, Bizer V (1972) Homotransplantation du tissu osseux en orthopédie infantile. Éditions de Moscou, Moscow
43. Imamaliev AS (1978) Homoplasty of the articular ends of bones. Mir, Moscow
44. Tomford WW, Thongphasuk J, Mankin HJ et al (1990) Frozen musculoskeletal allografts: a study of the clinical incidence and causes of infection associated with their use. J Bone Joint Surg Am 72:1137–1143
45. Greenwald AS, Boden SD, Goldberg VM et al (2002) Bone graft substitutes: facts, fictions and applications. Proceedings of the AAOS 69th Annual Meeting, Dallas
46. Warren SM, Fong KD, Nacamull RP et al (2004) Biomatériaux de réparation de la peau et de l'os en chirurgie plastique. Encycl Méd Chir (Chir Plast) 45–110, Elsevier, Paris
47. Meyrueis JP, Cazenave A, Le Saint B et al (1998) Utilisation d'unc céramique macroporeuse biphasée en traumatologie. À propos de 108 cas. Rev Chir Orthop 84[Suppl. 2]:59–64
48. Mont MA, Ragland PS, Biggins B (2004) Use of bone morphogenetic proteins for musculoskeletal applications. J Bone Joint Surg Am 86[Suppl. 2]:41–55
49. Calori GM, d'Imporzano M (2004) Fattori di crescita e bone morphogenetic proteins: storia e revisione della letteratura. Aggiorn Club Ital Osteosint 10:56–58
50. Johnson EE, Urist MR, Finerman GA (1988) Bone morphogenetic protein augmentation grafting of resistant femoral nonunions. A preliminary report. Clin Orthop Relat Res 230:257–265
51. Friedlaender GE, Perry CR, Cole JD et al (2002) Osteogenic protein-1 (bone morphogenetic protein-7) in the treatment of tibial nonunions. J Bone Joint Surg Am 84[Suppl. 1]:2123–2134
52. Lieberman JR, Daluiski A, Einhorn T (2002) The role of growth factors in the repair of bone: biology and clinical applications. J Bone Joint Surg Am 84:1032–1044
53. Ripamonti U, Pipino F (2003) Le bone morphogenetic proteins (BMPs). Dalla ricerca alla clinica. Giorn Ital Ortop Traumatol 29:124–140
54. Giltaji LR (2002) Osteogenic protein 1 (OP-1) in the repair of bone defects and fractures of long bones: clinical experience. In: Vukicevic S, Sampath KT (eds) Bone morphogenetic proteins: from laboratory to clinical practice. Birkhäuser, Basel, pp 193–205
55. Cherubino P, Ronga M, Baldo F et al (2004) Proteina osteogenica-1 (OP-1) nel trattamento delle pseudoartrosi e delle perdite di sostanza ossea. Esperienza preliminare. Giorn Ital Ortop Traumatol 30[Suppl. 1]:119–124
56. Marie P (1999) BMPs et réparation osseuse. Intérêt des facteurs de croissance dans la réparation osseuse. Proceedings of the 74e Réunion annuelle de la SOFCOT

57. Meyrueis JP, Cazenave A (2004) Consolidation des fractures. Encycl Méd Chir (App Locom) 14-031-A-20, Elsevier, Paris
58. Langenfeld EM, Langenfeld J (2004) Bone morphogenetic protein-2 stimulates angiogenesis in developing tumors. Mol Cancer Res 2:141–149
59. Yoshikawa H, Nakase T, Myoui A et al (2004) Bone morphogenetic proteins in bone tumors. J Orthop Sci 9:334–340
60. Hood AG, Biggi F (2003) The use of autologous growth factors to stimulate osteogenesis. Aggiorn Club Ital Osteosint 9:47–52
61. Mantelli P, De Girolamo L, Maggi F et al (2004) I fattori di crescita nel trattamento delle pseudoartrosi: studio clinico sperimentale. Arch Ortop Reumatol 115:20–21

Treatment of Infected Nonunions: Techniques Other Than Compression-Distraction Methods

REDENTO MORA, GABRIELLA TUVO, MILENA MICELI, STEFANO GILI

Introduction

Techniques for the management of infected nonunions of the long bones aim to solve three problems: infection, lack of bone continuity, and lack of skin coverage. These problems are always related to varying degrees: the lack of skin coverage can allow a superinfection; the persistence of infection damages the surrounding soft tissues; the lack of consolidation and the persistence of abnormal mobility improves infection [1].

Conventional treatment combines, in several operative stages, *débridement*, stabilization, and reconstruction. *Débridement*, associated with antibiotic therapy, attempts to sterilize the nonunion site. Stabilization aims to allow consolidation and to fight infection more effectively. Skin and bone grafts can be used for reconstruction.

Concerning bone grafts, there are two possibilities: corticocancellous bone grafting with skin coverage (the use of corticocancellous graft requires skin closing since the cortical bone suffers from air exposure) and cancellous bone grafting without skin coverage (Papineau method).

Débridement

Débridement should include accurate and complete excision of the sinus tract and all infected avascular tissues, i.e., avascular soft tissue bed (including skin, subcutaneous tissue, fascia, muscle, and scar tissue between bone ends) and avascular bone bed (avascular bone bed can result in persistent infection with drainage). Moreover, proximal and distal medullary canals must be curetted and reamed to remove all necrotic debris.

Repeated *débridements*, performed every 3–5 days, are often necessary because a complete removal of all dead bone and all infected tissues is mandatory [2–5]. The quality of the surgical *débridement* is the most critical factor for successful management of chronic orthopaedic infection [6].

Antibiotic therapy during treatment is established according to the results of susceptibility studies of the intraoperative cultures.

After *débridement*, treatment with closed suction-irrigation may sometimes be indicated (particularly in large cavities where an important bleeding can be expected) [4]. However, the irrigation system must not be used for more than 3 or 4 days in order to minimize the risk of superinfection.

Stabilization

Stability can be achieved by several means. Nonoperative techniques such as skeletal traction or cast immobilization cannot provide acceptable stability and should only be used as a temporary measure in selected cases. Therefore, internal or external fixation are usually employed to obtain adequate stability.

Plating, performed during *débridement* and irrigation or later (during the second or third *débridement*) in patients in whom local signs of inflammation are minimal or absent, is employed in combination with bone grafting and is considered by some authors a good method of treatment, with high success rates [4, 7]. The main risk of this technique is the possibility of spreading the infection.

Intramedullary nailing has been performed with discrete success rates by many authors. This technique has the risk of spreading infection to the entire medullary canal of the long bone, too. Furthermore, a particular surgical protocol (conversion protocol) has been suggested that involves the use of external fixation in the first phase of treatment and conversion to internal fixation by means of intramedullary nailing in the second phase (when the infection is under control) [8–12].

The advantages of using axial external fixation techniques are: insertion of the bone fixation elements far from the infected bone, easy care of the infected wound, and the possibility of further procedures such as bone and skin grafts without injuring the surrounding tissues [1, 10, 13].

Axial devices, therefore, have many important limitations compared to circular external devices (less stability, little versatility in axial or torsional deviations, and impossibility of immediate weight bearing). In brief, they do not allow a "dynamic" treatment of the infected nonunion (Figs. 1, 2).

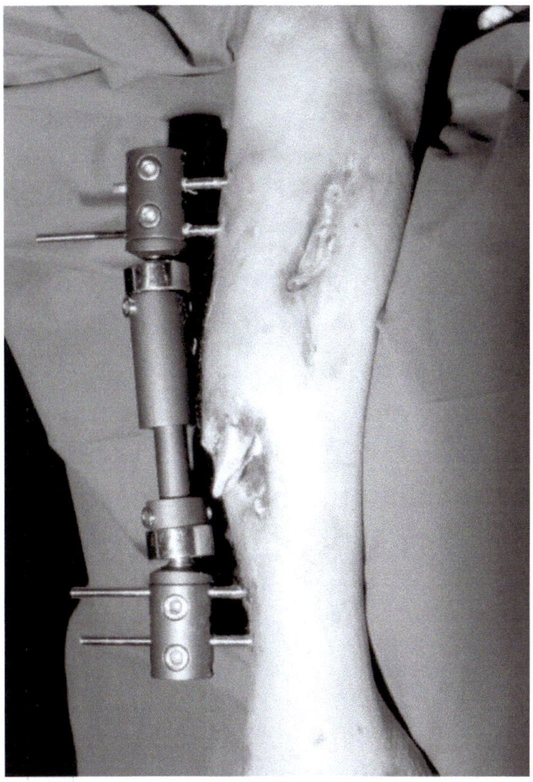

Fig. 1. Clinical feature of an infected tibial nonunion with bone loss in a 24-year-old man treated with axial external fixation

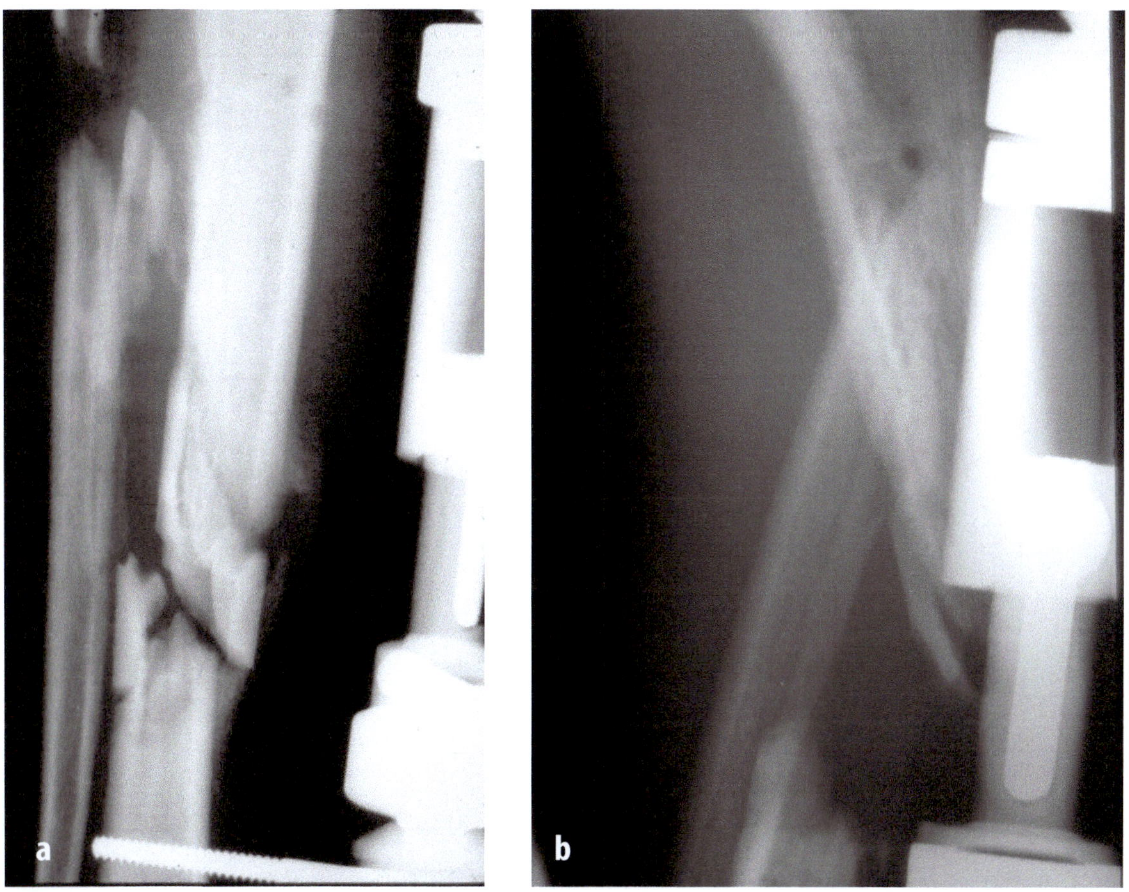

Fig. 2a, b. Same case as in Fig. 1. X-ray of the nonunion

Reconstruction

Soft Tissue Reconstruction

In most simple cases, in which skin and soft tissue *débridement* is minimal, wound closure can be delayed. However, in the majority of cases, open management with soft tissue reconstruction is necessary. This can be achieved by different means [1, 14–16]: simple split-thickness skin graft (not indicated in cases of poorly vascularized soft tissues or bone without periosteum), cross leg flap (rarely used today, due to the prolonged immobilization period required), shifting flap (only indicated for small local soft tissue coverage), fasciocutaneous flap and muscle flap (in which distant coverage is difficult or impossible), and free microvascularized graft (valid option for limb salvage, especially in the most severe cases, where an amputation might be considered) (Figs. 3–7).

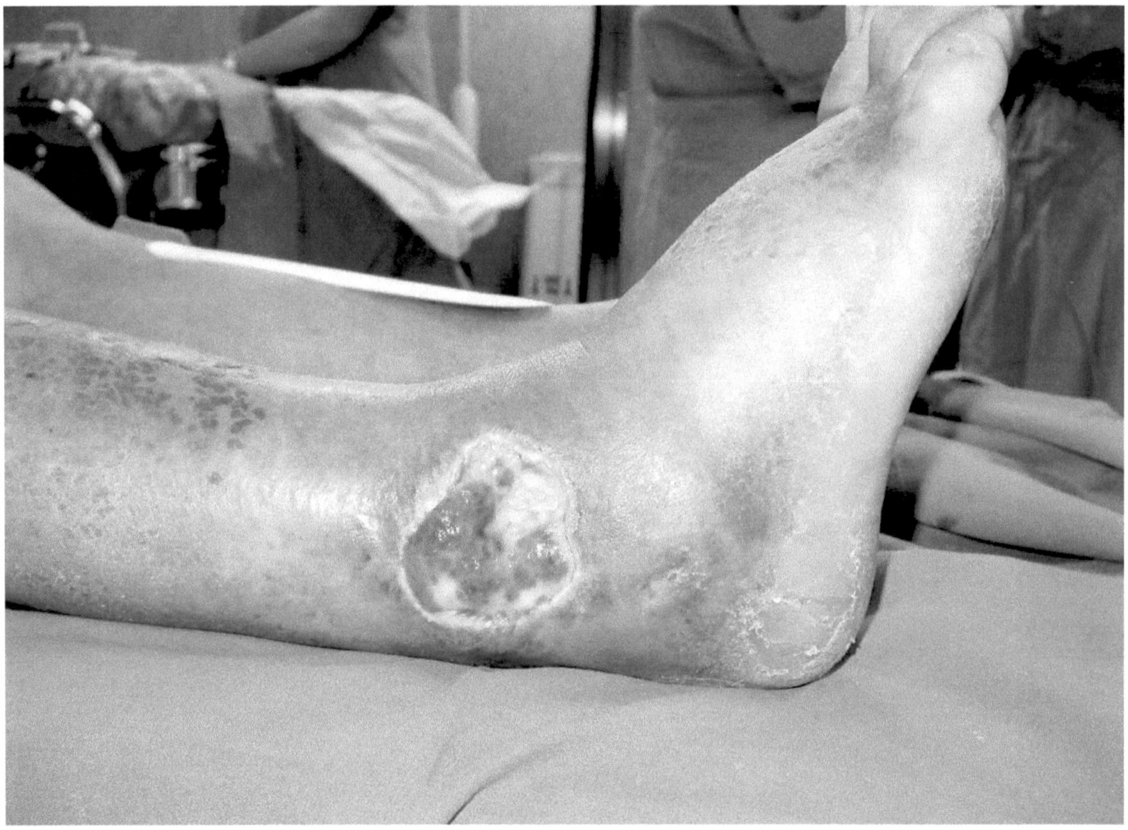

Fig. 3. Soft tissue loss in a 55-year-old patient with an infected nonunion of the right tibial pilon

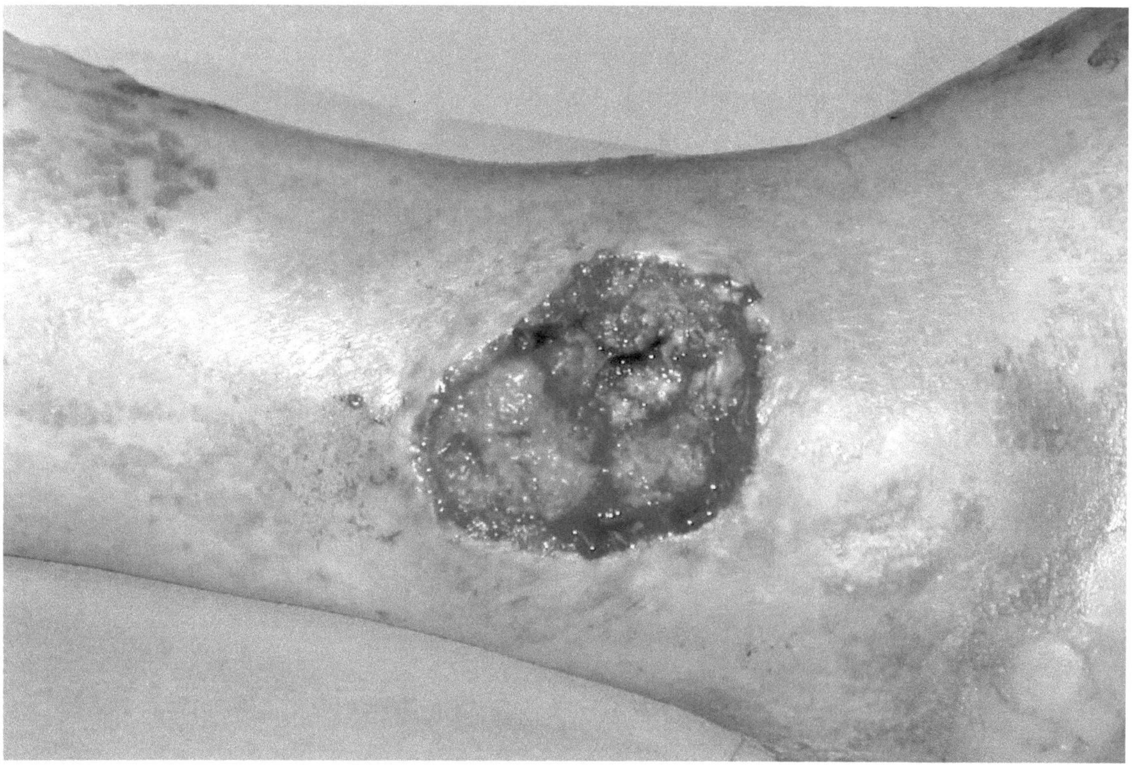

Fig. 4. Same case as in Fig. 3. *Débridement* of the infected and necrotic soft tissues

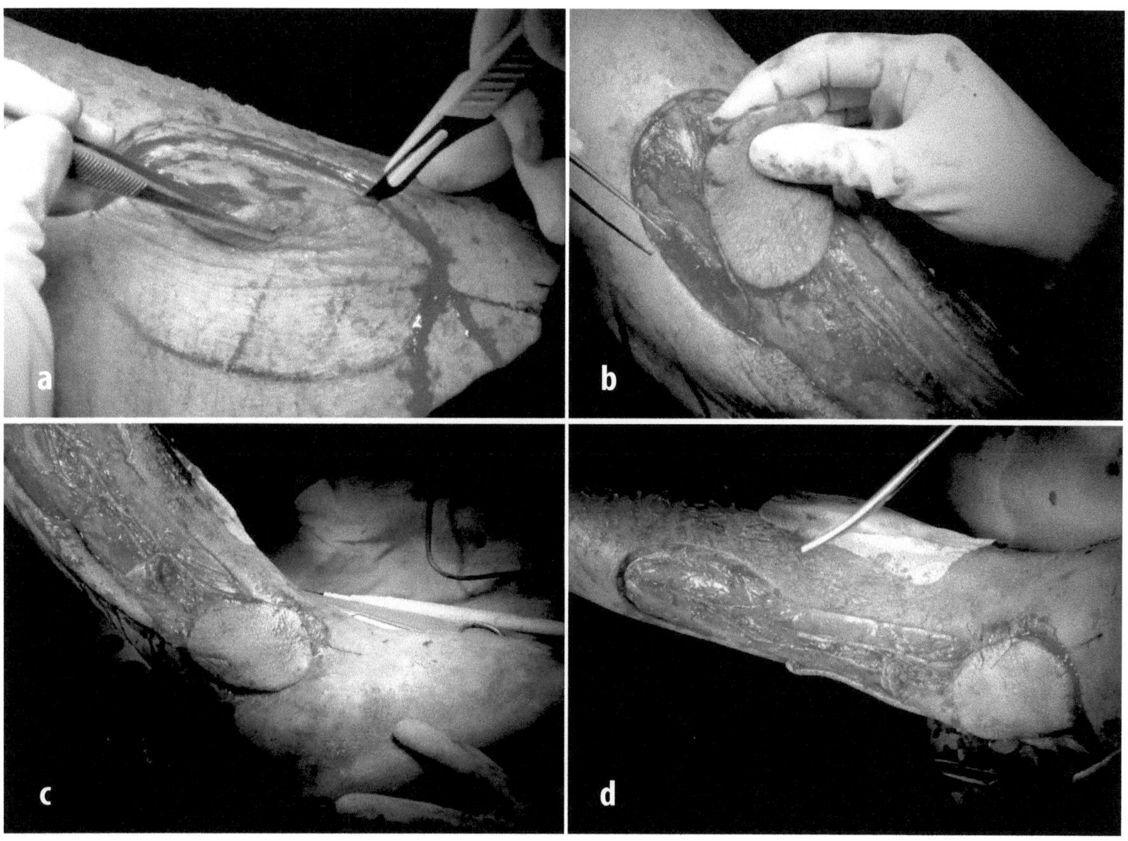

Fig. 5a-d. Same case as in Fig. 3. Fasciocutaneous flap

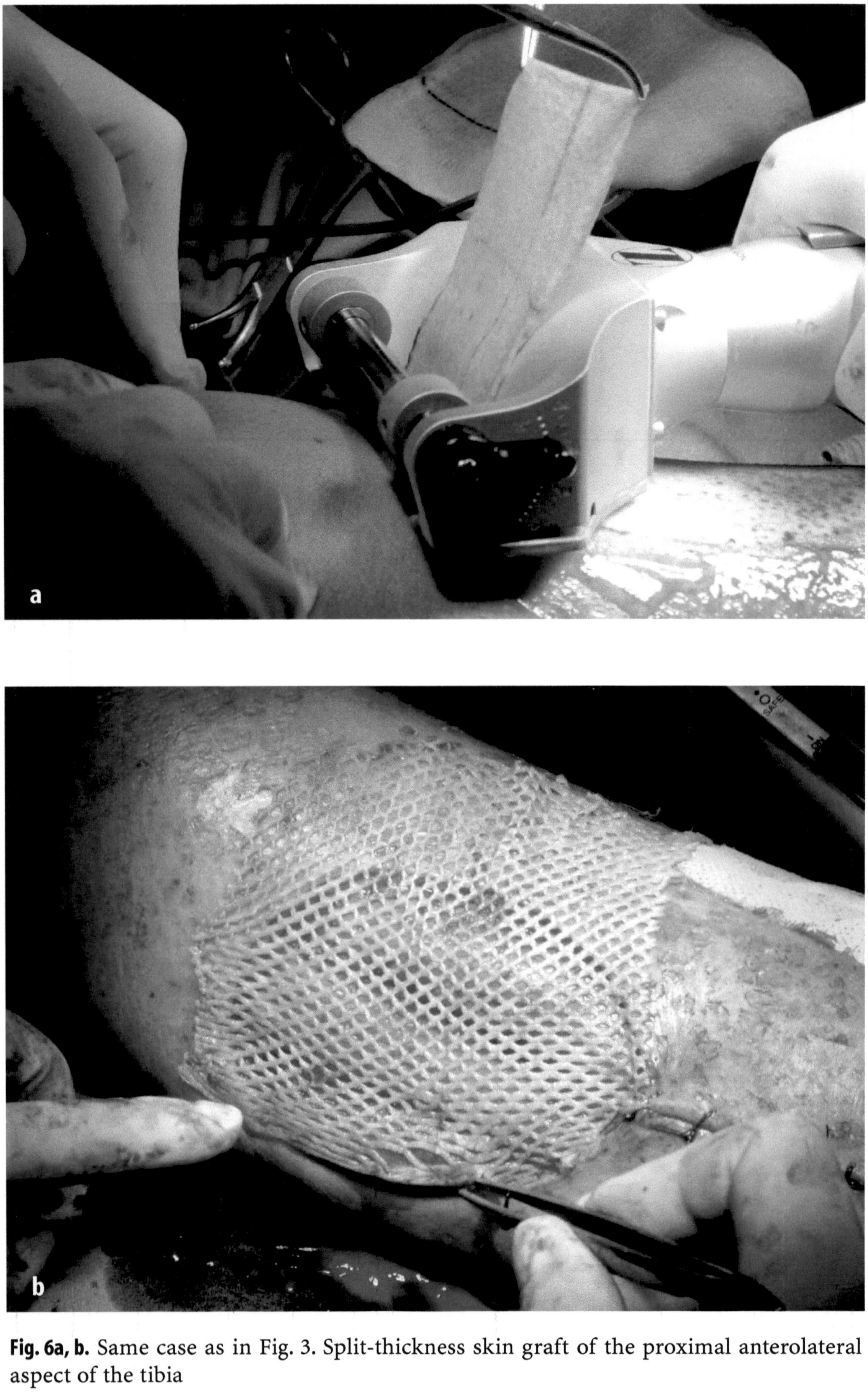

Fig. 6a, b. Same case as in Fig. 3. Split-thickness skin graft of the proximal anterolateral aspect of the tibia

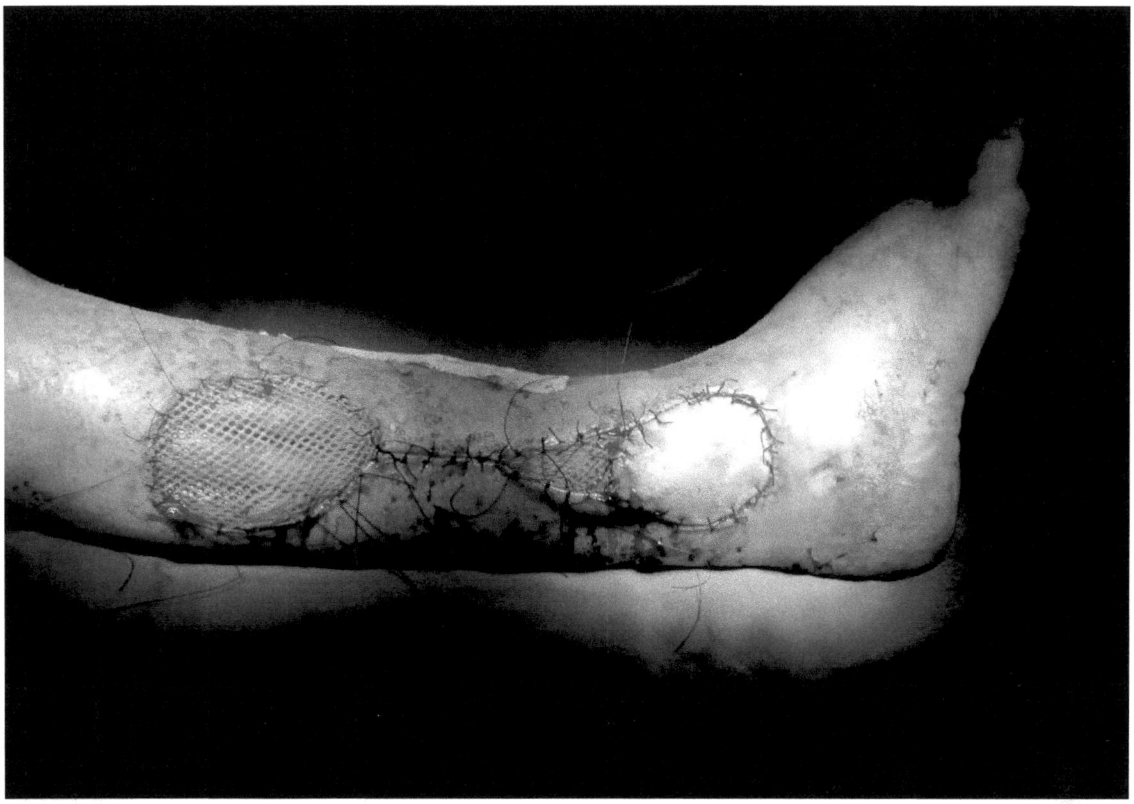

Fig. 7. Same case as in Fig. 3. Clinical feature at the end of the soft tissue reconstruction procedure

Bone Reconstruction

Different surgical treatments have been described and recommended.

Bone Reconstruction by Corticocancellous Bone Grafting

Bone grafts of adequate shape and size can be taken from iliac crest, and more rarely from the femur (great trochanter or distal metaphysis) or tibia (proximal metaphysis). If microvascularized bone grafts are required, ipsilateral or contralateral fibula [17] or iliac crest with soft tissue coverage (so-called composite grafts) is employed (Fig. 8).

Autoplastic bone grafts have some disadvantages and limitations, such as quantity of bone, immobilization, complications at the donor site (pain and infection) and at the recipient site (fractures, delayed union or nonunion, and nonunion at the graft-bone interface) [18].

In many countries, particularly in Russia, homoplastic bone grafts have been used for many years and are still successfully employed. This kind of graft, harvested under highly sterile conditions, is usually stored in special bone banks by deep refrigeration and can be employed as a massive bone graft or as thin sheets of cortical bone [19, 20].

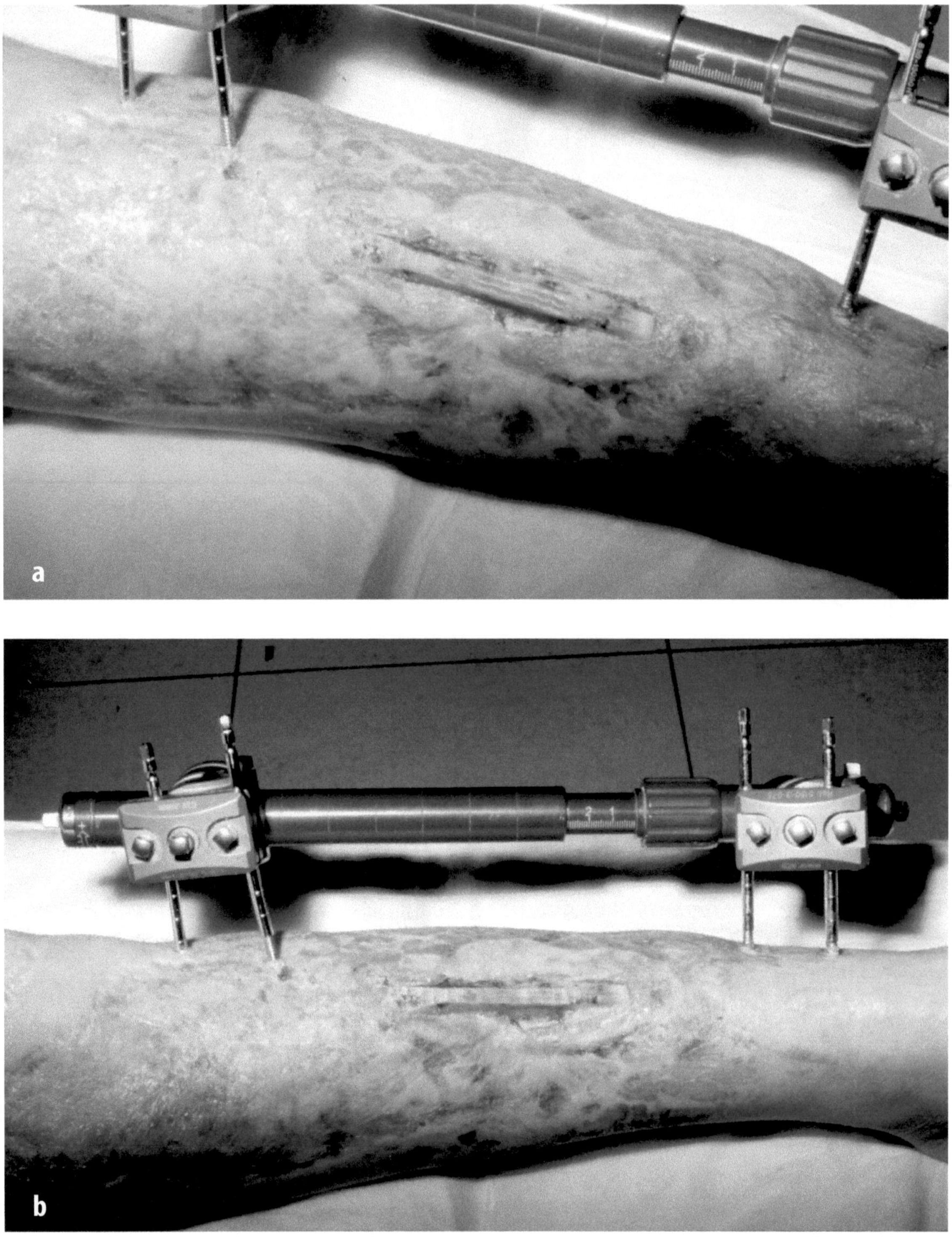

Fig. 8a, b. Nonunion at the graft-bone interface after microvascularized fibular grafting in a tibial infected nonunion in a 23-year-old woman

Bone Reconstruction by Cancellous Bone Grafting (Papineau Method)

With the Papineau method, morselized autologous cancellous bone grafts are used to obliterate bone defects in tibial infected nonunions [1, 10, 15, 21, 22]. The cancellous bone, usually harvested from the iliac crest, is reduced in bone chips and then packed into the bone cavity without leaving dead space. The dressing is changed every 4–5 days.

The graft is gradually incorporated and there is no need for soft tissue coverage: the wound heals spontaneously or is covered later, when granulation tissue grows through the bone graft, by split-thickness skin grafting. This technique is not very demanding and can be used in elderly patients or in patients with concomitant chronic diseases such as diabetes. The disadvantages are that the procedure can require many operative stages and prolonged periods of time for healing.

References

1. Lortat-Jacob A (1977) Principes de traitement chirurgical de l'infection osseuse. Infection sur os non solide. Encycl Méd Chir, Techn Chir-Orthop Traumatol 44–082 Elsevier, Paris
2. Morandi M, Zembo M, Ciotti M (1989) Infected tibial pseudoarthrosis. A 2-year follow-up on patients treated by the Ilizarov technique. Orthopaedics 12:497–505
3. Gustilo RB (1989) Orthopaedic infection. Saunders, Philadelphia
4. Connolly JF (ed) (1991) Tibial nonunions. Diagnosis and treatment. AAOS, Park Ridge (Illinois)
5. Biasibetti A, Aloj D, Gallinaro P (2000) Caratteristiche e confronto critico delle tecniche della ricostruzione ossea in traumatologia. Indicazioni alla tecnica di Ilizarov. Giorn Ital Ortop Traumatol 26[Suppl. 1]:302–308
6. Tetsworth K, Cierny G III (1999) Osteomyelitis debridement techniques. Clin Orthop Relat Res 360:87–96
7. Helfet DL, Jupiter JB, Gasser S (1992) Indirect reduction and tension band plating of tibial nonunion with deformity. J Bone Joint Surg Am 74:1286–1297
8. Gordon L, Chiu EJ (1988) Treatment of infected nonunions and segmental defects of the tibia with staged microvascular muscle transplantation and bone grafting. J Bone Joint Surg Am 70:377–386
9. Sledge SL, Johnson KD, Henley MB et al (1989) Intramedullary nailing with reaming to treat nonunion of the tibia. J Bone Joint Surg Am 71:1004–1019
10. Perry CR (1999) Bone repair techniques, bone graft and bone graft substitutes. Clin Orthop Relat Res 360:71–86
11. Sheperd L, Costigan WM, Gardochi R et al (1998) Local or free muscle flaps and unreamed interlocked nail for open tibial fractures. Clin Orthop Relat Res 350:90–96

12. Biggi F, Costacurta G, D'Andrea S et al (2001) Aspetti peculiari della traumatologia "ad alta energia". Giorn Ital Ortop Traumatol 27[Suppl. 1]:551–554
13. Marsh JL, Nepola JV, Meffert R (1992) Dynamic external fixation for stabilization of nonunions. Clin Orthop Relat Res 278:200–208
14. Weiland AJ, Russell Moore J, Hotchkiss RN (1983) Soft tissue procedures for reconstruction of tibial shaft fractures. Clin Orthop Relat Res 178:42–53
15. Stein H, Lerner A (2001) Advances in the treatment of chronic osteomyelitis. Curr Orthop 15:451–456
16. Meyer C, Schnettler R, Hartmann B et al (2004) Proximally based fasciocutaneous flaps of the lower leg for the coverage of soft tissue defects. Osteo Trauma Care 12:13–15
17. Gilbert A (1979) Surgical technique of vascularized transfer of the fibular shaft. Int J Microsurg 102:100–106
18. Khaleel A, Pool RD (2110) Bone transport. Curr Orthop 15:229–237
19. Volkov M, Bizer V (1972) Homotransplantation du tissu osseux en orthopédie infantile. Éditions de Moscou, Moscow
20. Imamaliev AS (1978) Homoplasty of the articular ends of bones. Mir, Moscow
21. Papineau LJ (1973) L'excision-greffe avec fermeture retardée délibérée dans l'ostéomyélite chronique. Nouv Presse Med 2:2753–2755
22. Roy Camille R, Reignier B, Saillant G et al (1976) Technique et histoire naturelle de l'intervention de Papineau. Excision-greffe de spongieux à l'air libre. Rev Chir Orthop 62:337–345

Treatment of Noninfected Nonunions: Hypertrophic Nonunions

Redento Mora, Luisella Pedrotti, Barbara Bertani, Gabriella Tuvo

Introduction

Nonunions are treated by compression-distraction techniques or any other surgical treatment, depending on the type (hypertrophic, normotrophic, or atrophic). In order to clearly identify the type of nonunion, a careful clinical and radiographic evaluation, including scintigraphic assessment, is crucial (Fig. 1).

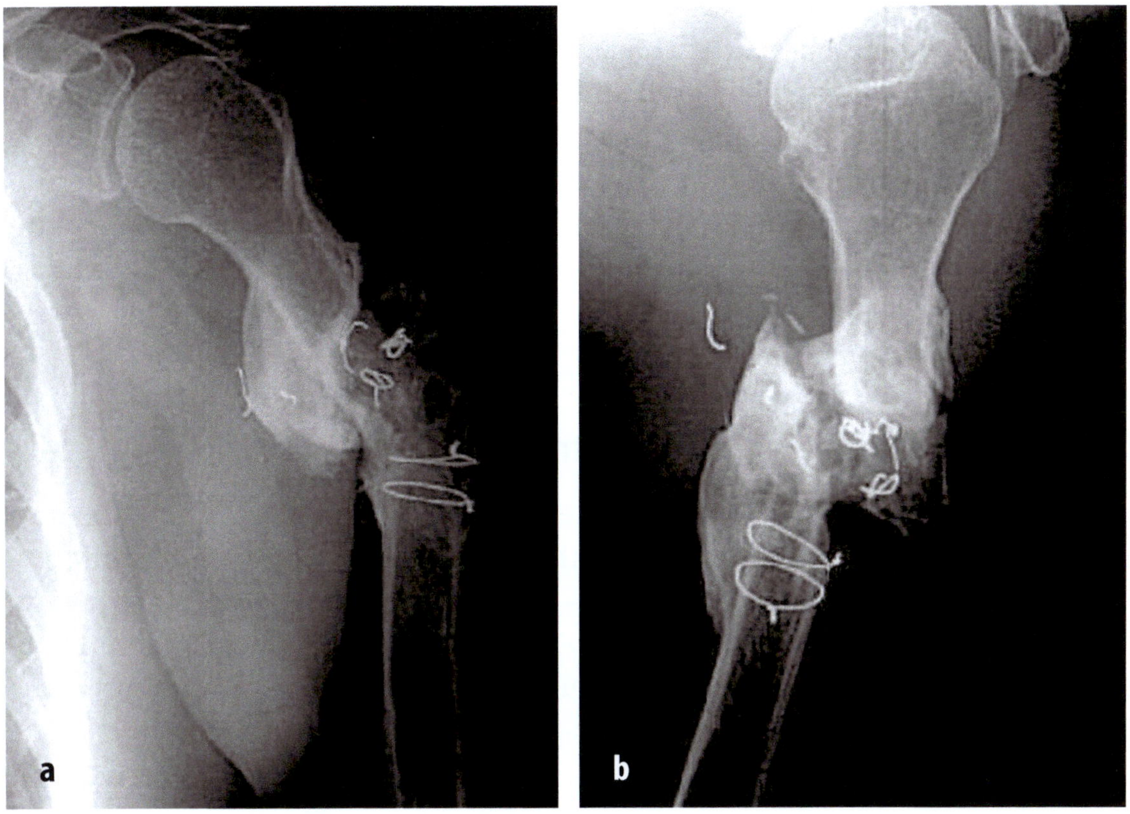

Fig. 1a, b. X-rays of a humeral hypertrophic nonunion

In the management of hypertrophic nonunions, compression-distraction techniques represent an evident improvement, especially considering that, in this type of nonunion, the lack of bone consolidation is associated with a deformity (mainly axial deviation and shortening) that can be treated at the same time as the nonunion using these techniques.

In atrophic nonunions, the gap between the bone fragments is filled by nonbiologically active smooth connective tissue whereas, in hypertrophic nonunions, the fibrous tissue or fibrocartilaginous tissue interposed between the bone fragments is biologically active.

The classic approach to nonunions is based on compression and rigid stabilization, and distraction is generally thought to be a predisposing factor for nonunion [1–4]. However, in hypertrophic forms of nonunion, gradual distraction acts as a stimulus on the tissue, which maintains its osteogenic potential.

For treating this type of lesion, compression or contact between the bone fragments is not strictly required because the true missing component is an appropriate mechanical environment, provided by stable osteosynthesis. These concepts are based on Ilizarov's "tension stress" theory [5].

Distraction osteosynthesis as the exclusive treatment for hypertrophic nonunions has been first described by some authors from Eastern Europe [6–9]; in Western Countries some other articles have been published dealing with this topic [10–24]. The fact that only few studies have been published on this topic has some important consequences. From a clinical point of view, this method is still not widely used and only few case histories have been published. Furthermore, the preoperative planning and the surgical technique are not strictly defined, and in different series the method of treatment varies in several significant aspects. Considering laboratory research, clear morphologic data are still not available, and in particular there is a lack of studies dealing with human samples.

Operative Technique (Monofocal Distraction Osteosynthesis)

The monofocal distraction osteosynthesis technique, developed in cooperation between the Department of Orthopaedics and Traumatology of the University of Pavia (at the Città di Pavia Institute) and the Central Institute of Traumatology and Orthopaedics (CITO) of Moscow, is particularly simple. In fact, this method merely provides adequate mechanical conditions to produce distraction osteogenesis.

The mechanical conditions consist of stable fixation with a circular external fixator and gradual distraction at a rate of 1.0 mm per day until the shortening has been corrected. Distraction is not administered in divided doses several times daily but as a single daily dose. Subsequently, a further distraction of 0.5 mm every 10 days is performed in order to maintain the tension effect on the nonunion during the whole period of treatment (Figs. 2–4).

In cases without shortening only periodic distraction is carried out in order to produce and maintain the tension effect during the treatment. Where angular deformity or other deformities are associated with dysmetria, treatment is modified in order to correct them.

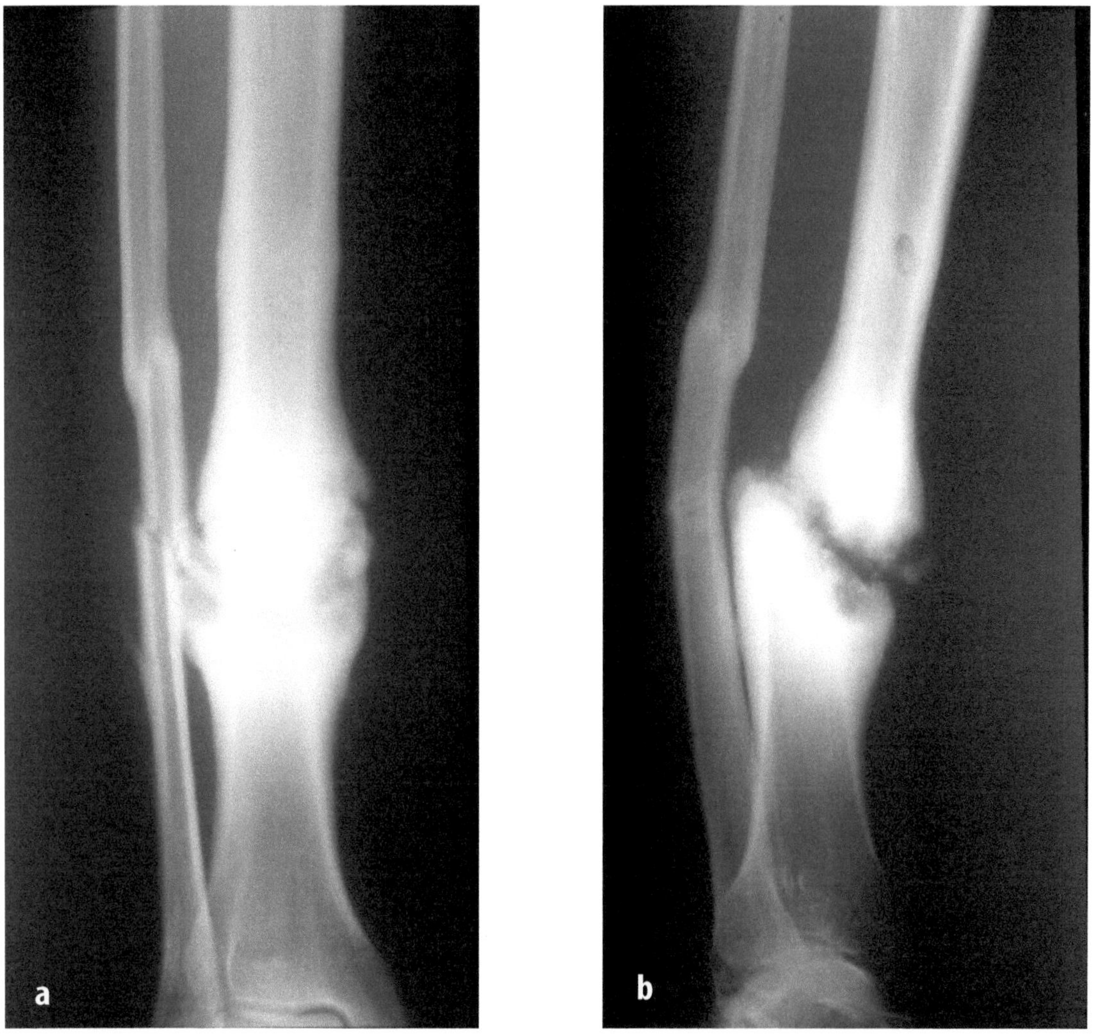

Fig. 2a, b. X-rays of a hypertrophic nonunion of the right tibia with leg length discrepancy of 2 cm in a 28-year-old man previously treated with three open surgical procedures

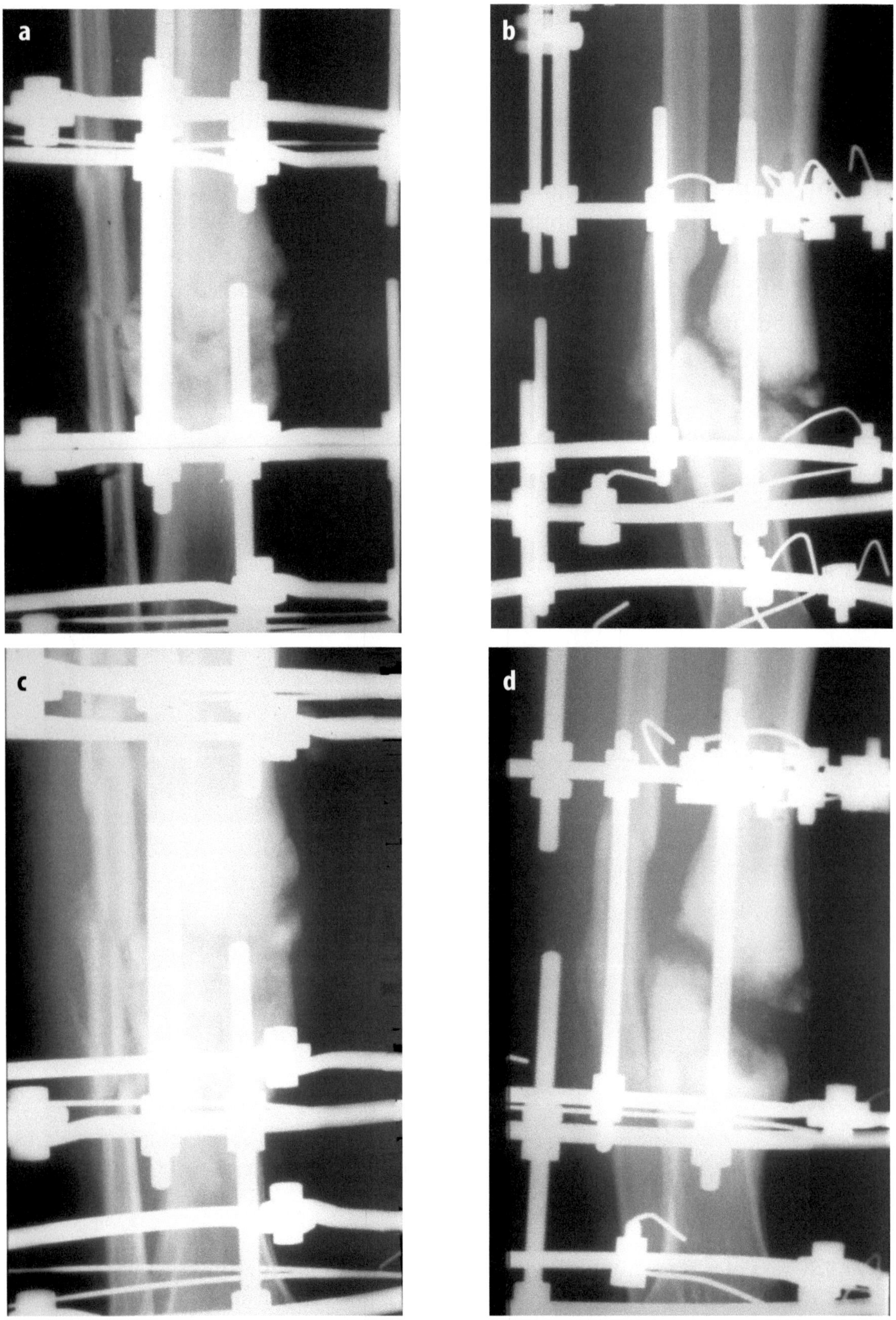

Fig. 3a-d. Same case as in Fig. 2. **a, b** X-rays at the beginning of treatment with distraction osteosynthesis. **c, d** X-rays at the end of the distraction phase

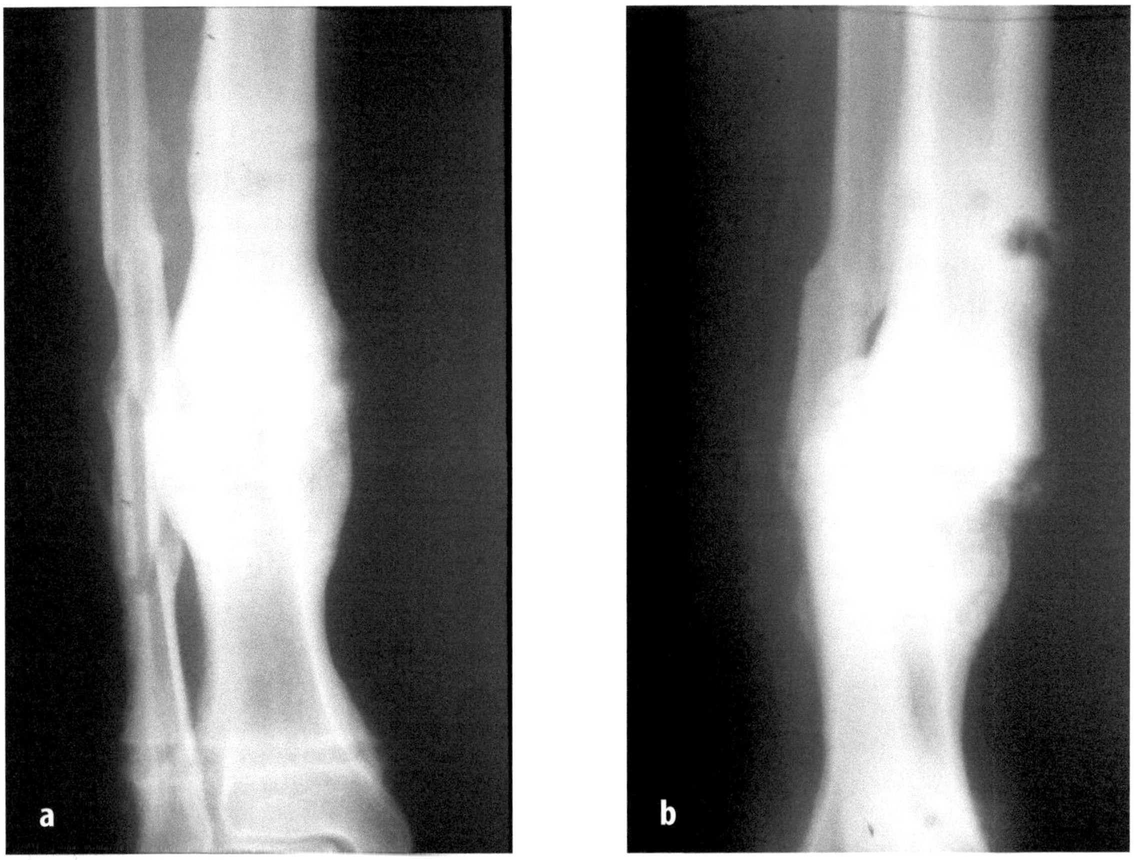

Fig. 4a, b. Same case as in Fig. 2. Healing of the nonunion with correction of leg length discrepancy after 4 months

Materials and Methods

Between 1986 and 2002, 347 hyperthrophic noninfected nonunions of long bones, assessed by means of x-rays and bone scan, were treated (with a minimal follow-up of 2 years). Among the patients were 234 men and 113 women ranging in age from 20 to 68 years (average age 31 years). The nonunion site was at the humerus in 41 cases, femur in 66, and tibia shaft in 240 cases. In 175 patients there was an open fracture (138 tibia, 24 femur, and 13 humerus). The time that had elapsed between the traumatic event and the treatment was from 5 to 46 months; 222 patients had previously received surgical treatment of the fracture; in 125 the fracture had been treated conservatively. A shortening deformity of the involved bone was present in 266 cases (ranging from 0.6 to 2.5 mm, average 1.5 mm). In 72 of these cases the shortening was associated with an angular deformity. Patients were treated with the "monofocal distraction osteosynthesis" technique combined with gradual correction of the angular deformity when required. In 289 cases the Ilizarov device and in 58 cases the Kalnberz device was employed. Patients were monitored clinically by means of radiographic, ultrasonographic, and extensimetric evaluation, and whenever possible by means of microscopic investigation.

Results

The average time of treatment was 5 months (range 3–10). There were no intraoperative complications. During the postoperative period some patients presented with minor complications. Superficial infections at the transfixion points of wires or screws were seen in 142 cases (with rapid resolution after local dressing and specific antibiotic therapy). One patient had a transient paresis of the common peroneal nerve, which resolved after 2 months.

In all patients treated bone consolidation was achieved. No angular deformity was observed at the end of treatment; a minimal residual shortening was seen in 12 patients (2–6 mm, average 3 mm).

The ROM of the proximal and distal joints was good during and after the treatment in all cases involving the tibial and humeral shaft. In patients with femoral nonunions knee stiffness was seen during treatment, which gradually resolved with the help of kinesitherapy after removal of the external circular fixator.

Discussion

Distraction is classically considered (as previously underlined) as one of the most frequent causes of nonunion and therefore it comes as a surprise that this technique can be used exclusively to cause the bone to consolidate. With this technique of osteosynthesis, based on the theory of "tension stress" proposed by Ilizarov [25], intensive osteogenesis is achieved by means of a very gradual distraction of the fibrous or fibrocartilaginous tissue at the nonunion site. This acts very similarly to the "interzone" located between the two ends of a corticotomy when bone lengthening is performed.

A distraction of 1 mm a day is considered the "standard" to be followed [26]. It should be underlined that this rate of lengthening, during the treatment, might be excessive or insufficient for different patients and often it needs to be reduced or increased accordingly.

Some Authors subdivide the distraction of 1 mm/day into several steps during the 24 h with the intent to give a minor trauma to the patient [27–29]. This does not seem to represent a real advantage for the speed of formation and consolidation of regenerating bone, however, considering that even distraction of 1 mm a day in one step is transferred to the bone very gradually. This is due to the elasticity of the compression-distraction device (especially using thin wires as bone fixation elements) and to the viscosity of soft tissues surrounding the bone. A very interesting clinical study based on 70 tibial lengthenings [30] showed that even using a very complex motorized system with which the distraction of 1 mm a day is subdivided in 1,440 steps, the new bone formation is not improved.

Our series is the largest among all those presented in Western Europe and it differs from other series in many respects. Other Authors give more attention to the clinical presentation of nonunions (no mobility at the site of nonunion) than to the functional features (hypertrophy and hypervascularity, which in our opinion are the main characteristics); as a consequence a fundamental preliminary assessment such as a bone scan (according to the studies of Weber and Cech [31]) is not mentioned in other papers.

Moreover, one particular aspect of the treatment is of utmost importance: the maintenance of a constant degree of tension at the nonunion site even after the distraction is achieved. This particular aspect of the technique is not mentioned in other papers, where it is simply recommended that the fixator should be "left in place" until bone consolidation is achieved.

The results obtained in our series confirm that in hypertrophic nonunions of long bones using a rigorous pre-, intra-, and postoperative technique, the bone consolidation can be achieved by simple gradual distraction (maintaining a tension effect during the entire treatment period), with simultaneous correction of shortening and of other deformities if present. Therefore, distraction osteosynthesis has been shown to be a powerful stimulus towards bone consolidation.

Monitoring of Distraction in Hypertrophic Nonunions

The individual steps in gradual distraction during the treatment of hypertrophic nonunions have been followed up at our department with radiographic, echographic, extensimetric, and histological studies. Therefore, qualitative morphological information provided by x-rays and ultrasound scans (and whenever possible by histological studies) were complemented by quantitative functional information provided by extensimetric data.

Some Authors have reported the use of additional methods of monitoring new bone formation during distraction. Mazess [32], Eyres et al. [33], and Reiter et al. [34] described a quantitative assessment of bone mineralization during the distraction procedure using dual photon or dual energy x-ray absorption, based on the measurement of the bone mineral density in the newly formed bone and in the adjacent bone. These studies provided a precise assessment of the mineralization, which is closely related to the stiffness, torsion, and stability of bone.

Tjernstrom et al. [35] and Iacobellis et al. [36] examined some anatomical characteristics and structural changes in the newly formed bone segments by means of CT and MRI evaluation. In comparison with the contralateral segment, CT showed variations in the dimensions and density of the cortical bone and the medullary canal [36].

These techniques may help to more accurately manage the distraction phases and reduce complications, but they are still quite difficult to use in routine clinical practice.

X-Ray Investigations

Evaluation by traditional radiographic methods shows the first signs of ossification as a slight, poorly defined, uniform opacity at the distraction site, crossed by longitudinal striations, 1 month after beginning the treatment. The opacity becomes darker between the first and second month while the longitudinal striations become wider and lean to fuse and the regenerating bone takes on the shape of an hourglass.

Radiographic investigations give only little information in the first stages (the first 4 weeks) but are nevertheless crucial in order to monitor the morphology of the bone during the lengthening period and to confirm the right connection between the bone extremities.

After 3 months from the beginning of treatment, a thin shell of cortical bone appears, becoming gradually thicker. The external fixator can be removed on average after 5 months (Figs. 5–12).

The device can be removed once the new bone formed in the distraction gap demonstrates bridging neocorticalization on at least three sides on orthogonal radiographs [15, 20, 37, 38].

Ultrasound Scan

The need to reduce the high dose of radiation while at the same time obtaining clear information about the earliest phases of development of the bone regeneration makes ultrasound evaluation especially useful [20, 38–44]. During the first phases of bone distraction, a *hypoechogenic* band is found between the bone extremities. After nearly 3 weeks the process of bone regeneration can be seen as an *echogenic* signal. Later (nearly 2 months afterwards) transmission of the ultrasound waves is reduced by this *echogenic* material; after 3 months the regenerating bone appears as an *echogenic* stripe between the two extremities of the cortical bone. In the last part of the treatment period (4 months from the beginning, on average) the cortex appears uninterrupted (Figs. 13–15).

Once treatment is completed, ultrasound is less relevant due to the fact that the wave given from the probe is highly reflected from the mineralized bone.

The ultrasound evaluation is important also to identify any abnormality in regenerating bone. Three types of regenerating bone formation can be observed by ultrasound [44] (Figs. 16, 17).

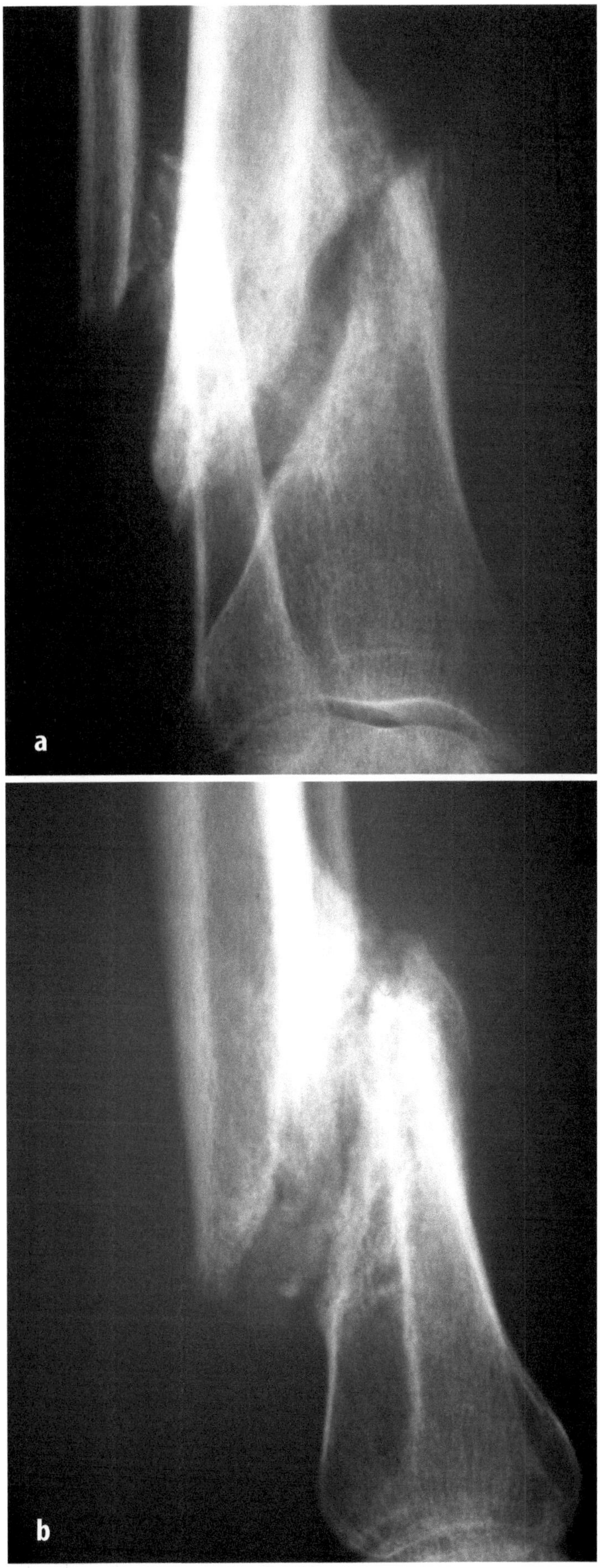

Fig. 5a, b. X-rays of a hypertrophic nonunion of the right tibia in a 68-year-old woman

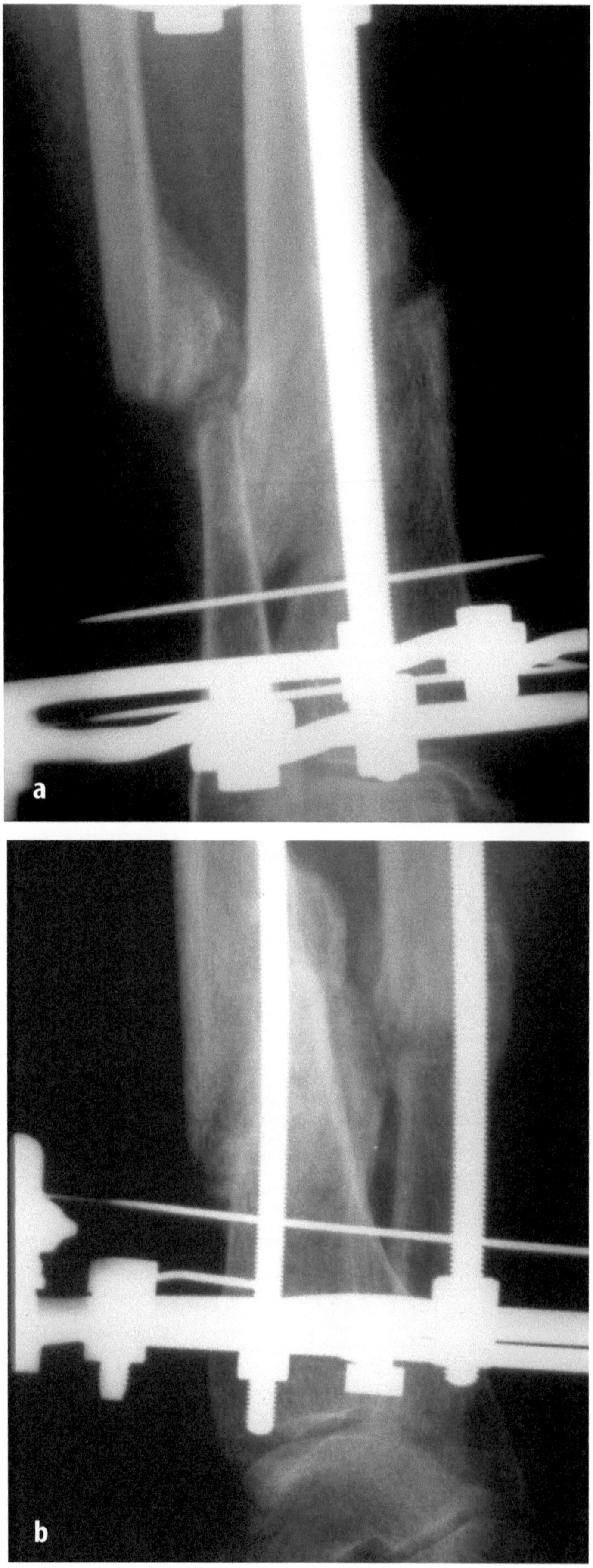

Fig. 6a, b. Same case as in Fig. 5. Stabilization with an Ilizarov device and gradual distraction of the nonunion site

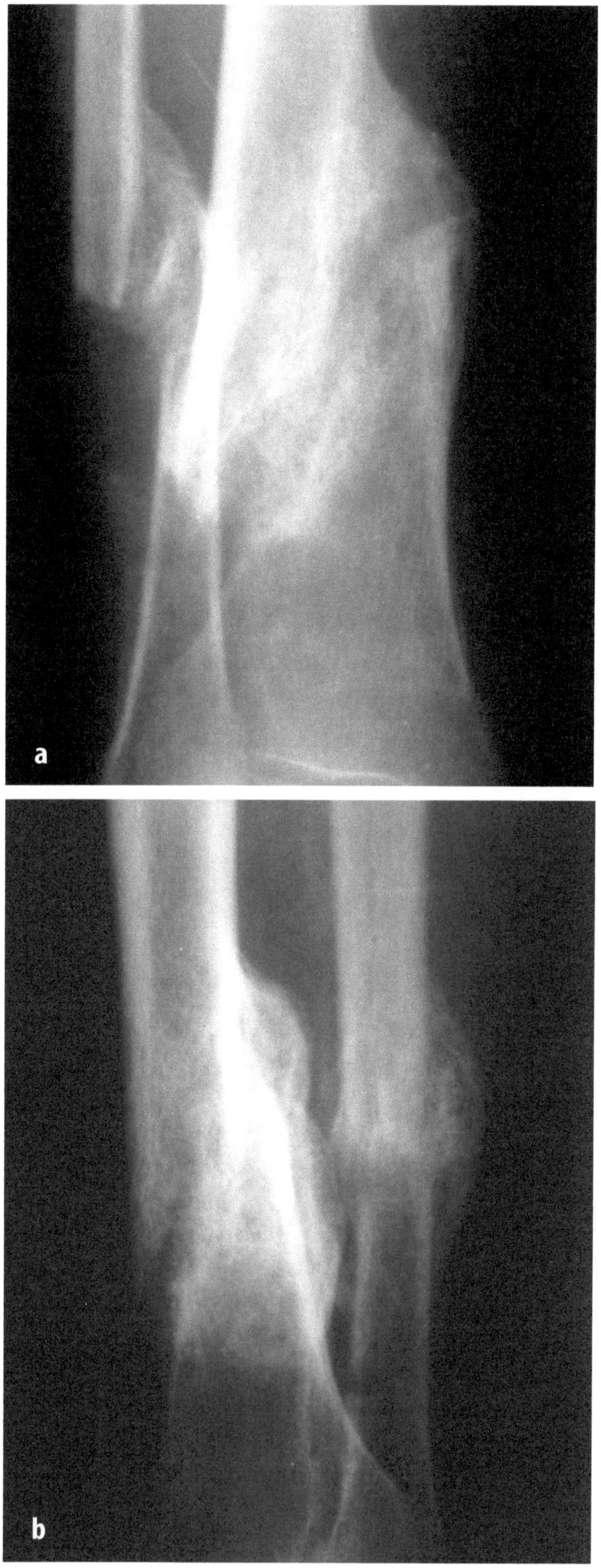

Fig. 7a, b. Same case as in Fig. 5. Healing of the nonunion after 2 months and 20 days

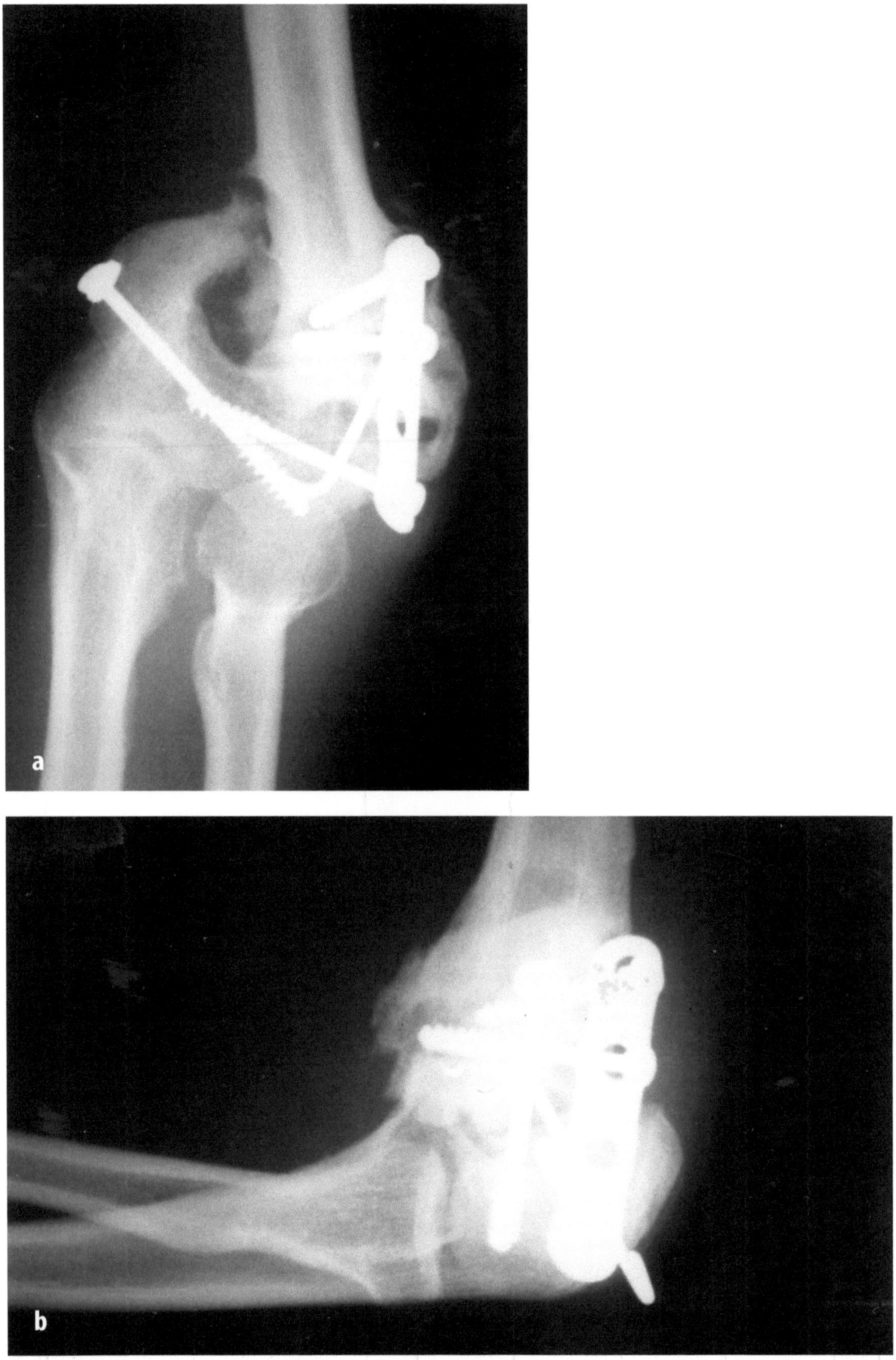

Fig. 8a, b. X-rays of a hypertrophic nonunion with shortening after open reduction and internal fixation of a fracture of the distal third of the left humerus

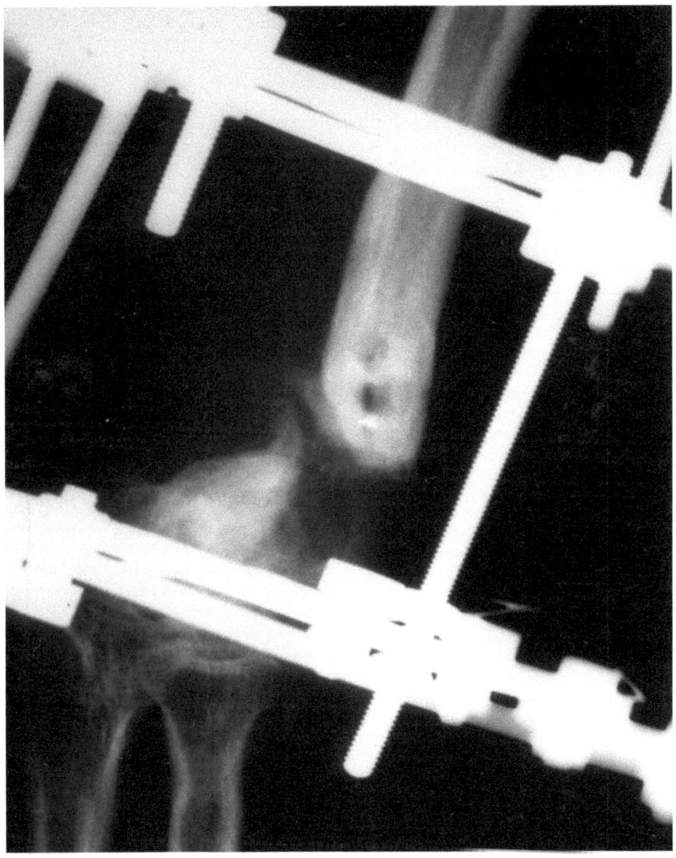

Fig. 9. Same case as in Fig. 8. After the removal of plate and screws an Ilizarov circular external fixator was applied and then gradual distraction was started.

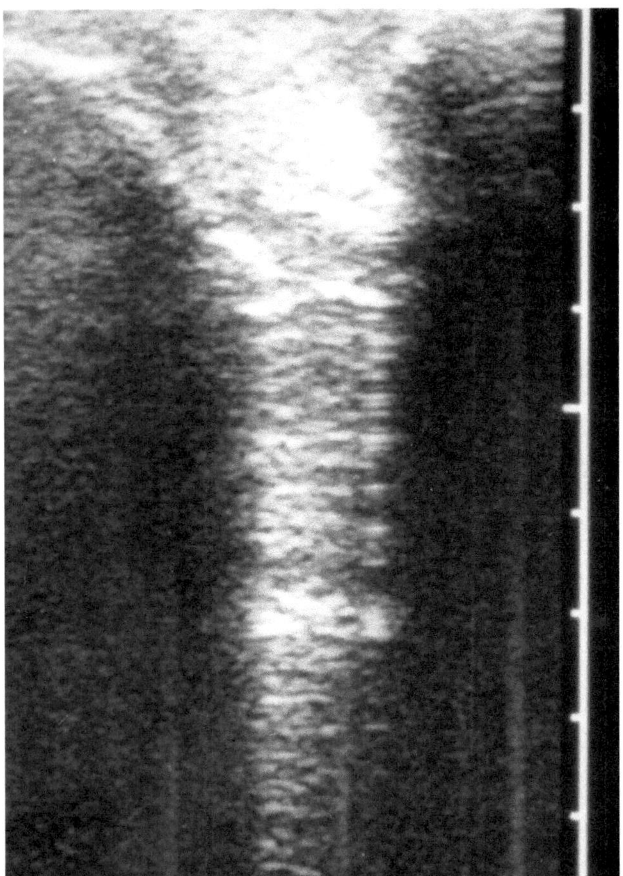

Fig. 10. Same case as in Fig. 8. Sonographic control at the same time of the radiographic control shown in Fig. 7

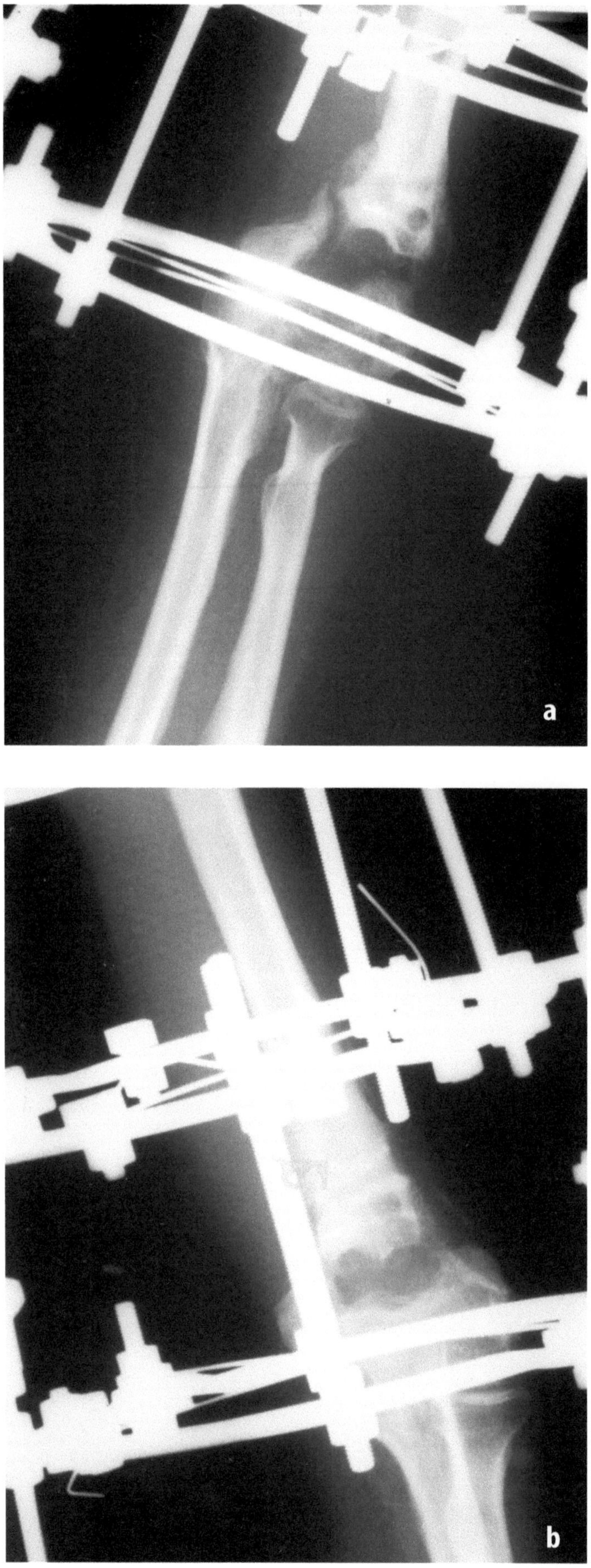

Fig. 11a, b. Same case as in Fig. 8. **a** X-ray 2 weeks after the beginning of distraction. **b** X-ray at the end of the distraction phase

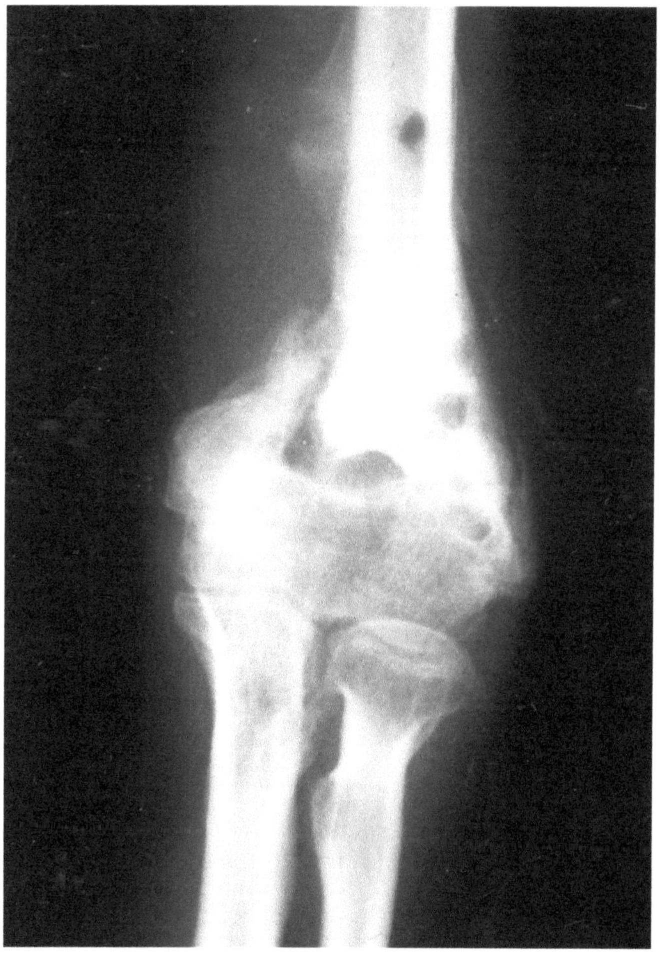

Fig. 12. Same case as in Fig. 9. Healing of the nonunion after 3 months

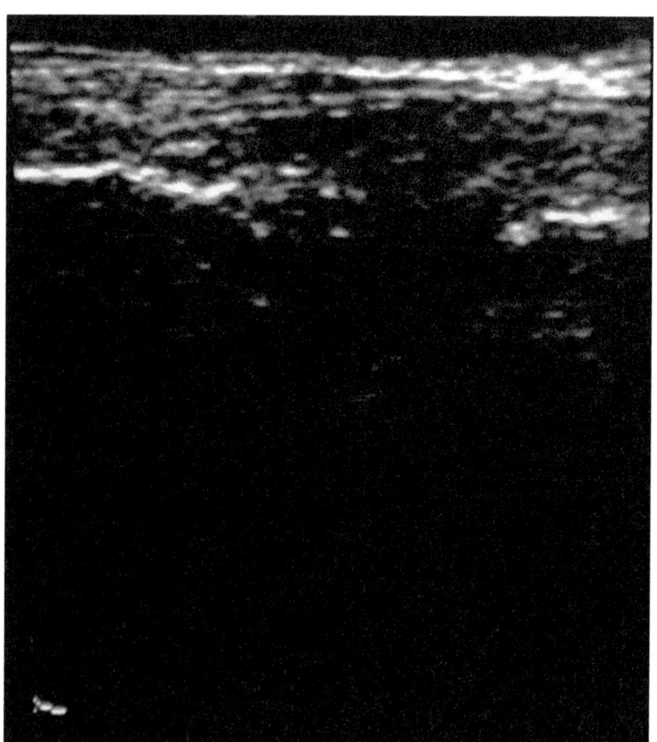

Fig. 13. Sonographic features of the initial phases of bone distraction: an hypoechogenic band between the bone extremities is seen

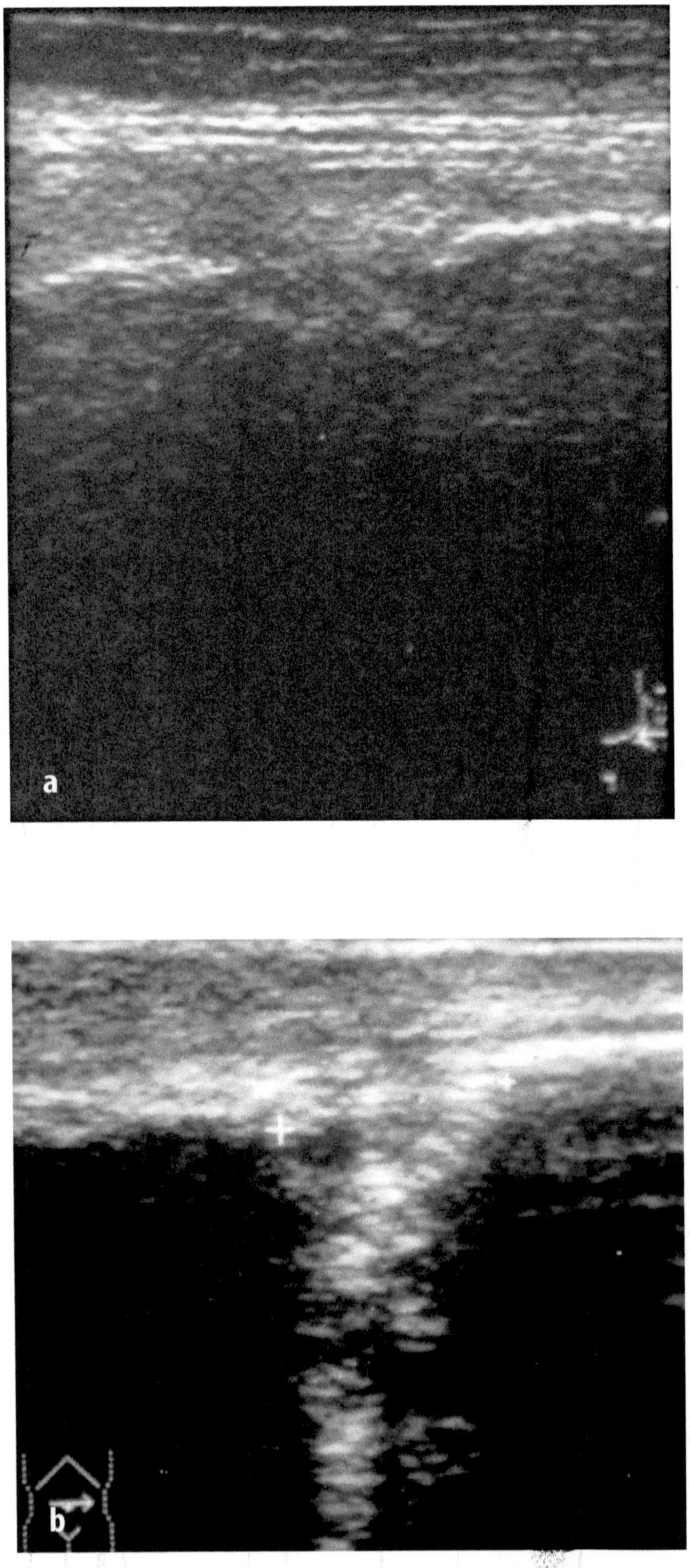

Fig. 14a, b. **a** Echogenic material is observed 3 weeks after the beginning of the distraction. **b** After 2 months, transmission of ultrasounds is reduced

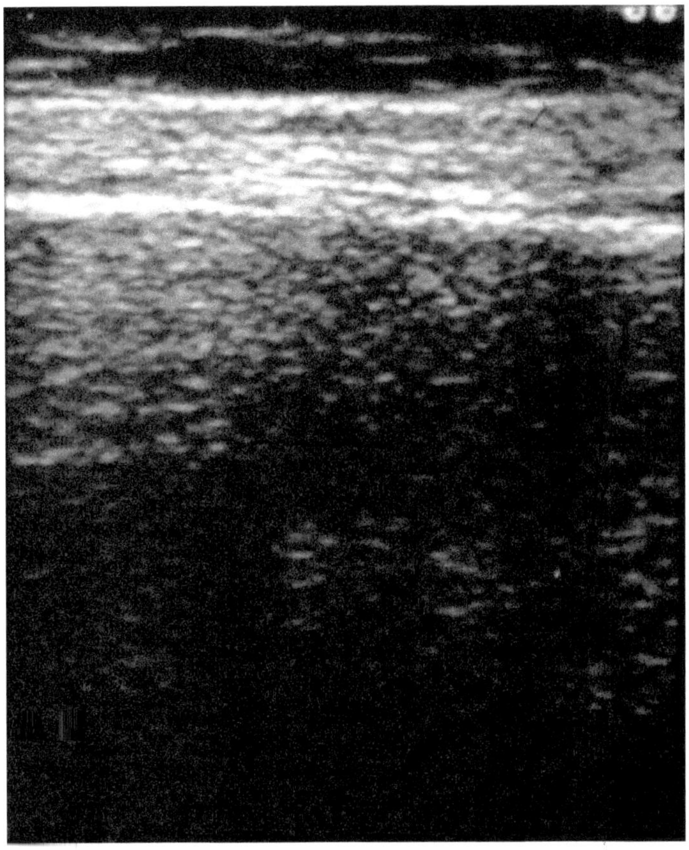

Fig. 15. After 3 months an echogenic stripe between the bone ends is seen

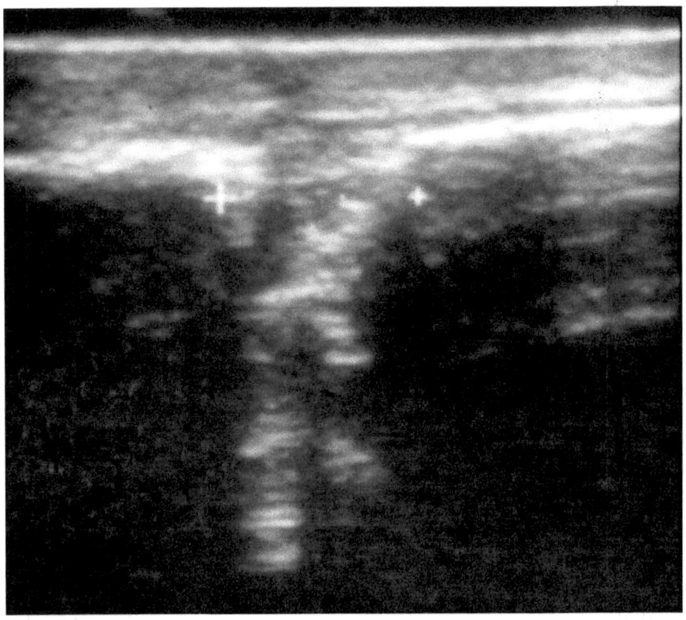

Fig. 16. Sonographic features of normal bone regeneration

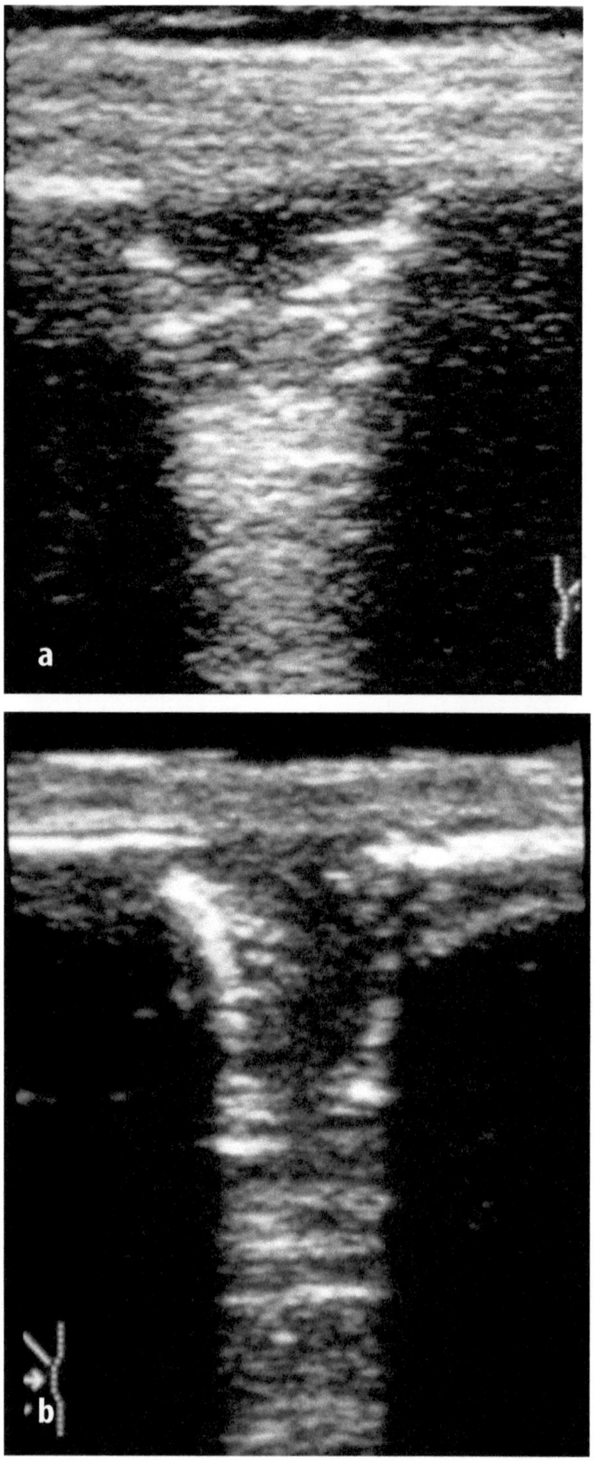

Fig. 17a, b. Sonographic features of hypotrophic (cystic) distraction osteogenesis (**a**), and of hypertrophic bone regeneration (**b**)

In the first phase of distraction normal regeneration shows an abundant presence of fibrous tissue, followed by a normal beginning of mineralization after the first 30–40 days. In hypotrophic (cystic) regeneration, a narrowing of the regenerating bone and a lacunar image in the regenerated bone is observed. Then the distraction must be stopped or slowed to obtain a gradual disappearing of the cyst and to avoid an insufficient or delayed consolidation.

In hypertrophic regeneration an abnormal abundance of fibrous tissue is observed, and a sonographic gap that is smaller than the radiographic gap is seen between the bone ends. In these cases the distraction speed must be increased for 7–10 days in order to prevent an early consolidation.

Extensimetry

Using extensimetry, the mechanical properties of the regenerating bone can be quantified by evaluating the deformation of the system bone-fixator at different stages of bone consolidation [20, 45, 46] (Fig. 18).

During fracture healing, an increase in mechanical resistance is observed at the same time as consolidation of the regenerating bone. This increased resistance is related to the progression of regenerating bone through different mechanical phases that correspond to specific biologic phases. They can be detected with tests such as flexo-extension, bending, and walking (periodically performed every 20 days):

1. Initial phase (different deformation according to the different kind of assembly;
2. Phase of maximal deformability, which corresponds to a maximum plasticity of the regenerating bone;
3. Phase of reducing the deformation, related to progressive calcification;
4. Phase of mechanical stability, which shows minimal readings of deformation and correspond to corticalization of the regenerating bone;
5. Final phase of secondary deformability (due to the process of bone remodeling).

Morphologic Study

In eight cases, material for morphological examination of the nonunion site could be obtained at different time intervals from the beginning of distraction treatment and while associated lesions requiring a surgical approach were being treated. Biopsy material was in part fixed in 4% phosphate-buffered formaldehyde, pH 7.2, at room temperature and dehydrated in graded series of ethanol. After embedding in paraffin, blocks were serially sectioned at 7 μm and the sections stained with hematoxylin-eosin. Some of the specimens were fixed in 2.5% glutaraldehyde, pH 7.3, and postfixed in OsO4. The tissues were dehydrated in graded series of ethanol and embedded in Epon 812 resin. Semithin sections were then stained with Rosenqvist silver stain.

In the very first phases, nonunion tissue is seen histologically as hypovascular fibrous or fibrocartilaginous tissue with very few capillaries and nearly always empty. The aspect of the nonunion tissue contrasts with the hypervascular bone ends on either side.

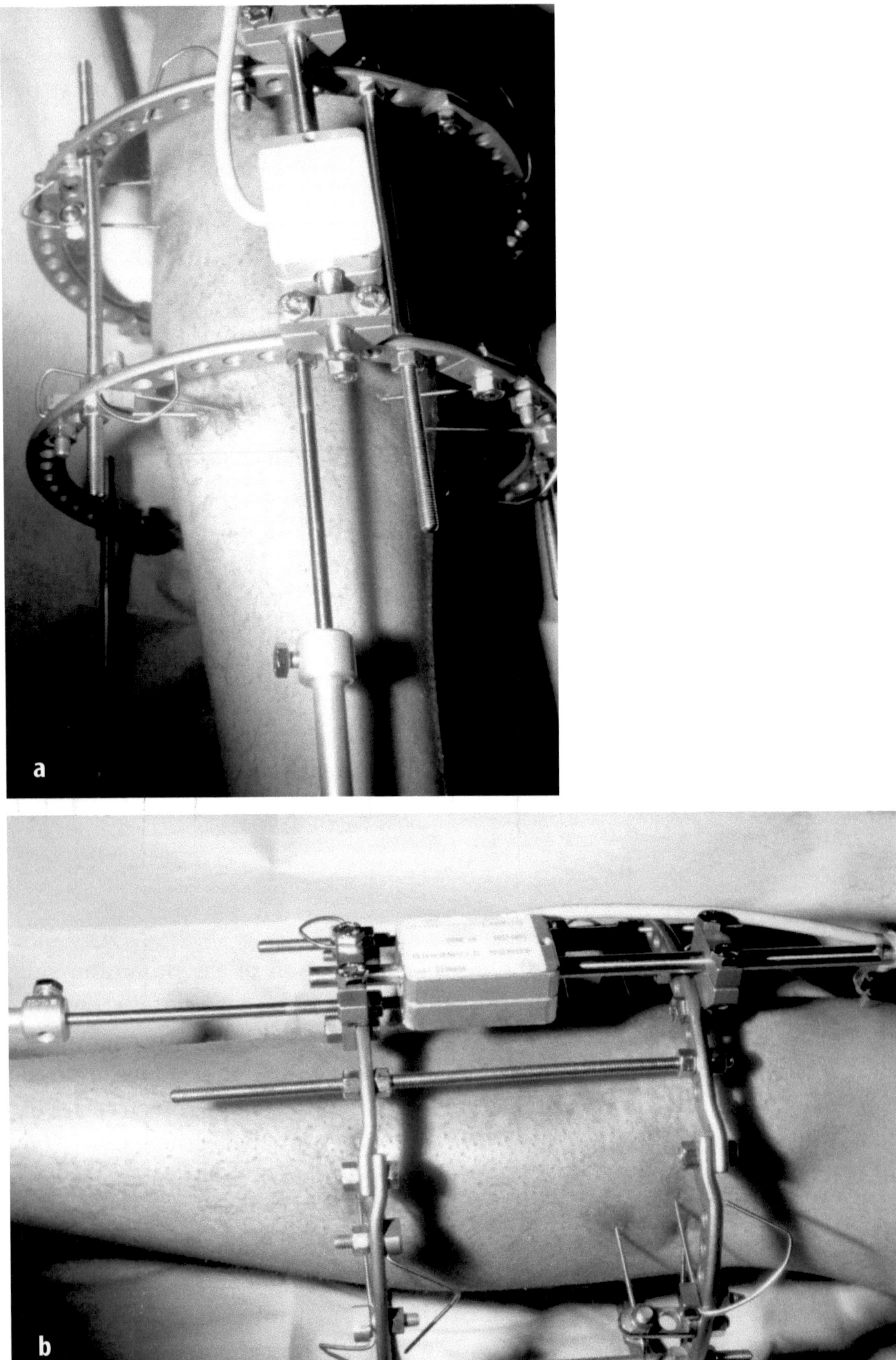

Fig. 18 a, b. Extensimetric device applied to an Ilizarov apparatus, in order to evaluate the mechanical properties of the regenerating bone

Ten days after the beginning of distraction, there is a high proliferation of capillaries that form a vascular net and they are no longer empty but rather are filled by red blood cells. After 20 days there are fascicles of fibroblasts parallel to the lines of distractional stress.

In more advanced phases there is a gradual differentiation of osteoblasts that start to form osteoid tissue and then deposits of calcium salt are observed between the collagenic fibers and inside the organic matrix of the osteoid. Two months and half after after distracton is applied, the new bone trabeculae can be readily identified (Figs. 19–27).

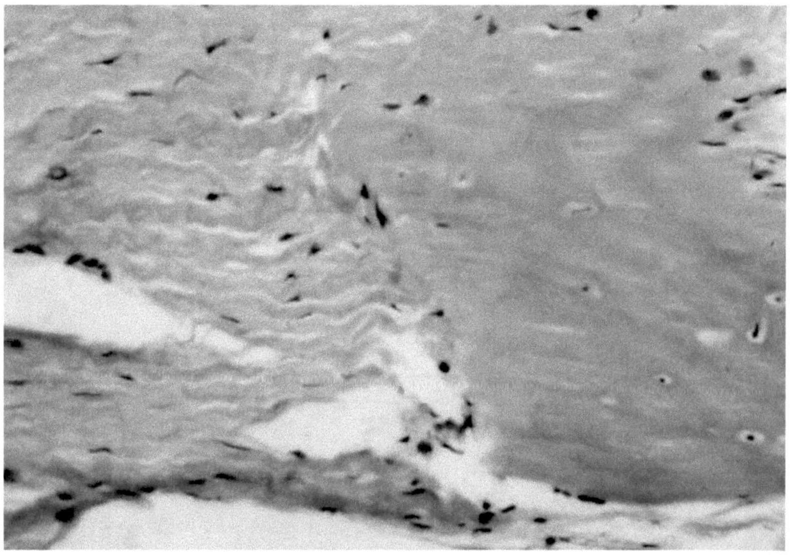

Fig. 19. Micrograph of an hypertrophic nonunion. The nonunion tissue (on the left side) appears as a fibrous hypovascular tissue (Hematoxylin and Eosin, original magnification: x 100)

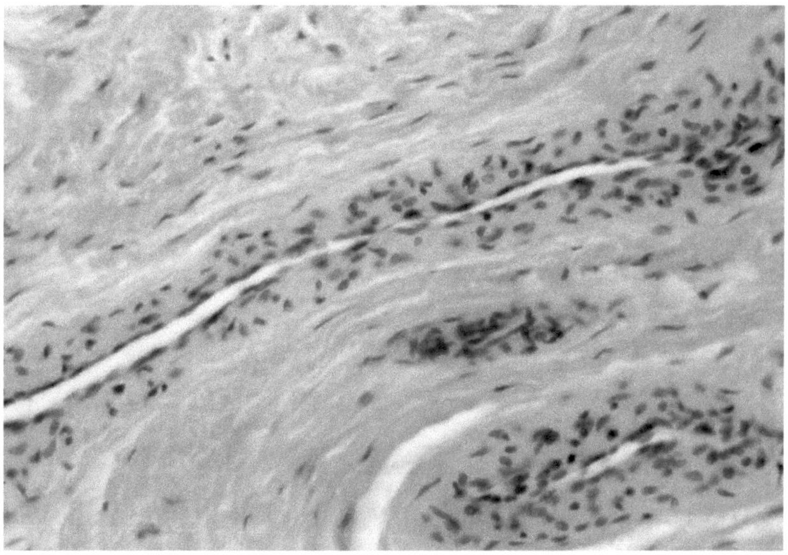

Fig. 20. In the fibrous tissue of the nonunion very few capillaries are seen (Hematoxylin and Eosin, original magnification: x 250)

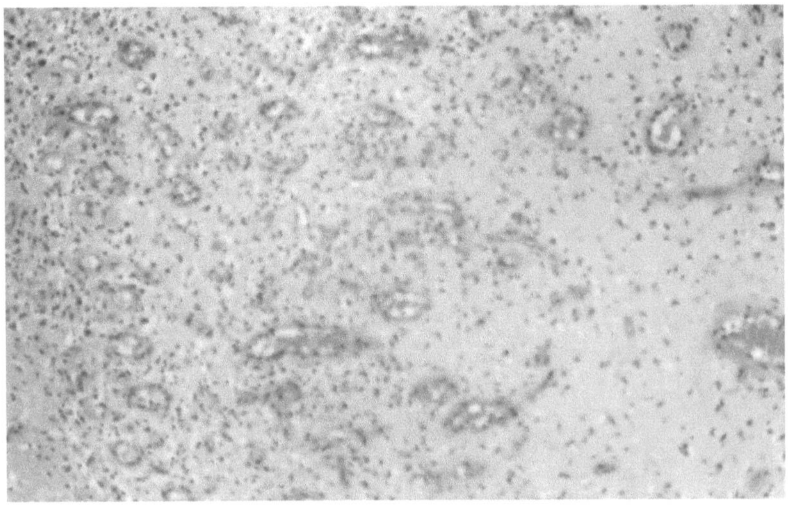

Fig. 21. Proliferation of capillaries 10 days after the beginning of distraction (Hematoxylin and Eosin, original magnification: x 250)

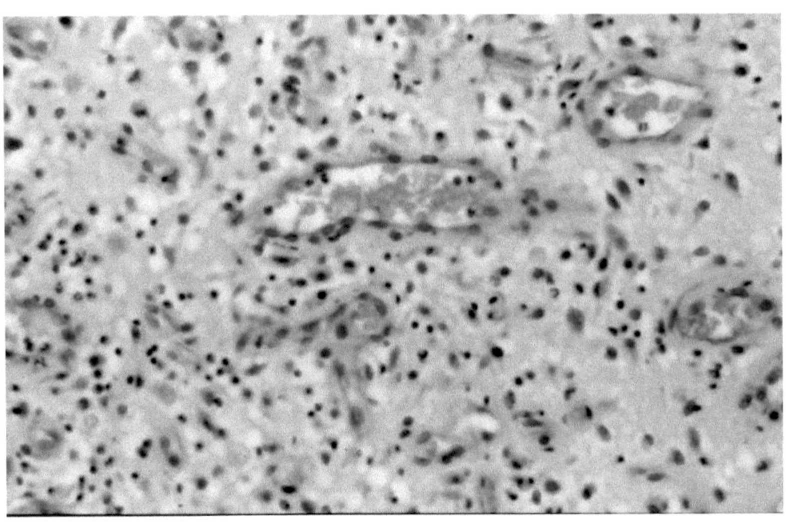

Fig. 22. At higher magnification, capillaries appear filled by red blood cells (Hematoxylin and Eosin, original magnification: x 400)

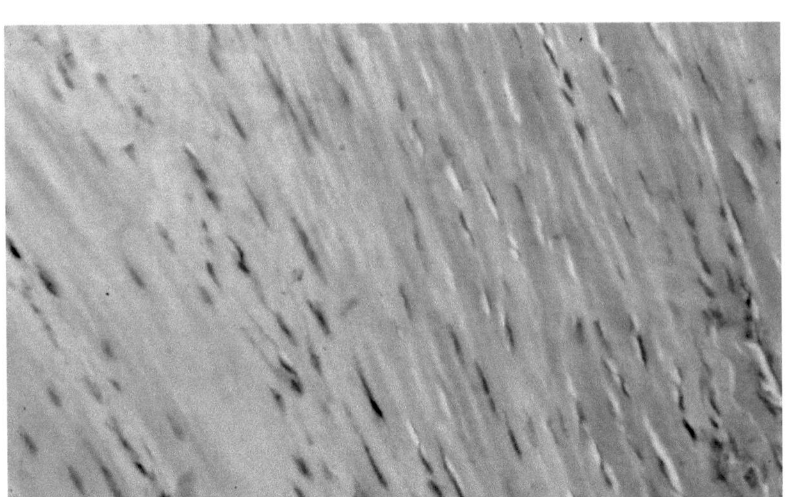

Fig. 23. Twenty days after the beginning of distraction, fascicles of fibroblasts parallel to to the lines of distractional stress are seen (Hematoxylin and Eosin, original magnification: x 250)

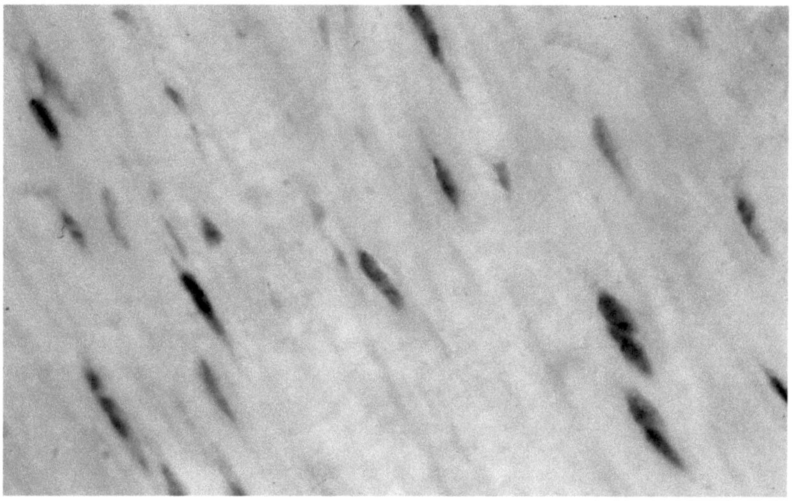

Fig. 24. Same field as in Fig. 16 at higher magnification (Hematoxylin and Eosin, original magnification: x 400)

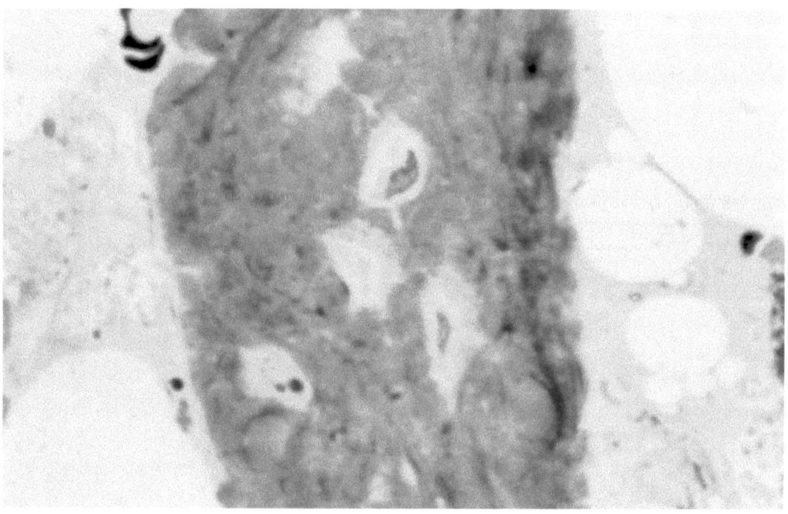

Fig. 25. Differentiation of osteoblasts (with deposition of osteoid substance and calcium salts) and gradual transformation into osteocytes. (Rosenqvist silver stain, original magnification: x 1250)

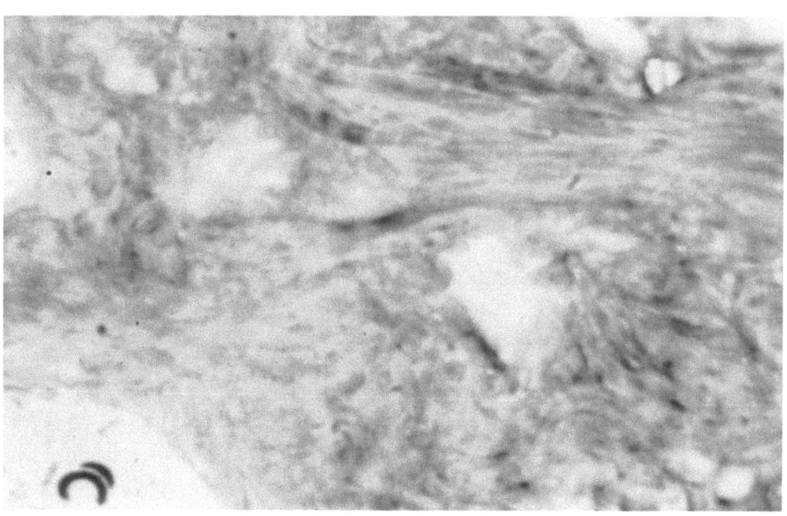

Fig. 26. Osteoid substance with osteocytic lacunae (semi-thin section, Rosenqvist silver stain, original magnification: x 1250)

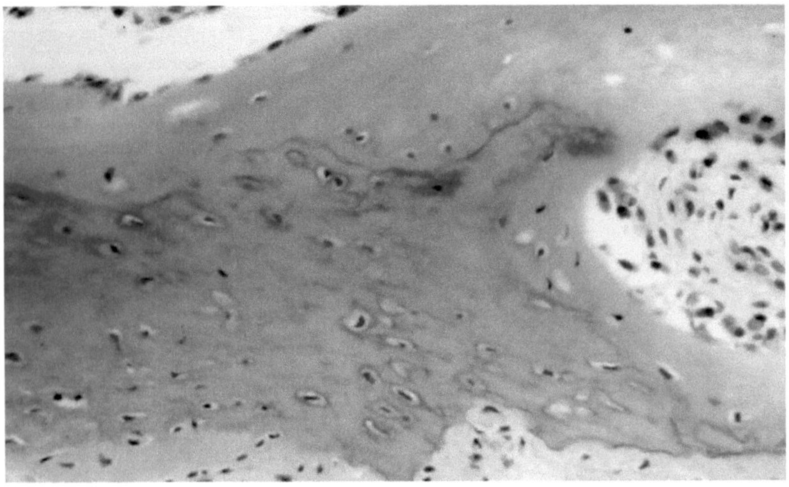

Fig. 27. New bone trabeculae are clearly seen 2 months after the beginning of distraction (Hematoxylin and Eosin, original magnification: x 100)

This morphologic study, performed for the first time on human specimens (from eight patients), has clarified some obscure and controversial points regarding the evolution of the nonunion site under the action of tension forces. In particular it has shown the intensive stimulus to neoangiogenesis (seen from the first days of the distraction treatment).

The study has also shown the absence of a cartilaginous stage between the initial tissue and the new bone, and so the process can be considered as a membranous ossification and not an enchondral ossification. Moreover, the evaluation of the histological patterns confirmed that the process of osteogenesis does not proceed in a sequential manner but evolves in stages that overlap, as underlined by Tajana et al. [47], so that it is possible to observe different stages in one specimen.

References

1. Bohler L (1951) Tecnica del trattamento delle fratture. Vallardi, Milano
2. Monticelli G, Boni M (1955) Il callo osseo normale e patologico. Atti del 40° Congresso SIOT, Roma
3. Heiple K, Herndon C (1965) The pathologic physiology of nonunion. Clin Orthop Relat Res 43:11–21
4. Song HR, Cho SH, Koo KH et al (1999) Spontaneous healing of an atrophic pseudoarthrosis during femoral lengthening. Int Orthop 23:126–127
5. Ilizarov GA, Green SA (1992) Transosseous osteosynthesis. Springer, Berlin Heidelberg New York
6. Ilizarov GA, Kaplunov AG, Grachova VI et al (1971) Closed compression-distraction osteosynthesis of the tibial pseudoarthroses with Ilizarov method. Kniiekot, Kurgan
7. Kravchuk VI (1976) Clinico-roentgenographic dynamics of the reparative regeneration in conditions of distraction in pseudoarthroses of tubular bones of the lower extremities. Ortop Travmatol Protez 36:28–35
8. Gyulnazarova SV, Shtin VP (1983) Reparative bone tissue regeneration in treatment of pseudoarthroses with simultaneous elongation in the pathologic focus region

(experimental study). Ortop Travmatol Protez 4:10–15
9. Umiarov GA (1986) Classification of nonunions of the long bones complicated by infection, and principles of treatment. Sborn Trud CITO 30:5–9
10. Mora R, Soldini A, Raschellà F et al (1989) Le traitement des pseudoarthroses infectées du tibia selon la technique d'Umiarov. Z Unfallchir Vers Berufs 82:187–190
11. Mora R, Benazzo F, Ceciliani L (1990) Bone regeneration with compression-distraction devices. In: Bonucci E (ed) Biology and pathology of cell-matrix interactions. CLEUP, Padua
12. Paley D (1990) Treatment of tibial nonunions and bone loss with the Ilizarov technique. AAOS Inst Course Lect 39:185–197
13. Schwartsman V, Choi SH, Schwartsman R (1990) Tibial nonunions. Treatment tactics with the Ilizarov method. Orthop Clin North Am 21:639–653
14. Catagni M, Probe R, Cattaneo R (1990) Ilizarov distraction osteogenesis in the treatment of stiff hypertrophic nonunions. Proceedings of the Second Meeting ISFR, Rochester
15. Catagni M, Guerreschi F, Holman J et al (1994) Distraction osteogenesis in the treatment of stiff hypertrophic nonunions using the Ilizarov apparatus. Clin Orthop Relat Res 301:159–163
16. Mora R, Ceciliani L (1992) Classificazione delle pseudoartrosi e principi di trattamento mediante sistemi di compressione-distrazione. Atti, I Corso: La fissazione esterna nella traumatologia degli arti inferiori. Ospedale San Giovanni, Roma
17. Mora R, Benazzo F, Pedrotti L (1996) L'osteosintesi in distrazione nel trattamento delle pseudoartrosi ipertrofiche. Minerva Ortop Traumatol 47:255–257
18. Saleh M, Royston S (1996) Management of nonunion of fractures by distraction with correction of angulation and shortening. J Bone Joint Surg Br 78:105–109
19. Marsh DR, Shah S, Elliott J et al (1997) The Ilizarov method in nonunion, malunion and infection of fractures. J Bone Joint Surg Br 79:273–279
20. Mora R, Pedrotti L, Benazzo F et al (2000) Stimolazione meccanica della consolidazione nelle pseudoartrosi ipertrofiche mediante osteosintesi in distrazione. Giorn Ital Ortop Traumatol 26:3–5
21. Gordon JE, Jani M, Dobbs M et al (2002) Treatment of rigid hypertrophic posttraumatic pseudoarthrosis of the tibia in children using distraction osteogenesis. J Pediatr Orthop 22:419–423
22. Rozbruch R, Herzenberg J, Tetsworth K et al (2002) Distraction osteogenesis for nonunion after high tibial osteotomy. Clin Orthop Relat Res 394:227–235
23. Kocaoglu M, Eralp L, Sen C et al (2003) Management of stiff hypertrophic nonunions by distraction osteogenesis: a report of 16 cases. J Orthop Traumatol 17:543–548
24. Mora R, Pedrotti L, Bertani et al (2003) Treatment of osteolysis: the state of the art. Bone regeneration. J Orthop Traumatol 4:155–156
25. Ilizarov GA (1971) Basic principles of transosseous compression-distraction osteosynthesis. Ortop Travm Protez 31:7–15
26. Peretti G, Peretti GM, Romanò F (1999) Pianificazione degli interventi chirurgici nella correzione delle differenze di lunghezza degli arti inferiori. Minerva Ortop Traumatol 50:107–116
27. Ilizarov GA (1989) The tension-stress effect on the genesis and growth of tissues. Part I: The influence of stability of fixation and soft tissue preservation. Clin Orthop Relat Res 238:249–281
28. Ilizarov GA (1989) The tension-stress effect on the genesis and growth of tissues. Part II: The influence of the rate and frequency of distraction. Clin Orthop Relat Res 239:263–285

29. Peretti G (1989) Lower limb lengthening by means of external circular stabilizer. Sperri, Casiacco
30. Bright AS, Weiner L, Paley D et al (1995) Preliminary experience with motorized distraction for tibia lengthening. Proceedings of the EOA, 26th Annual Meeting, Rome
31. Weber BG, Cech O (1976) Pseudoarthrosis. Huber, Berne
32. Mazess RB (1983) Non-invasive bone measurements. In: Kunin A (ed) Skeletal research. Academic, New York
33. Eyres KS, Bell MJ, Kanis J (1993) Methods of assessing new bone formation during limb lengthening. J Bone Joint Surg Br 75:358–364
34. Reiter A, Sabo D, Pfeil J et al (1997) Quantitative assessment of callus distraction usinf dual energy X-ray absorpiometry. Int Orthop 21:35–40
35. Tjernstrom B, Thoumas KA, Pech P (1992) Bone remodeling after leg lengthening: avaluation with plain radiographs and computed tomography and magnetic resonance imaging scans. J Pediatr Orthop 12:751–755
36. Iacobellis C, Bulzacchi A, Rioda A (2004) CT evaluation of regenerated osseous segments following bone transport. J Orthop Traumatol 5:178–184
37. Monticelli G, Spinelli R (1986) L'osteogenesi riparativa in corso di distrazione. Giorn Ital Ortop Traumatol 12:45–54
38. Peretti G, Ippolito E (1990) Il comportamento dell'osso, della cartilagine articolare e delle parti molli durante l'allungamento degli arti. Giorn Ital Ortop Traumatol 16[Suppl. 2]:87–104
39. Memeo A, Marinoni EC, Di Lelio A et al (1989) Monitoraggio ecografico del rigenerato osseo in pazienti sottoposti ad allungamento degli arti inferiori con fissatore esterno circolare. Minerva Ortop Traumatol 40:451–453
40. Rengo C (1991) Ultrasound evaluation of regenerate bone. In: Bianchi Maiocchi A, Aronson J (eds) Operative principles of Ilizarov. Williams and Wilkins, Baltimore
41. Maffulli N, Hughes T, Fixsen J (1992) Ultrasonographic monitoring of limb lengthening. J Bone Joint Surg Br 74:130–132
42. Eyres KS, Bell M, Kanis J (1993) Methods of assessing new bone formation during limb lengthening. J Bone Joint Surg Br 75:358–364
43. Boero S, Dell'Acqua A (1995) Monitoraggio ecografico del rigenerato in corso di allungamento con fissatore esterno. Giorn Ital Ortop Traumatol 21:365–372
44. Iacobellis C, Bulzacchi A, Rioda A (2002) The ultrasound scan in monitoring regenerate bone. J Orthop Traumatol 3:41–48
45. Ceffa R, Perissinotto A (1994) Strain analysis. In: Catagni M, Malzev V, Kirienko A (eds) Advances in Ilizarov apparatus assembly. Medicalplastic, Milan
46. Ceffa R, Bombelli M, Boero S et al (1997) Extensimetric monitoring of healing in the treatment with the lizarov apparatus. Bull Hosp Joint Dis 56:41–45
47. Tajana GF, Morandi M, Zembo M (1989) The structure and development of osteogenetic repair tissue according to Ilizarov technique in man: characterization of extracellular matrix. Orthopaedics 12:512–523

Treatment of Noninfected Nonunions: Normotrophic Nonunions

GABRIELLA TUVO, REDENTO MORA, GIOVANNI BATTISTA GALLI

Introduction

In normotrophic nonunions (the intermediate category between hypertrophic and atrophic nonunions), vascularization at the nonunion site is poor but exists, and on the bone scan detection of the tracer is poor.

The biological activity of the connective tissue in the interfragmentary gap is low but not absent. Therefore, the aim of the treatment is to increase this capability and enhance the osteogenic properties of the tissue.

Operative Technique (Monofocal Compression-Distraction Osteosynthesis)

The monofocal compression-distraction osteosynthesis technique consists of alternating phases of compression and distraction of the nonunion site, generally performed with a cycle of gradual compression of 4–5 mm at the rate of 1 mm per day in only one session, followed by a gradual distraction of 4–5 mm and a rest period of 4–5 days (Figs. 1–3).

The cycle is then repeated two or three times. These "gymnastics" revive, in most cases, the osteogenic capacity at the nonunion site and consolidation is achieved [1]. In patients in whom a dysmetria or an axial deviation are present, the treatment is appropriately modified to correct the deformity.

Materials and Methods

In the period 1894–2002, 74 normotrophic nonunions were treated. The minimum follow-up time was 2 years. Of the patients, 51 were men and 23 women. Age ranged from 30 to 72 years (average 38 years). The affected bone was the humerus in 10 cases, the femur in 18, and the tibia in 46. An open fracture was present in the history of 19 patients.

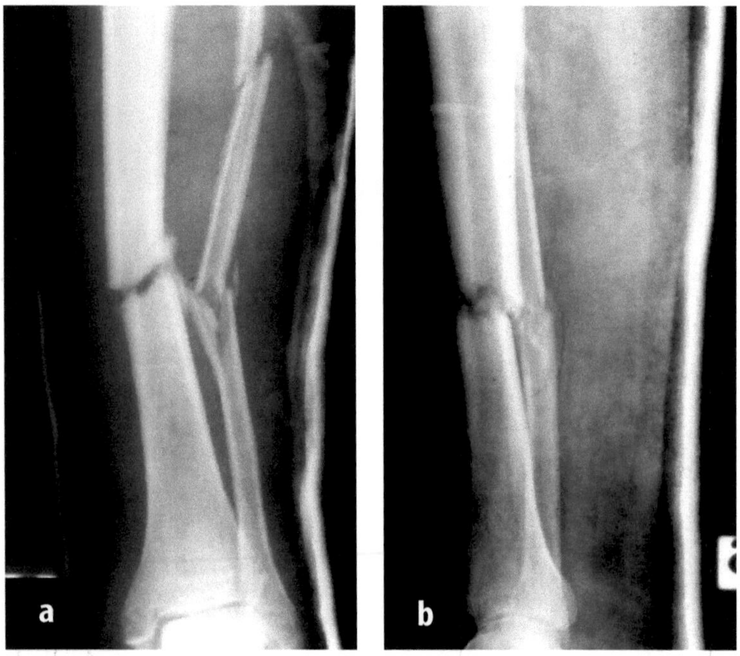

Fig. 1a, b. X-rays of a non-union of the left leg in a 65-year-old man

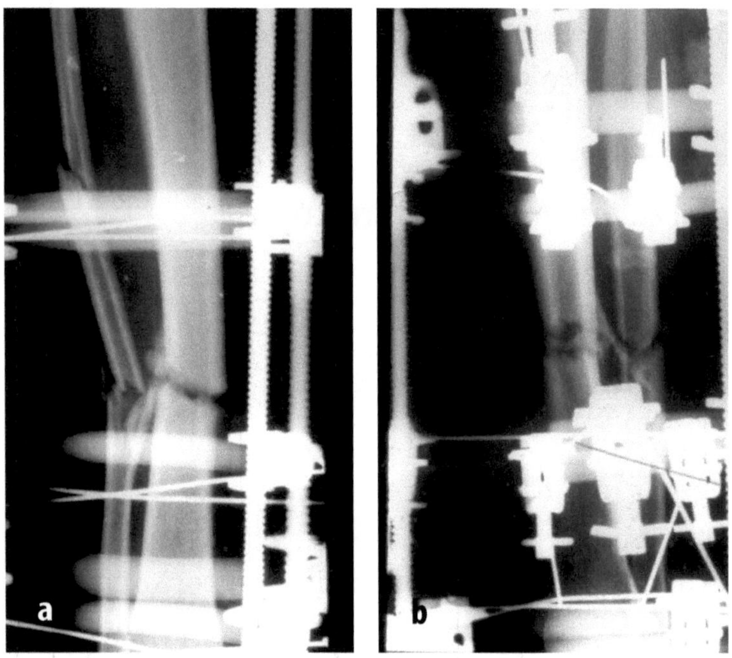

Fig. 2a, b. Same case as in Fig. 1. Treatment with monofocal compression-distraction osteosynthesis by means of a Kalnberz "Rigid Simplex" external fixator

The period between the trauma and the treatment with compression-distraction methods was 6–50 months. Previously, 31 patients had received conservative treatment and 43 patients surgical treatment. A limb shortening was evident in nine cases, an axial deviation in six. Patients were treated with the monofocal compression-distraction osteosynthesis technique, correcting both dysmetria and axial deviation when these deformities coexisted. For the treatment the Ilizarov system was used in 66 cases and the Kalnberz system in eight cases.

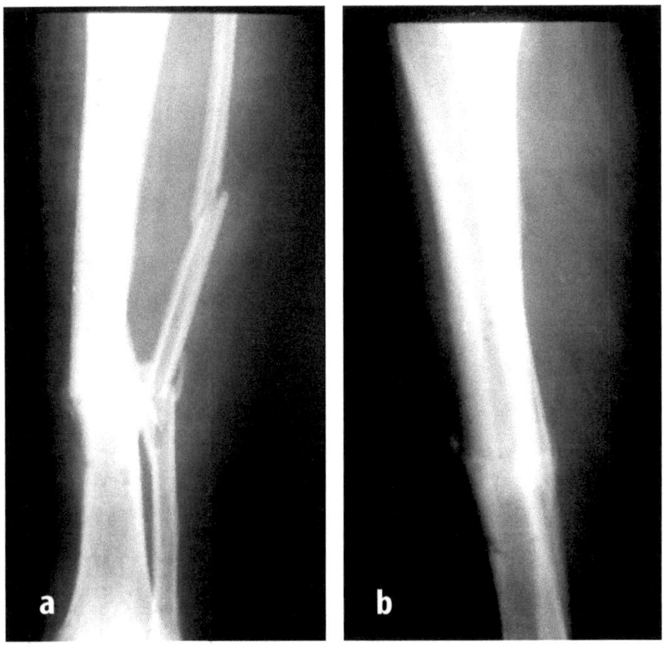

Fig. 3a, b. Same case as in Fig. 1. Healing of the nonunion after 3 months

Results

The average time of treatment was 4 months (2.5 to 6 at most). No intraoperative complications developed. Among the minor postoperative complications, there were 27 cases of superficial infection at the entry site of wires or screws (treated with local medication and antibiotic therapy) and two cases of wire breaking (substituted in one case). No vascular or nervous complications were observed.

Consolidation was obtained in all but four cases, which were then treated with autologous bone grafting. No residual deformity was observed. The articular function (reduced during the treatment of femoral nonunions) appeared to be normal after fixator removal and kinesitherapy.

Discussion

Alternating compression-distraction stimulation of the nonunion site has proven to be very effective in the management of normotrophic nonunions, where biological activity of the connective tissue in the gap is poor [2–4].

The favorable effect on bone formation can be explained by Leung's hypothesis [4], which is based on experimental data on weight bearing during distraction osteogenesis. According to this hypothesis, it is likely that, in normotrophic nonunions, the tensile stress on the biologic tissue induced by distraction initiates osteogenesis and also creates microstrain across the distraction site. The compression across the distraction site induces changes in microstrain and causes an additive effect with enhancement of osteogenesis and mineralization, provided that, according to Kenwright et al. [5], the change in strain is the most effective kind of stimulation for bone formation.

References

1. Ilizarov GA, Green SA (1992) Transosseous osteosynthesis. Springer, Berlin Heidelberg New York
2. Paley D (1990) Treatment of tibial nonunions and bone loss with the Ilizarov technique. AAOS Inst Course Lect 39:185–197
3. Mora R (2000) Tecniche di compressione-distrazione. Amplimedical, Milano
4. Leung K, Cheung W, Yeung H et al (2004) Effect of weightbearing on bone formation during distraction osteogenesis. Clin Orthop Relat Res 419:251–257
5. Kenwright J, Richardson JB, Cunningham JL et al (1991) Axial movement and tibial fractures. A controlled randomised trial of treatment. J Bone Joint Surg Br 73:654–659

Treatment of Noninfected Nonunions: Atrophic Nonunions

Redento Mora, Luisella Pedrotti, Barbara Bertani, Milena Miceli

Introduction

In atrophic nonunions vascularization of the bone ends is almost absent, and the scintigraphic images do not detect anything. In this kind of nonunion the interfragmentary gap is filled with loose connective tissue, unable to express any biological activity: thus, further stimulation with gradual distraction cannot lead to bone regeneration.

Operative Technique (Biofocal Compression-Distraction Osteosynthesis)

The operative technique with compression-distraction systems (bifocal compression-distraction osteosynthesis) acts at two levels [1]: at the nonunion site (where a reshaping of the hypotrophic-hypovascularized bone ends is performed) and at the proximal or distal metaphysis of the long bone (where a corticotomy is performed in order to allow a gradual distraction with "bone transport" or "internal lengthening" at the rate of 1 mm per day in only one daily session).

The bone fragment, which is gradually transported, comes into contact with the other bone end at the resection site; then interfragmentary compression is performed at the docking site to achieve consolidation (Figs. 1–7).

The shape of the bone ends must be considered. In most cases the segmental excision technique is the best choice in order to achieve a wide area of bone contact on both bone ends. In particular cases, bone contact may be improved by modifying the bone ends: with the invagination technique one of the fragments is fitted into the other; with the reshaping technique the two fragments are surgically molded in complementary shapes [2, 3].

Bone can be transported using transversely oriented, obliquely oriented, or longitudinally oriented transport wires. The first technique is the simplest, but actually the most troublesome for the patient, so it is rarely used. We pre-

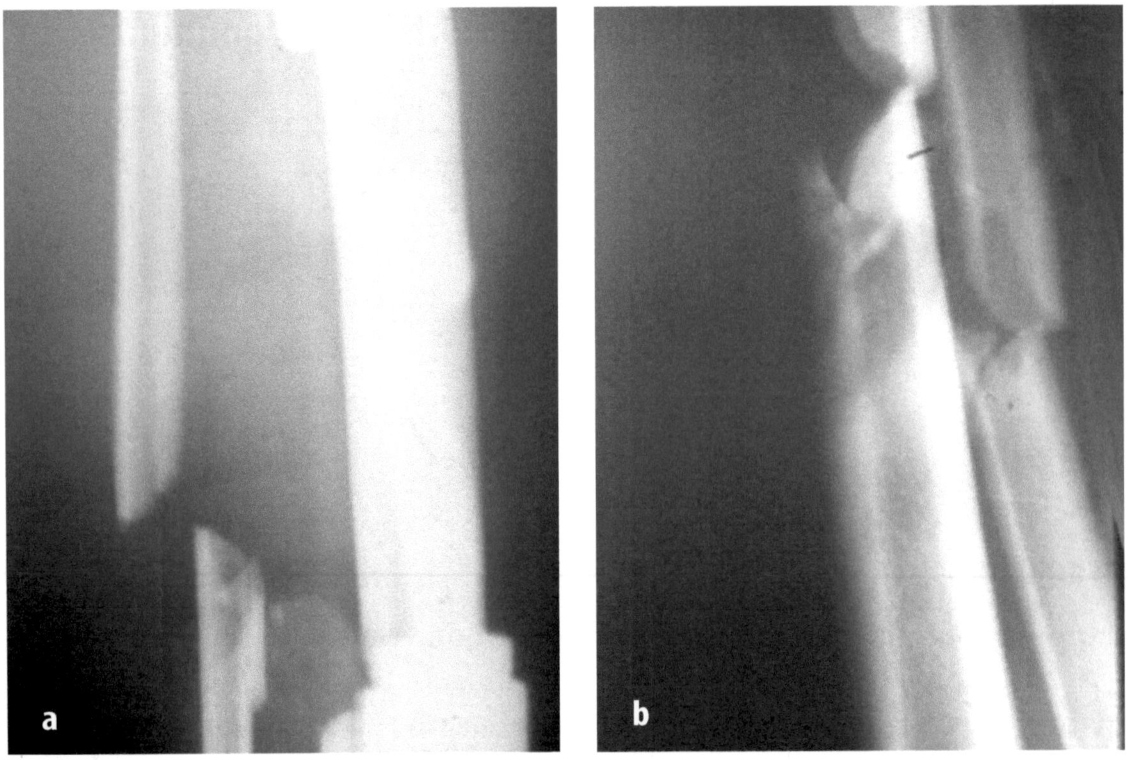

Fig. 1a, b. X-rays of an atrophic nonunion of the distal third of the right tibia in a 34-year-old man

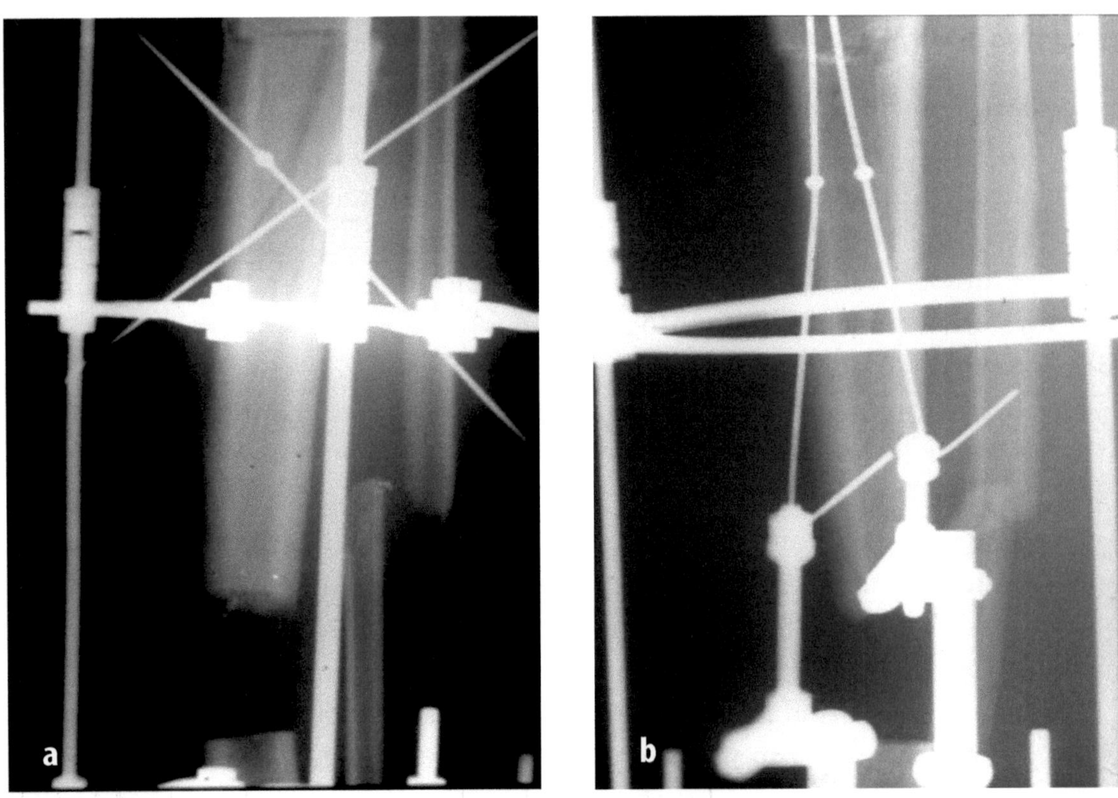

Fig. 2a, b. Same case as in Fig. 1. Treatment with reshaping of the bone ends, proximal metaphyseal corticotomy, bifocal compression-distraction osteosynthesis performed with an Ilizarov apparatus

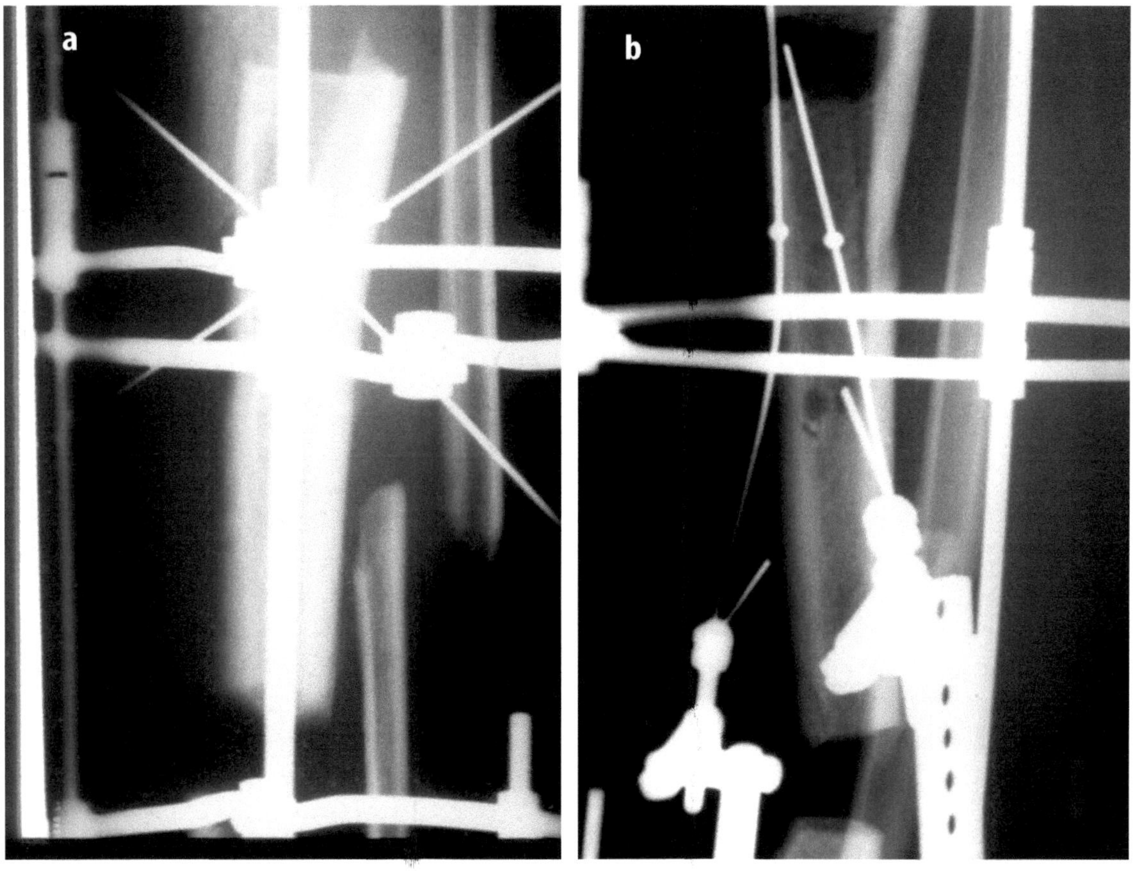

Fig. 3a, b. Same case as in Fig. 1. Bone transport with the oblique wire system. X-rays performed 2 months after transport has begun

fer the oblique wire transport system, which shows the best compromise between functionality and tolerability. The longitudinal wire transport system proposed by Umiarov [4] is described in Chapter 16 ("Treatment of Infected Nonunions"): the bulking and the discomfort of this system (in the early stages of treatment) are balanced by the accuracy of the transported fragment movement.

Distraction performed at two sites within the bone can help shorten total treatment time. Three forms of this kind of treatment can be determined [3]:

1. "Unilateral" bone transport: the kind of transport described above.
2. "Contralateral" bone transport: a corticotomy is performed both proximally and distally and two bone segments are transported centripetally.
3. "Ipsilateral" bone transport: the segment is divided in two (or more) parts and each part is transported towards the next one (Figs. 8–10).

Delayed consolidation or lack of consolidation of the nonunion site can be observed. Opening the nonunion site and once again reshaping the bone ends or bone grafting at the site of the delayed consolidation is sometimes necessary [2, 3].

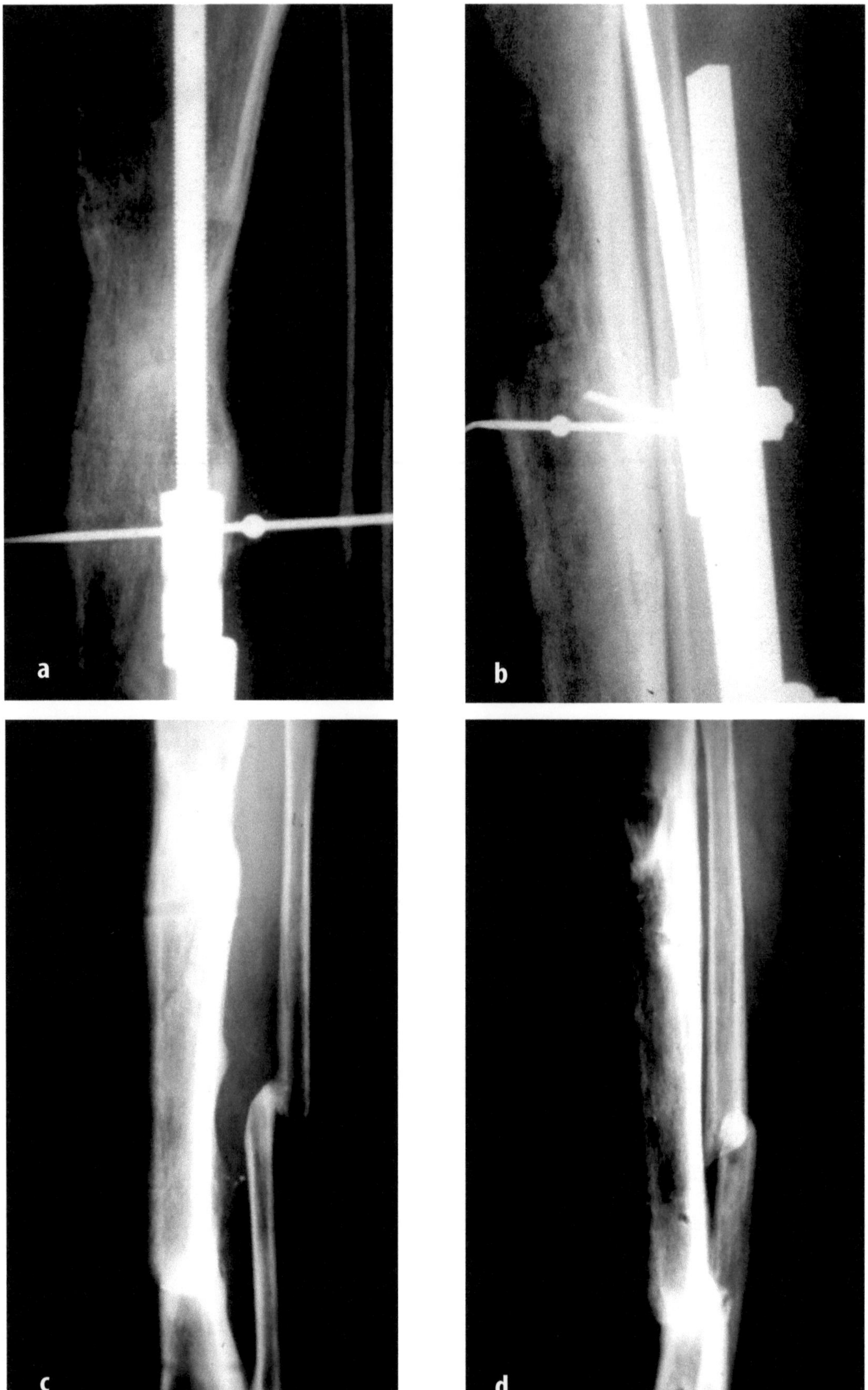

Fig. 4a-d. Same case as in Fig. 1. At the end of the treatment (6 months), proximal bone is well regenerating (**a, b**) and the docking site is consolidated (**c, d**)

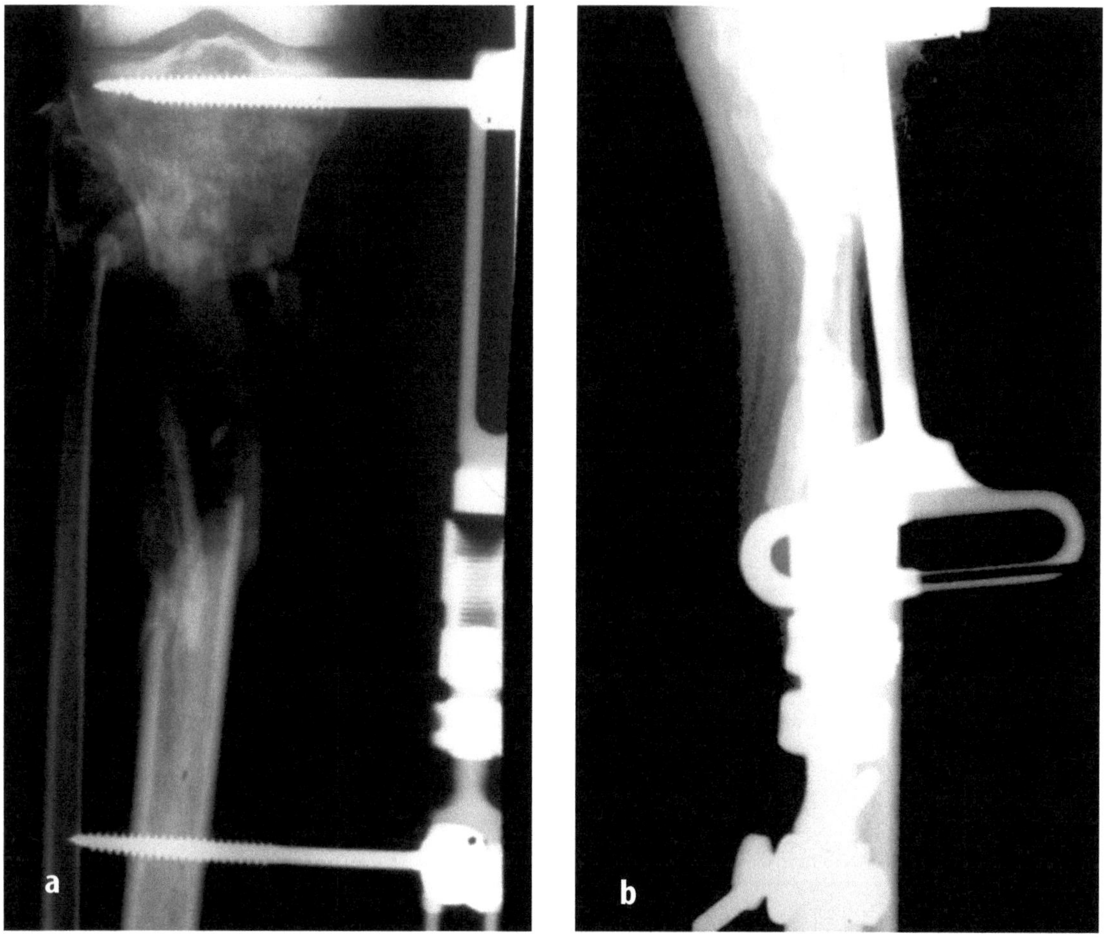

Fig. 5a, b. X-rays of an atrophic nonunion of the proximal third of the left tibia in a 57-year-old woman

Materials and Methods

Between 1984 and 2002, 61 noninfected atrophic nonunions were treated with a follow-up of at least 24 months. There were 38 men and 23 women, with an average age of 33 years (range 26–45 years).

In all cases the nonunion site was the tibia. In 43 cases there was an open fracture at the moment of the trauma. The average time from the injury to the treatment with compression-distraction systems was 6 months (range 4–12). Almost all patients had previously received surgical treatment (n=52).

Leg shortening was evident in 25 patients; axial deviation was observed in 19 patients. The surgical treatment used was bifocal or multifocal compression-distraction osteosynthesis technique, reshaping bone ends and correcting dysmetria and angular deformity when necessary. In all patients the Ilizarov system was employed.

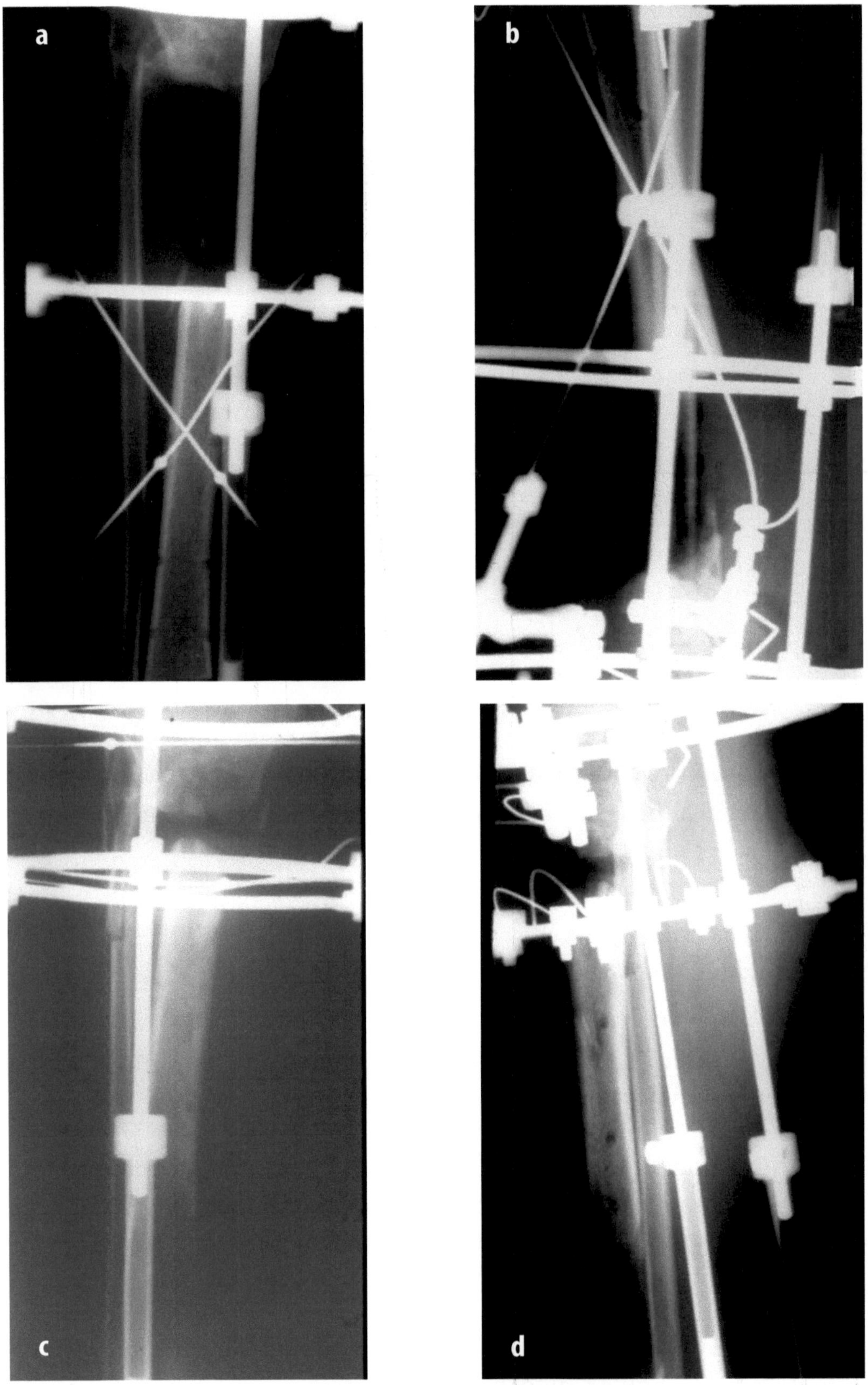

Fig. 6a-d. *Same case as in Fig. 5.* **a, b** Treatment with reshaping of the bone ends, distal metaphyseal corticotomy, bifocal compression-distraction osteosynthesis by means of an Ilizarov apparatus. **c, d** Bone transport with the oblique wire system. X-rays performed 3 months after transport has begun

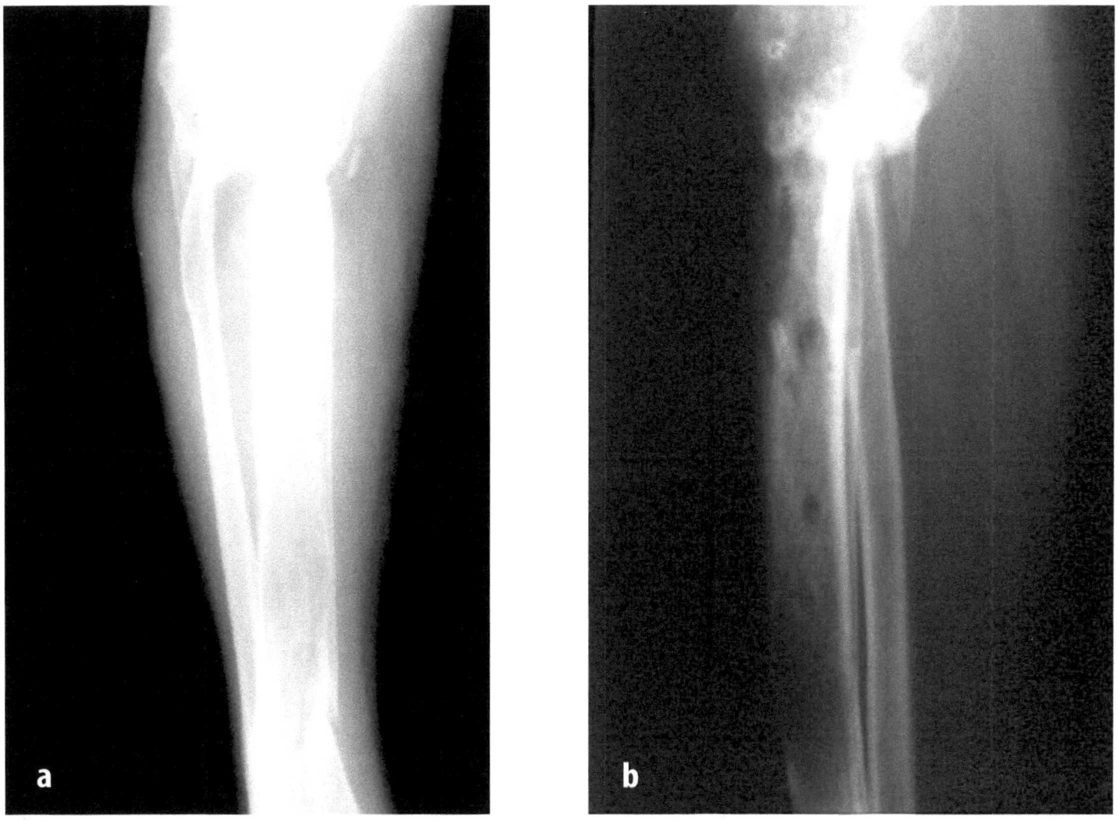

Fig. 7a, b. Same case as in Fig 5. X-rays at the end of the treatment (7 months): distal bone is well regenerated and the docking site is consolidated

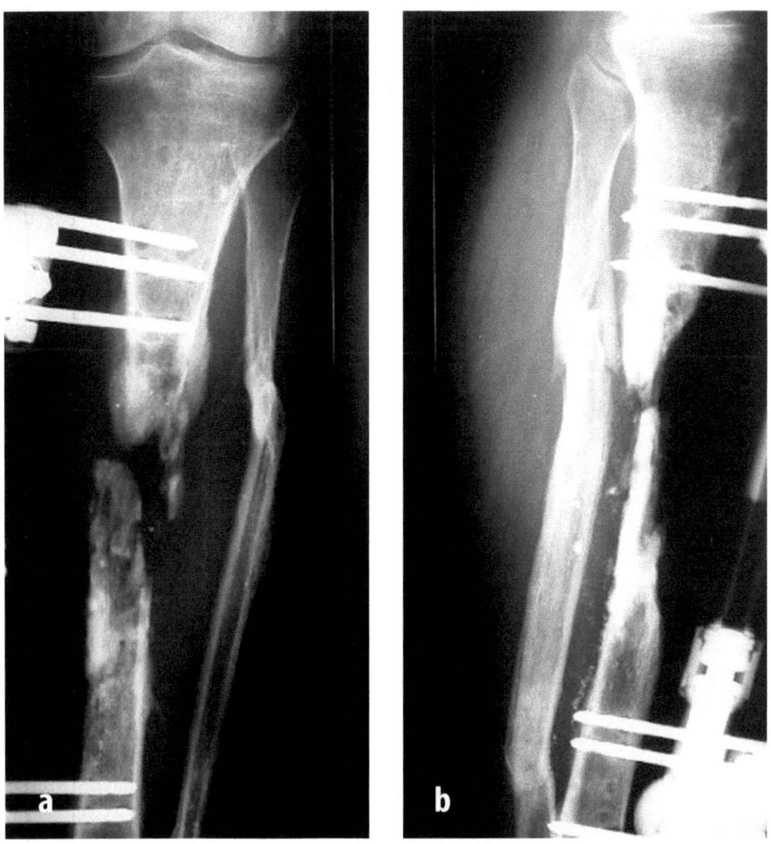

Fig. 8a, b. X-rays of an atrophic nonunion of the left tibia in a 24-year-old man

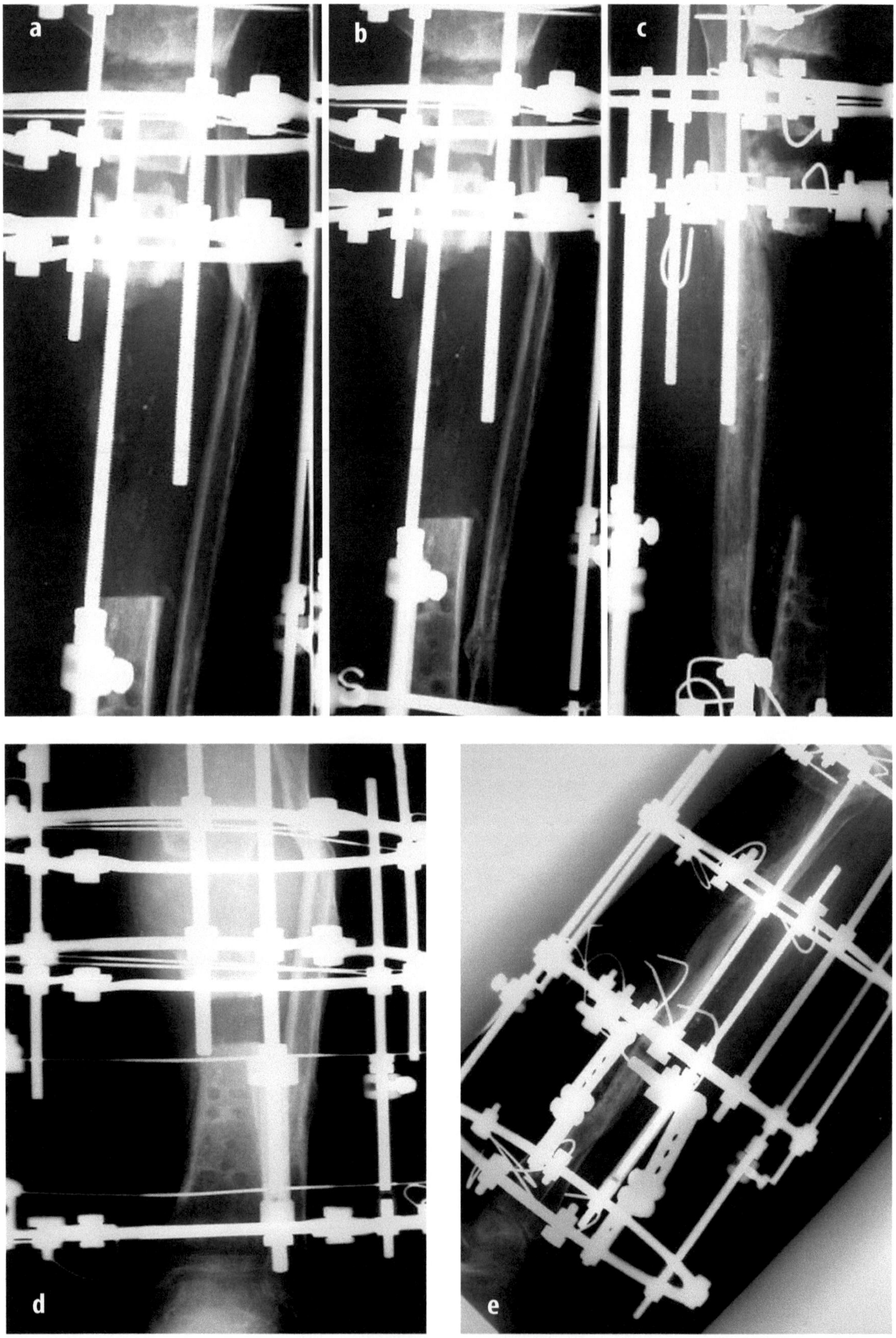

Fig. 9a-e. *Same case as in Fig. 8.* **a-c** Treatment with wide resection (12 cm) of the atrophic ends and "double level" bone transport. **d, e** Multiple simultaneous distraction of the two parts of the intermediate fragment

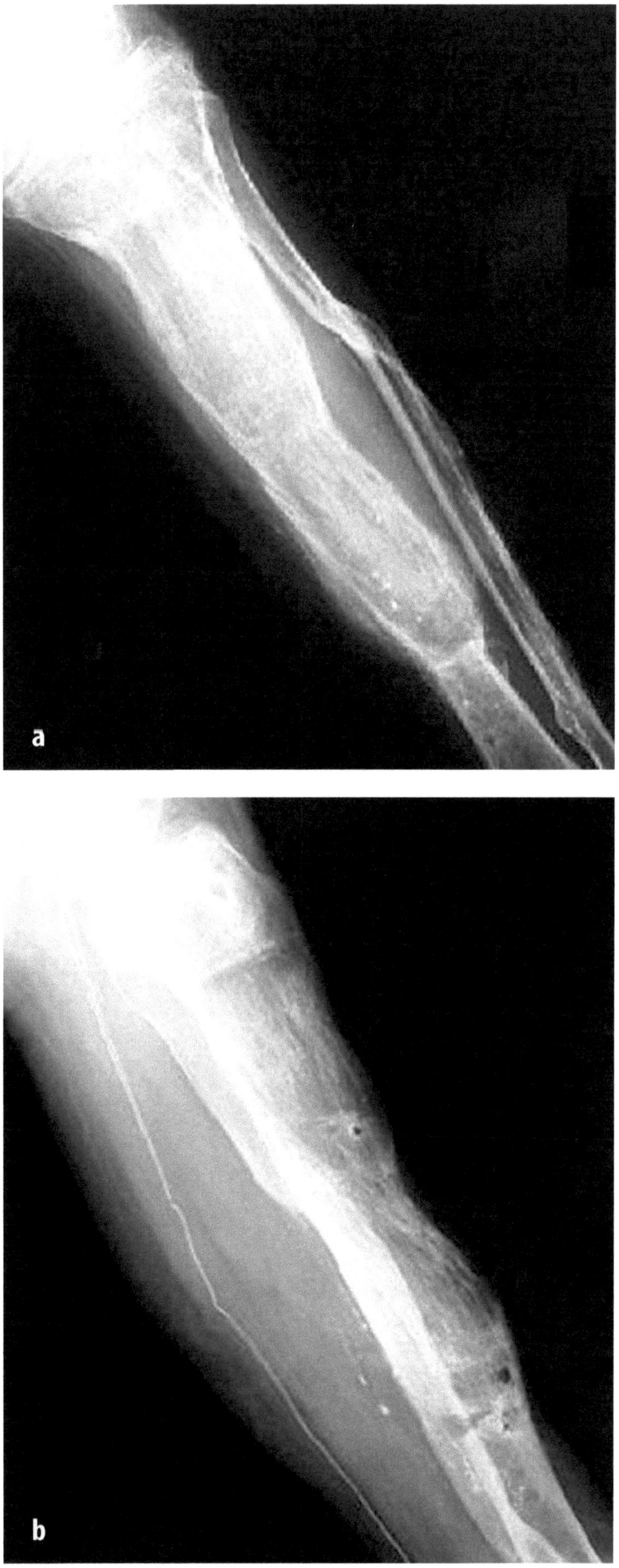

Fig. 10 a, b. Same case as in Fig. 8. X-rays at the end of the treatment (after 8 months) show formation of two bone regenerates of very good quality and consolidation at the docking site

Results

The average period of treatment was 7 months (range 5–11 months). No intraoperative complications developed. Postoperative complications were: superficial infection in 15 cases and wires breaking in five cases; no vascular or nervous complication were observed.

Consolidation at the docking site was achieved in 57 cases; formation of regenerating bone was regular in all these patients. In the four patients in whom consolidation was delayed, a bone grafting was performed.

A residual deformity, represented by a slight angular deformity at the previous nonunion site (max 4°), was observed in five cases. The articular function was good during the treatment, with a moderate limitation of knee flexion, and ankle flexion and extension. It had become almost normal a few weeks after the treatment ended and the fixator was removed.

Discussion

Corticotomy creates an important effect, which has been well described by some Authors who studied and employed the parafocal osteotomy techniques [5–7] and then the corticotomy techniques [3, 8, 9]. Vascularization of the whole bone segment increases greatly, enabling a good quality of regenerating bone (even in elderly patients) at the distraction site, and the development of bone callus at the previous nonunion site. Moreover, it has a stimulating effect on the surrounding soft tissues.

References

1. Ilizarov GA, Green SA (1992) Transosseous osteosynthesis. Springer, Berlin Heidelberg New York
2. Schwartsman V, Choi SH, Schwartsman R (1990) Tibial nonunions. Treatment tactics with the Ilizarov method. Orthop Clin North Am 21:639–653
3. Paley D (1990) Treatment of tibial nonunions and bone loss with the Ilizarov technique. AAOS Inst Course Lect 39:185–197
4. Umiarov GA (1982) Epidermato-fascial-osteoplasty of tibial defects under conditions of purulent infection. Ortop Travmatol Protez 6:65–66
5. Paltrinieri M (1961) Osteotomia nel trattamento dei ritardi di consolidazione e nelle pseudoartrosi di tibia. Atti e Mem Sotimi 6:11–12
6. Kenig I, Radojevic B, Stevanovic M et al (1983) Traitement des pseudoarthroses des os longs par ostéotomie parafocale. In: Campanacci M, Del Monte A (eds) Modern trends in orthopaedic surgery. Gaggi, Bologna
7. Pilnacek J (1998) The role of osteotomies in the healing of nonunions. Proceedings of the 3rd European Traumatology Congress, Amsterdam

8. Ilizarov GA (1989) The tension-stress effect on the genesis and growth of tissues. Part I: The influence of stability of fixation and soft tissue preservation. Clin Orthop Relat Res 238:249–261
9. Choi IH, Ahn JH, Chung CY et al (2000) Vascular proliferation and blood supply during distraction osteogenesis: a scanning electron microscopic observation. J Orthop Res 18:698–705

Treatment of Noninfected Nonunions: Parafocal Osteotomy

Barbara Bertani, Luisella Pedrotti, Stefano Gili, Giovanni Battista Galli, Redento Mora

Introduction

Osteotomies performed in the management of nonunions can be classified into three types [1]:

- Intrafocal osteotomy (performed at the nonunion site: it consists essentially of the resection of the entire area around the nonunion);
- Transfocal osteotomy (performed through the nonunion site to reshape the bone ends: it is indicated for nonunions with a longitudinal or oblique fracture line);
- Parafocal osteotomy (Paltrinieri's osteotomy, performed some centimeters from the nonunion site).

In this chapter the original idea by Paltrinieri (parafocal osteotomy) and the indications for this technique are described and discussed.

Parafocal Osteotomy

In the 1960s Paltrinieri described a personal operative technique that had not previously been described in the literature [2, 3]. According to this technique, it was possible to stimulate the osteogenic potential of the bone in cases of delayed union or nonunion and obtain healing of the nonunion through a single or double osteotomy performed some centimeters away from the nonunion level, proximal or distal to the lesion.

In such cases osteotomy has a dual role: (1) to remove all mechanical stimulation from the nonunion site, transferring it to the osteotomy, and (2) to reestablish the axis to normal by correcting single or complex deformities. In this manner well-vascularized bone tissue can be deposited, substituting the formerly nonvascularized connective tissue interposed between the bone ends.

Paltrinieri developed this technique when attempting to treat a tibial nonunion in a 48-year-old man. This patient was affected by a left tibial nonunion, as a consequence of an open fracture sustained 2 years previously during a road accident, and had previously been treated with osteosynthesis, without healing. That nonunion caused a severe varus and recurvation leg deformity.

Paltrinieri performed a tibial osteotomy to correct the deformity and immobilized the limb in a cast. Three months later, he surprisingly noticed that the nonunion had healed, refuting the dominant idea that nonunions are irreversible. In Paltrinieri's opinion the mechanical moment is the main event in determining the lack of fracture consolidation, and therefore healing could be achieved by resting the nonunion site. The operation indeed produces a perfect immobilization of the nonunion site, protecting it from any mechanical stress; moreover, it facilitates the contact between the bone ends and the renewal of the physiologic pressure stimulus, and eliminates flexion and torsion tibial movement (improved by fibular integrity, which works as a lever), which have a detrimental effect on bone healing. To this mechanical or passive effect, a biological or active effect was added, consisting in stimulation of osteogenic mesenchyma.

In brief, the bone healing process ends at the nonunion site, but the creation of a new fracture site stimulates the regenerative capability of the former site.

Surgical Technique

The operative technique for parafocal osteotomy is simple: for tibial nonunion a short skin incision is performed, taking care not to tear soft tissues; then the periosteum is cut and carefully separated from the cortical bone. For nonunion of other long bones, the technique is similar, but the soft tissues must be carefully dissected to reach the bone.

The osteotomy is performed 3–6 cm away from the nonunion site and preferably with an osteotome rather than a motorized saw, to avoid the risk of bone tissue necrosis. The osteotomy level is chosen according to certain considerations: areas of dystrophic skin and areas with phlogosis or infection are to be avoided. Moreover, the osteotomy must be performed at a healthy bone level, and radiograms may help exclude areas involved in nonunion or those with osteoporosis, sclerosis, with a closed medullary canal, or previously affected by inflammation.

The osteotomy requires immobilization so that the anatomical axis of the bone segment is maintained during healing. For this, Paltrinieri used a cast. Umiarov [4] suggested the use of a parafocal osteotomy associated with immobilization by means of a compression-distraction device, to combine the advantages of these techniques.

Indications

Parafocal osteotomy is indicated in delayed unions and nonunions where the mechanical moment is predominant (hypertrophic or normotrophic nonunions). It is also indicated for treating nonunions with simple or complex deformities and is useful in nonunions with skin lesions at the affected site.

Parafocal osteotomy is contraindicated for infected nonunions with extensive tissue loss.

This treatment is particularly indicated for lower limb nonunions. In upper limb nonunions, whose origin is more biological than mechanical, and where traction or compression forces depending on weight bearing are lacking, this technique is less useful.

Patients and Methods

Between 1984 and 2002, 10 patients affected by tibial nonunion were treated with Paltrinieri parafocal osteotomy. Among the patients there were eight men and two women with a mean age of 32 years (range 25–50 years). We began employing this technique at the Department of Orthopaedics and Traumatology of the University of Pavia in 1996, so the real period the cases refer to is 1996–2002.

Eight patients had been previously treated with osteosynthesis for the former fracture (intramedullary nailing in four cases, plating in two, and external axial fixation in two). Two patients were treated conservatively with a cast.

Nonunions were normotrophic in six patients and hypertrophic in four. Each case was associated with a simple or complex bone deformity: four patients had a varus deformity, three a valgus deformity, two had a recurvation deformity, and one a proximal varus and a distal valgus-recurvation deformity. All patients were treated 8–17 months after the fracture had occurred (mean: 10 months).

The operation consisted of osteotomy, performed as a corticotomy close to the nonunion site, 3–6 cm away from the nonunion. The osteotomy was usually performed distal to the nonunion site. The double complex tibial deformity was treated with a double (proximal and distal) parafocal osteotomy. In all cases both nonunion and osteotomy were stabilized with an Ilizarov apparatus.

The postoperative plan required an immediate rehabilitation program and early weight bearing. From the second postoperative day, gradual corrective maneuvers were performed at the corticotomy site until the deformity was corrected and a good axis restored. At the end of the correction phase, moderate compression was given at at the nonunion level. Nonunion and corticotomy healing processes were radiographically, sonographically, and extensimetrically monitored.

Results

Patients were followed up up for 3–9 years. No vascular or nervous lesions were observed in this period. During treatment, wires broke in two cases (treated with wire substitution). Four patients developed superficial infection at some wire tracts, which healed with local dressing and antibiotic therapy.

Nonunion healing, with simultaneous consolidation of the corticotomy and correction of the deformity, was obtained in all patients in an average of 110 days (range 90–155 days) (Figs. 1–3).

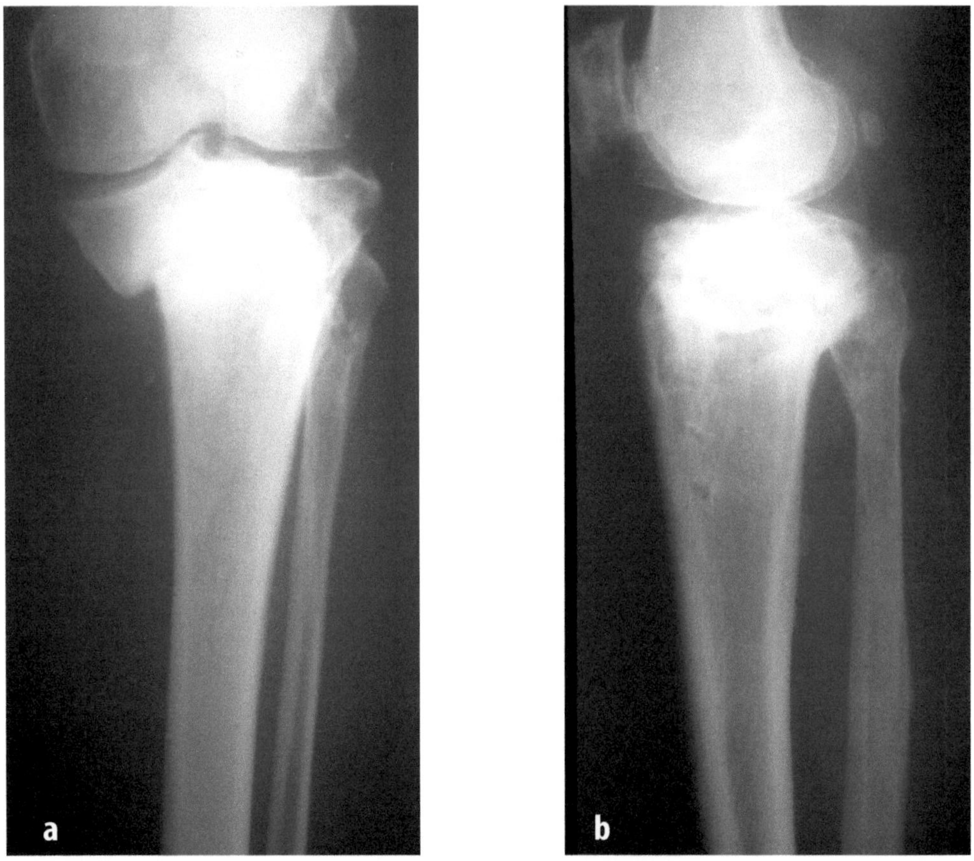

Fig. 1a, b. X-rays of a proximal metaphyseal nonunion with axial and translational deformity of the left tibia in a 45-year-old man

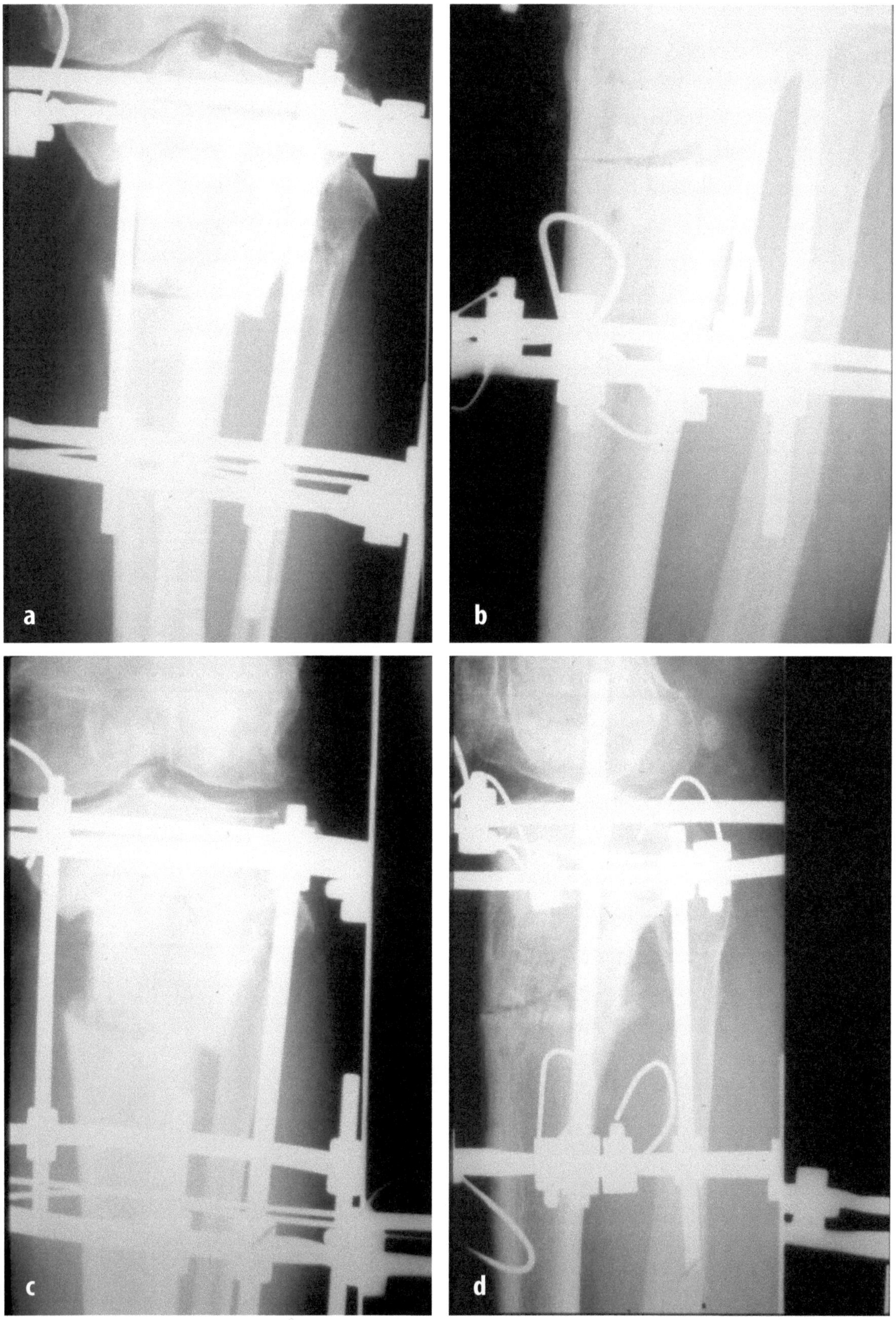

Fig. 2a-d. Same case as in Fig. 1. **a, b** Treatment with Paltrinieri's technique. A corticotomy was performed 5 cm distal to the nonunion level and axial and translational deformities were corrected. Stabilization wad obtained by means of an Ilizarov device. **c, d** X-rays after 45 days

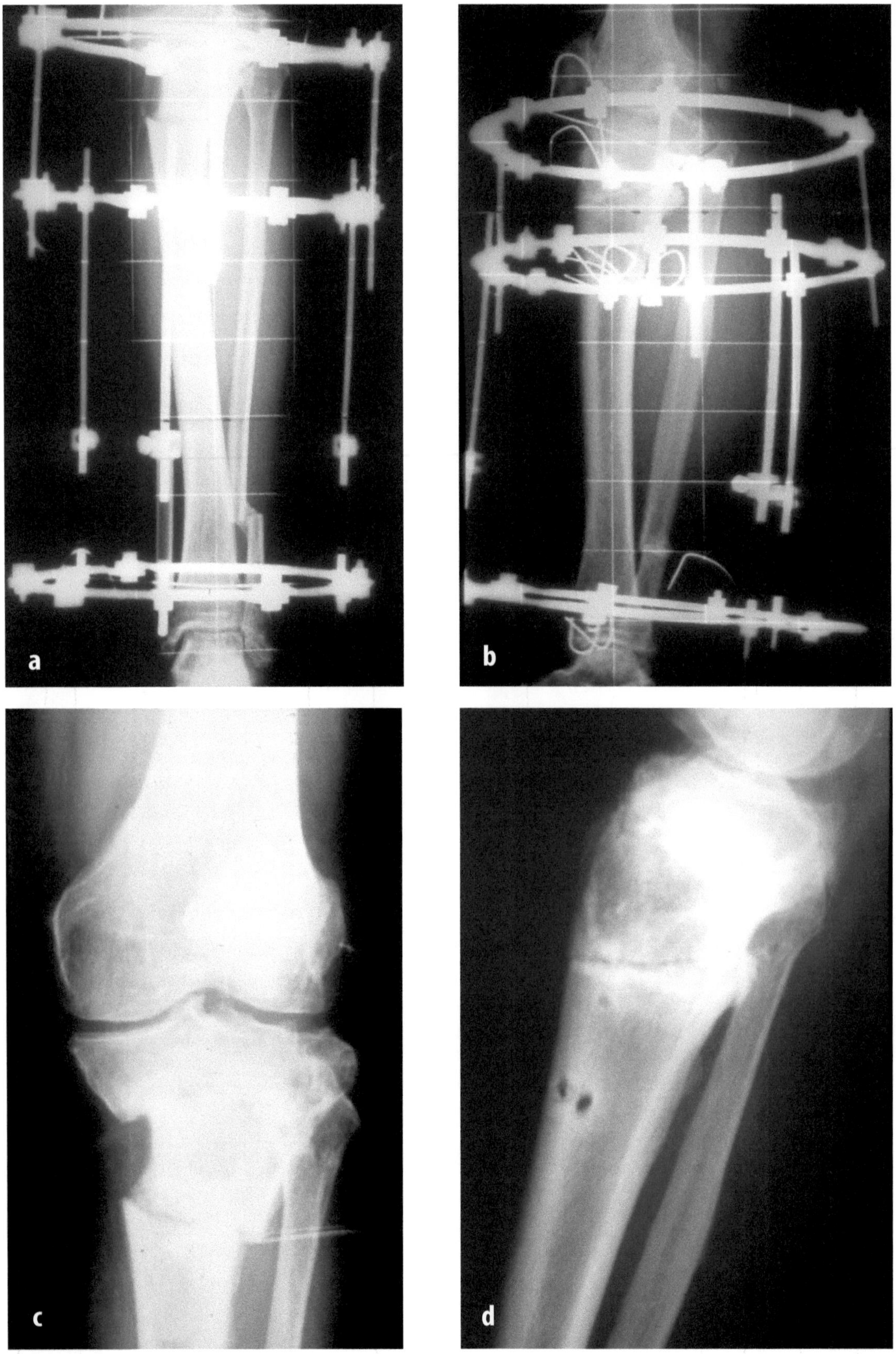

Fig. 3a-d. Same case as in Fig. 1. **a, b** X-rays after 90 days. **c, d** X-rays at the removal of the compression-distraction device (after 4 months), showing healing of the corticotomy, consolidation of the nonunion, and complete correction of the deformity

At the end of treatment no worsening of the knee or ankle range of motion was observed. Hypotrophy of the femoral quadriceps muscle was initially observed, but rapidly improved with physiotherapy. All patients were able to walk without canes.

Discussion

Paltrinieri thought that trophic and reactive alterations of bone tissue occur at the nonunion site. This would explain the not infrequent failure of local treatments, such as bone grafting. Failure risk increases in the management of open or infected fractures, even after the phlogosis ended, because of the latent microbial colonization.

The osteotomy performed at the fracture site has the ideal effect of perfectly interfacing the opposite fragments, anatomically reconstructing the morphology and completely resolving the mechanical aspect of the problem. However, this method fully ignores the biological aspect: it acts on bone tissue that generally is sclerotic and not entirely suitable for undergoing a new regenerative process.

To solve the biological problem, the osteotomy is indicated at a site away from the original fracture. Biologically, the metaphysis offers the best result; here the cortical bone is sharp, with a lot of spongy tissue and the possibility of obtaining wide contact surfaces. The metaphyseal osteotomy, however, has limited indications both in femur and tibia, because it is not suitable from the mechanical point of view.

If the indications for osteotomies at the fracture site and at a distance conflict, the former with the biological factor and the latter with the mechanical factor, it is logical to assume that an osteotomy performed as close as possible to the fracture site would successfully solve the problem. The parafocal osteotomy acts on a normal bone tissue with normal osteogenic capacities and achieves a good correction both aesthetically and mechanically.

As for the convenience of performing the osteotomy proximal or distal to the nonunion site, some biological and mechanical aspects should be considered. Biologically, vascularization by the feeding artery must be considered. The osteotomy must be performed in respect of vascularization proximal or distal to arterial penetration into the diaphysis. From the mechanical point of view, parafocal osteotomy aims to correct angular displacements. The irregular weight distribution on abnormally oriented articular surfaces causes degenerative alterations over time: it is then necessary to ensure that the articular lines are parallel. The closer the osteotomy is to the fracture line, the less difference there will be between the nonunion angle and the osteotomy angle.

Paltrinieri evaluated the possibility of performing a double osteotomy, proximal and distal to the lesion, on the basis of the hypothesis that complete rest at the site of delayed union or nonunion can only be achieved with this solution. The results obtained in his series do not confirm this hypothesis; on the contrary, they failed to show any advantage over the single osteotomy.

Paltrinieri's technique was successfully employed later by other authors [1, 4, 5–15]. In particular, the stabilization with circular external fixation systems, suggested by Umiarov [4], shows many favorable aspects: stability, assembly modularity, multiplanar control, and the possibility of gradually correcting deformities.

Therefore compression-distraction techniques seem to represent a natural complement to Paltrinieri's technique: the elasticity of these systems allows easy control of mechanical stress, taking away the cut and torsion forces and maintaining and improving the compression and distraction forces at the corticotomy site. This represents a further stimulus to healing and helps improve weight transfer from the fixator to the bone as the consolidation proceeds.

References

1. Pilnacek J (1998) The role of osteotomies in the healing of nonunions. Proceedings of the 3rd European Traumatology Congress, Amsterdam
2. Paltrinieri M (1961) Osteotomia nel trattamento dei ritardi di consolidazione e nelle pseudoartrosi di tibia. Atti e Mem SOTIMI 6:11–12
3. Paltrinieri M (1966) L'osteotomia parafocale nel trattamento dei ritardi di consolidazione e delle pseudoartrosi delle ossa lunghe dell'arto inferiore. Chir Organi Mov 55:15–39
4. Umiarov GA (1986) Parafocal osteotomy. Vestn Khir 136:63–64
5. Maldarelli GF, Ponti G (1967) L'osteotomia parafocale nella correzione delle deviazioni assiali delle fratture diafisarie viziosamente consolidate. Minerva Ortop 18: 14–21
6. Ranieri L (1968) L'osteotomia parafocale nei ritardi di consolidazione. Chir Organi Mov 57:146–156
7. Trentani C (1971) Le osteotomie parafocali. Chir Organi Mov 60:305–311
8. Traina GC, Flores G (1972) L'osteotomia parafocale: quando e perchè. Minerva Ortop Traumatol 23:333–338
9. Figna P, Demartin F (1973) L'osteotomia parafocale nel trattamento chirurgico dei ritardi di consolidazione delle fratture di gamba. Contributo clinico-statistico. Chir Organi Mov 62:161–168
10. Gusta A, Matwiejko L, Krolewski J (1976) Treatment of delayed union and nonunion of the long bones and pseudoarthroses by means of Paltrinieri's method. Chir Narzadow Ruchu Ortop Pol 41:631–635
11. Matasovic T (1978) Parafocal osteotomy in the treatment of nonfused fractures and pseudoarthroses of the long bones. Acta Chir Yugosl 25:95–100
12. Burghele N, Troianescu O, Serban N et al (1979) The Paltrinieri operation in treatment of pseudoarthroses of the leg. Rev Chir Oncol Radiol 28:443–448

13. Kenig I, Radojevic B, Stevanovic M et al (1982) Traitement des pseudoarthroses des os longs par ostéotomie parafocale. In: Campanacci M, Del Monte A (eds) Modern trends in orthopaedic surgery. Gaggi, Bologna
14. Iacobellis C (2000) Parafocal osteotomy and the Ilizarov method in the treatment of femoral pseudoarthrosis. Case report. Chir Organi Mov 85:79–83
15. Mora R, Pedrotti L, Bertani B et al (2001) Role of parafocal osteotomy in the management of nonunions with compression-distraction techniques. Proceedings of the 2nd International Meeting of the ASAMI, Rome

Treatment of Infected Nonunions

REDENTO MORA, LUISELLA PEDROTTI, BARBARA BERTANI, FABRIZIO QUATTRINI

Treatment

Among infected nonunions, treatments are based on the classification and on the therapeutic principles developed by Umiarov at the Central Institute of Traumatology and Orthopaedics (CITO) of Moscow [1–3] (Table 1).

Table 1. Classification of infected nonunions and principles of treatment according to Umiarov [1]

Types	Treatment
Normotrophic nonunion without shortening	*Débridement*, monofocal osteosynthesis (compression-distraction)
Hypertrophic nonunion with shortening	*Débridement*, monofocal osteosynthesis (distraction)
Atrophic nonunion with shortening	*Débridement*, bifocal osteosynthesis (compression-distraction)
Nonunion associated with bone and soft tissue loss	*Débridement*, bone resection without soft tissue coverage, bone transport

The first three types of the classification outlined in Table 1 are the "infected variety" of the three corresponding types of noninfected nonunion, whose morphologic and functional features and whose principles of treatment have already been discussed. Their treatment is similar to that of the noninfected variety, but commences after accurate *débridement* and adequate specific antibiotic therapy. Only on rare occasions does "infection burn on the fire of the bone regenerate", as Ilizarov mentioned with a sort of optimism

[4], and it is better not to rely only on this "fire" but rather to trust in modern antibiotic therapy, carefully planned in collaboration with the infectious diseases specialists.

The fourth type of this classification includes nonunions with bone and soft tissue loss, which are usually observed after open fractures with large soft tissue damage, complicated by infection and bone loss.

It should be stressed that bone and soft tissue loss is only directly produced by trauma in a small number of patients; most often it is due to the wide surgical *débridement* performed, usually during numerous operations in an attempt to eliminate the necrotic and infected areas [2]. In these cases the choice of treatment requires previous evaluation of all the possible options, according to the trauma and the features in the individual patient [5].

The possible options are:

- Amputation and prosthesis;
- Reconstructive treatment.

Amputation rather than reconstruction may be indicated by certain local features, such as posterior tibial nerve damage, severe vascular lesion, and severe contamination, and by features relating to the patient, such as old age, chronic diseases (diabetes or peripheral arteriopathy), smoking, and inability to take part in the treatment.

In theory, the evaluation and the treatment decision may be helped by one of the "Scoring Systems" developed in the past few years (Mangled Extremity Syndrome Index, Mangled Extremity Severity Score, Predictive Salvage Index, or Limb Salvage Index); however, these tests have not shown any clinic usefulness [6].

If reconstruction is chosen, a very complex treatment is usually necessary to solve three related problems: infection, lack of bone continuity, and lack of skin coverage. The essential aims of the treatment are then represented by: infection healing, soft tissue reconstruction, and bone consolidation with preservation of the limb length, the most important stage in the therapeutic planning being the accurate *débridement* [7].

The first stage of the reconstructive methods is bone stabilization. The indication, according to most authors [5] and also in our opinion, is always the external osteosynthesis due to the high infection rate associated with endomedullary nailing. In particular, in spite of the (theoretical) simplicity of application and the (theoretically) better access to soft tissues allowed by the axial fixation, we prefer circular fixation due to its intrinsic advantages (stability and immediate functional weight bearing and easy removal at the end of the treatment) [2].

Soft tissue reconstruction can be achieved by different means [8]: a split-thickness skin graft is rarely used because it would surely fail if the graft is applied on poorly vascularized soft tissues or bone without periosteum. Therefore, alternative methods are usually employed. A cross-leg flap is also rarely used because of the prolonged period of immobilization and the many aesthetic problems that it produces. Local muscle flap has the advantage of self-vascularization: it allows a firm coverage and can also be covered by a skin graft as an immediate or delayed procedure; however, distant coverage often is difficult, and it is often impossible to perform because of the extent of the lesion to the whole limb. An important improvement has been achieved with the use of free microvascularized grafts [9], with which the graft can be sampled from areas spared by the trauma. Among the most frequently used microvascularized grafts are the groin flap, the latissimis dorsi flap, and the tensor fasciae latae flap. One very particular kind of flap is the composite bone-muscle-skin graft, composed of iliac crest and soft tissues (composite osteocutaneous groin flap) based on the deep circumflex iliac artery, and which is indicated in the treatment of combined defects of both bone and soft tissue.

The reestablishment of bone continuity can be achieved with autoplastic bone graft, most often taken from the iliac crest, or sometimes from femoral great trochanter, femoral distal metaphysis, or tibial proximal metaphysis. Here, it has been observed that bone of membranous origin (iliac bone) shows better osteoinductive activity than bone of endochondral origin (tibia and femur) [10].

A particular surgical technique employing autoplastic bone graft is the Papineau method [11], which consists of excision, stabilization, and reconstruction by cortical spongy bone graft without skin coverage. This procedure has the severe disadvantage of being performed in many operative stages and requires prolonged periods of time to heal.

The microvascularized autoplastic bone graft [12] is based on the employment of ipsilateral or contralateral fibula or, more rarely, the iliac crest with soft tissue coverage (composite graft as previously described).

The disadvantages of the autoplastic graft are mainly due to the quantity of bone tissue needed, the prolonged immobilization, the complications at the sampling site (morbidity and pain) and graft site (absence of healing and fractures), the frequent need for many operations, and prolonged period to achieve graft hypertrophy.

In particular in the microvascularized graft the length of the operation and the risks in cases where there is only one vascular axis must be considered [13].

It is necessary to remember that good outcome is also produced by homoplastic grafts [14, 15], which are generally stored by refrigeration and employed as massive bone graft or as thin sheets of cortical bone. Obviously the use of homoplastic bone presumes a perfectly functional bone bank for both sampling and storing bone grafts. The complications most often described in this kind of treatment are infection and graft fracture.

A good alternative to bone graft is represented by the compression-distraction techniques, mainly developed by Ilizarov [4], in the form of bifocal (or multifocal) compression-distraction osteosynthesis, also known as bone transport technique. The advantages consist of lack of morbidity at the sample site, lack of limits to the dimensions of bone defect, width of regenerated bone (which does not become hypertrophic), and easiness of soft tissue lesion healing if the temporary shortening techniques are used. The disadvantages are the necessity of "compliance" by the patient and the possible complications (angular deformities in the regenerated bone, delayed consolidation at the docking site). Therefore a very accurate evaluation of the case is needed before beginning such a treatment. The use of the compression-distraction systems [16–19] offers an important contribution to solving the severe problems related to these lesions.

In some papers describing monofocal or bifocal osteosynthesis techniques by means of compression-distraction devices, good results are usually reported in the treatment of infected nonunion with tissue loss. However, the problem of the correction of bone defect is always well stressed, but little attention is directed to the problems of treating infection and soft tissue loss [17, 20–23].

In Umiarov type 4 infected nonunion of the tibia, the method of epidermofascioosteoplasty, developed by Umiarov (from the CITO of Moscow), offers the essential advantage of precisely classifying the operative phases and the stages of simultaneous bone and soft tissue regeneration and eliminating wide tissue losses without previous sterilization of the infected site and closure of the soft tissue or the use of any kind of graft [24–30].

Operative Technique

The first step consists in performing a corticotomy at the proximal or distal tibial metaphysis according to the resection site, distal or proximal (Figs. 1, 2a).

Then an accurate *débridement* of the infected nonunion site, with bone end resection until healthy bone is observed and complete excision of the infected and necrotic soft tissues are performed (Figs. 2b, 3a). The soft tissue resection level must correspond to the bone resection level; otherwise, a new infection will develop. The wide *débridement* area is then kept open.

At this time a compression-distraction device is applied to the leg (Fig. 3). The assembly must be extended to the hindfoot in patients in whom a loss of tissue in the distal tibia requires extensive resection and the length of the distal tibial fragment is only few centimeters in length.

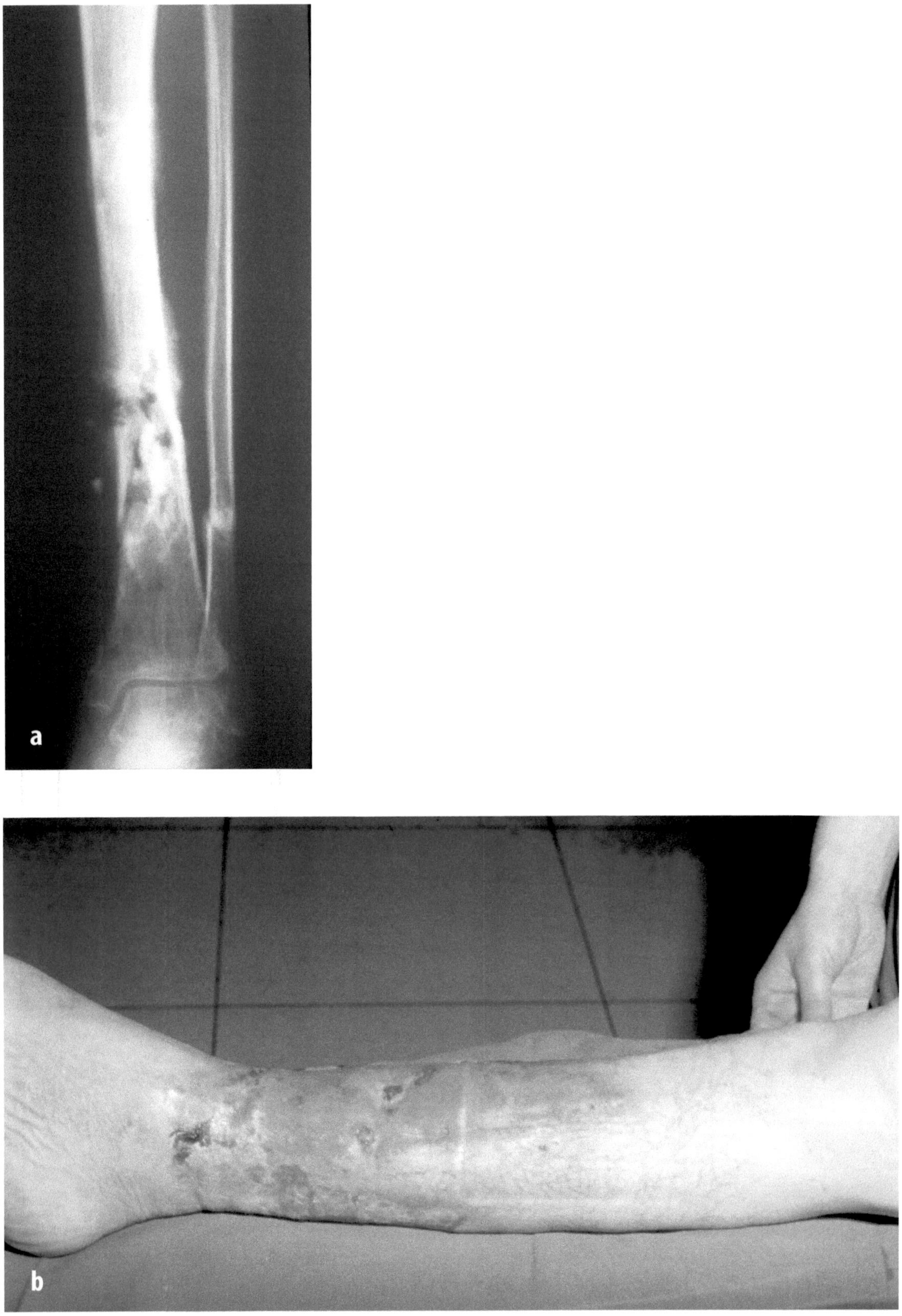

Fig. 1a, b. a X-ray of an infected nonunion of the left tibia with bone and soft tissue loss in a diabetic 38-year-old man previously treated with external osteosynthesis by means of an axial device. **b** Clinical feature of the left leg

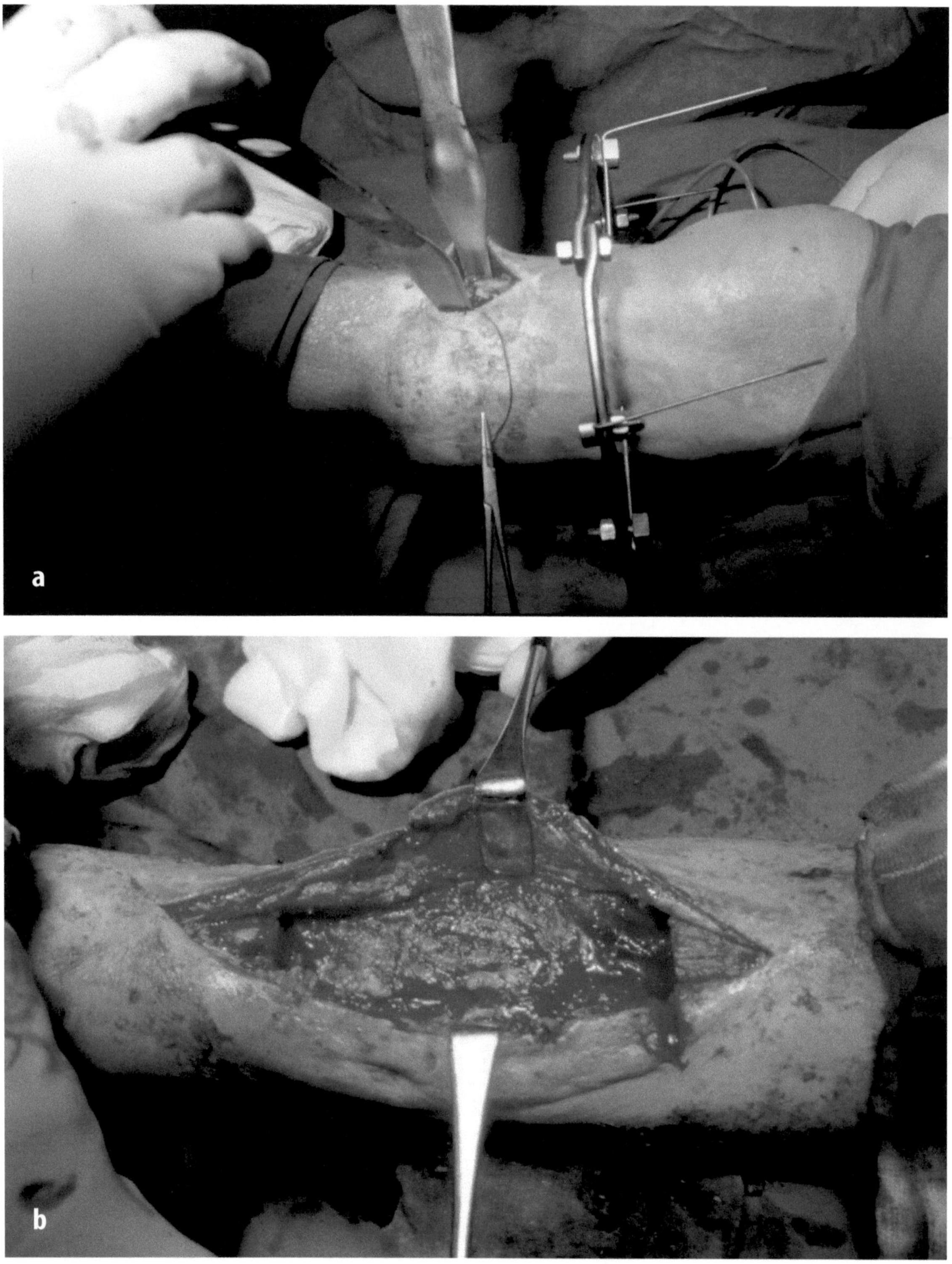

Fig. 2a, b. Same case as in Fig. 1. **a** Treatment with Umiarov's technique: tibial proximal corticotomy. **b** Excision of infected and necrotic tibial segment and soft tissue

A system of gradual distraction is applied to the tibial fragment designed to be transported, which is made up of two oblique wires with a support base connected to the apparatus or of one wire (only for proximal corticotomy),

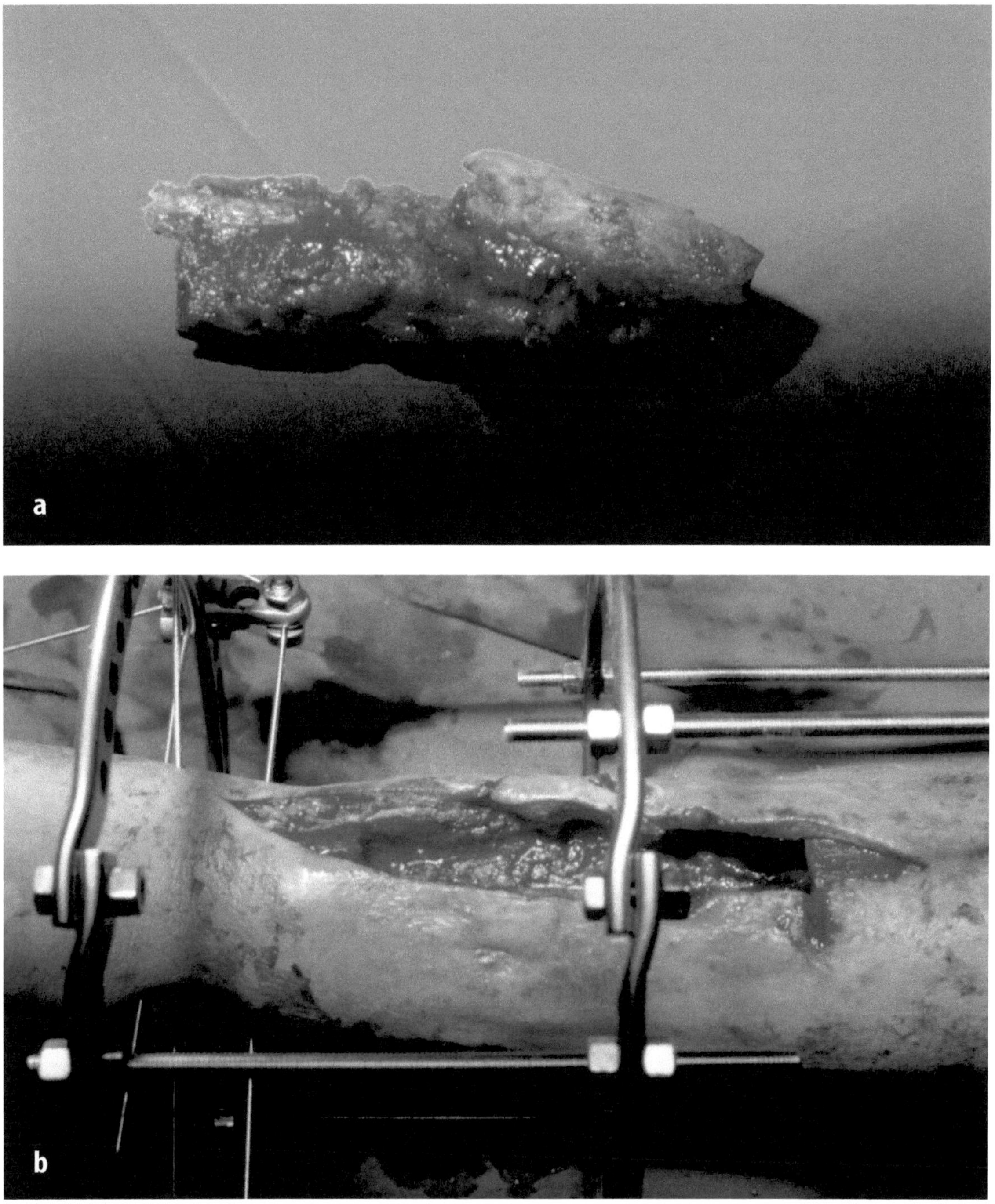

Fig. 3a, b. Same case as in Fig. 1. **a** Resected bone (length: 18 cm). **b** Mounting of the compression-distraction device is almost completed

whose end, bent like a hook, is supported on the cortical edge. This wire is passed through the medullary canal, the talus, and the calcaneus, ultimately protruding from the middle of the sole, and is then fixed by a progressive traction device to the distal ring of the apparatus. The transverse wire transport technique should only be employed, in our opinion, when multilevel transport is performed (Figs. 4, 5).

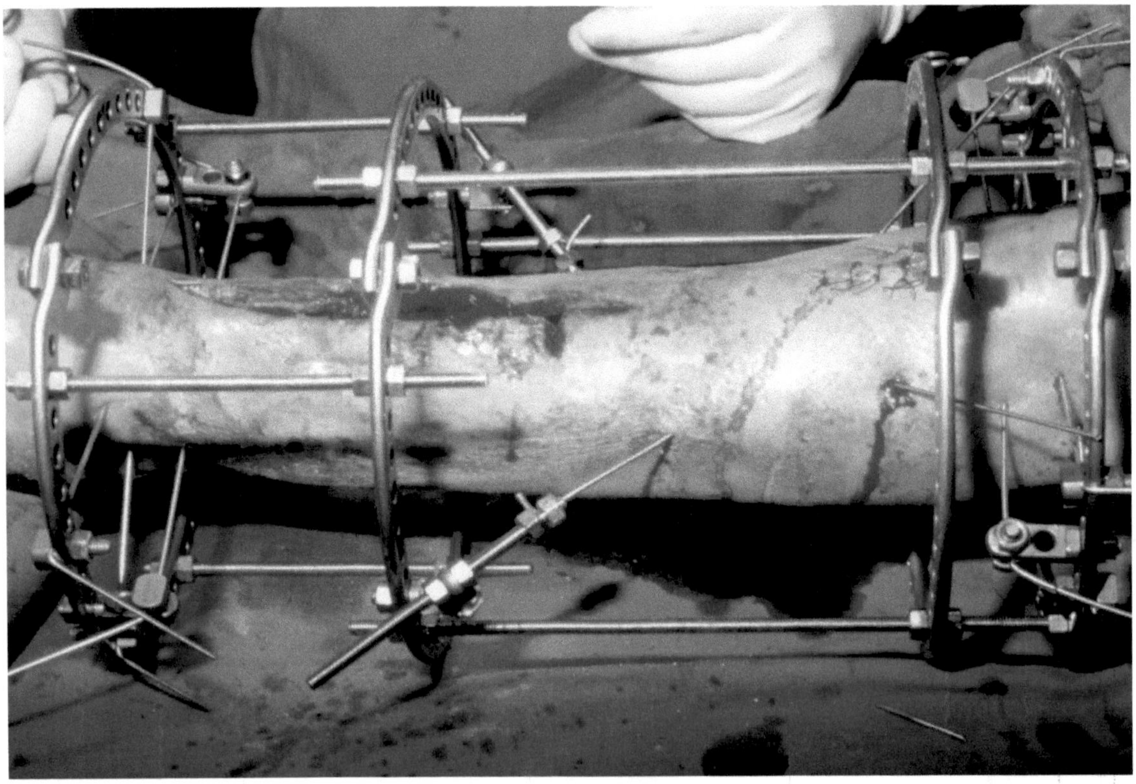

Fig. 4. Same case as in Fig. 1. Clinical features at the end of the surgical procedure. The wound is kept open

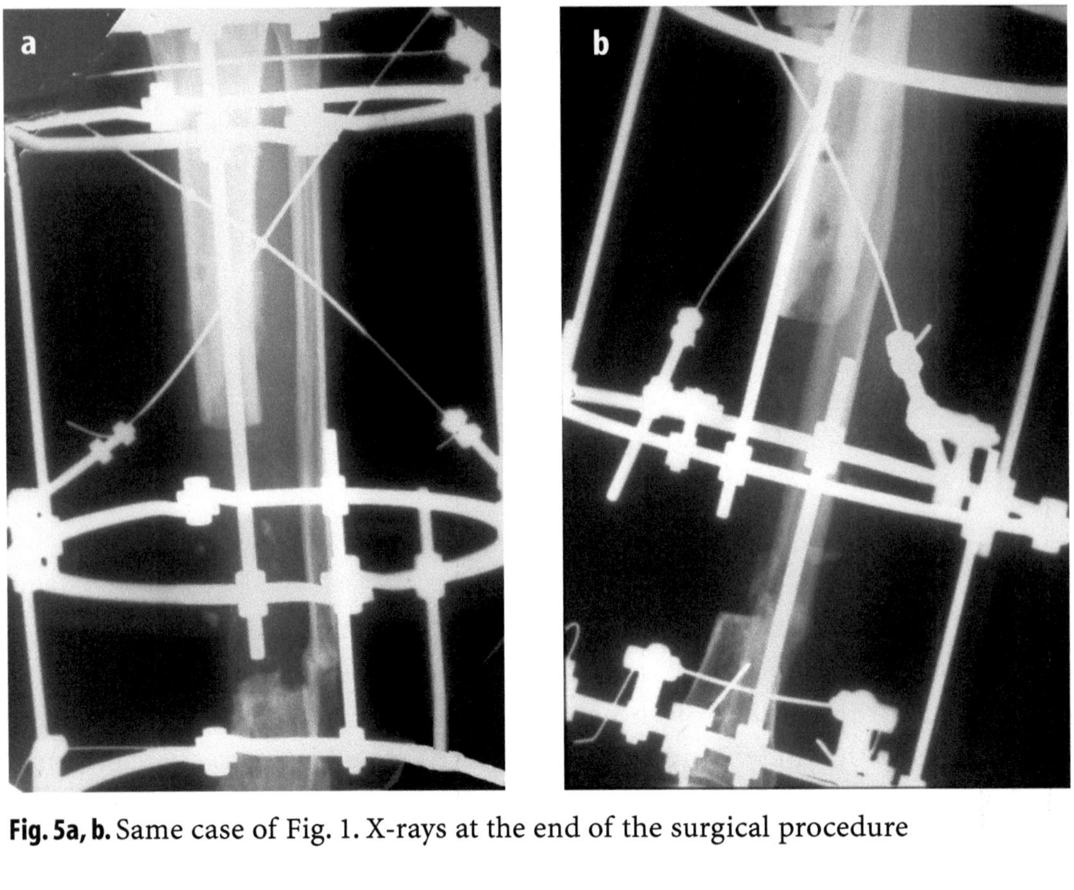

Fig. 5a, b. Same case of Fig. 1. X-rays at the end of the surgical procedure

In the postoperative phase the patient receives specific antibiotic therapy [30] and daily dressings. After 2 weeks a granulation tissue covers the bone segment surfaces. From this moment, the transport of the bone fragment at 1 mm daily causes a progressive distraction with regenerating bone formation at the corticotomy site and a gradual narrowing of the gap between the fragments at the nonunion site (Fig. 6). Simultaneously, the gradual approach

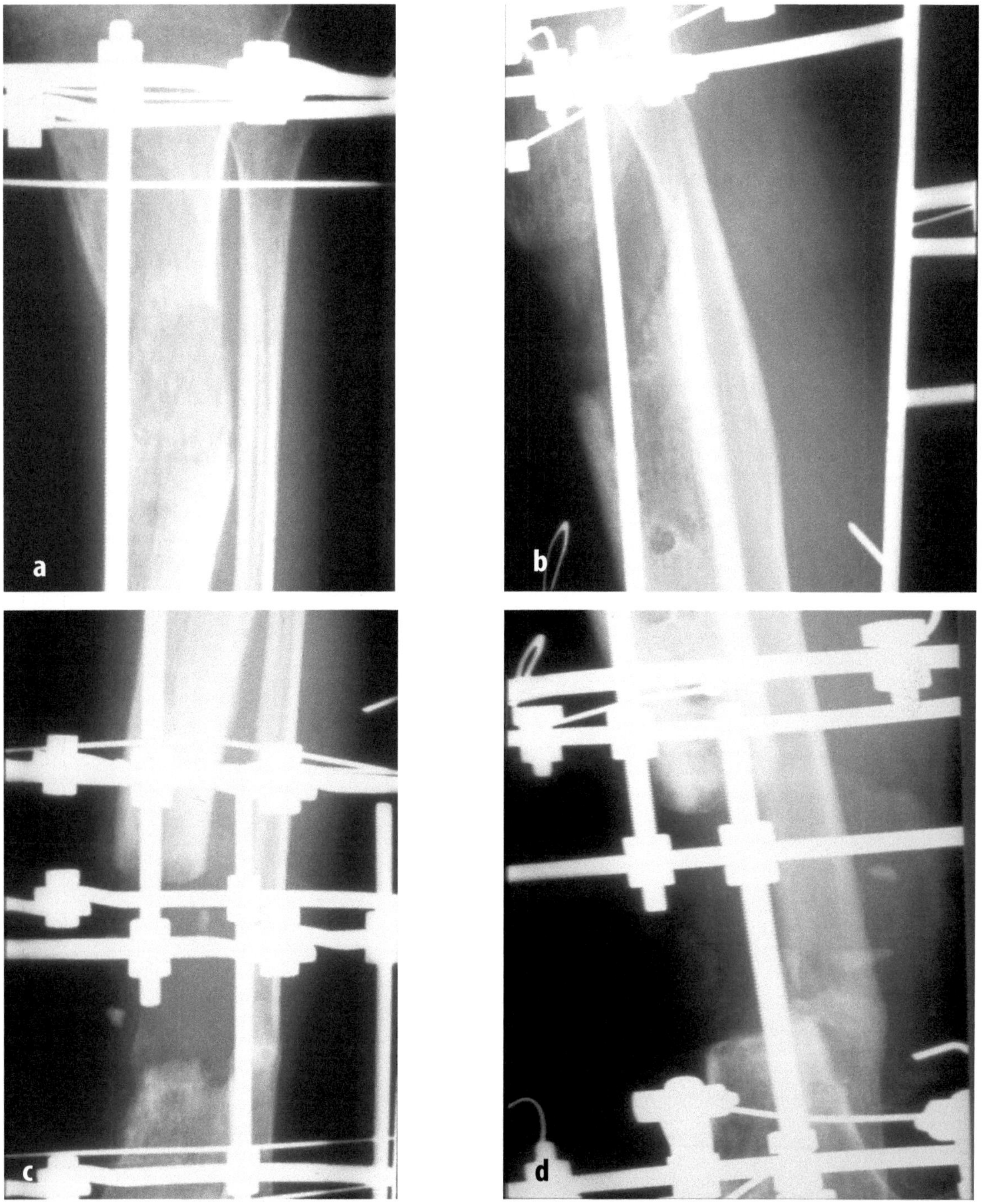

Fig. 6a-d. **a**, **b** X-rays after three months shows good formation of proximal regenerating bone. **c**, **d** X-rays after 3 months: the bone transport is in progress

of the tibial fragments closes the edges of the soft tissue gap until the epidermic and fascial reconstruction is complete because the tibial fragment takes the fascia and the skin, both closely connected to the bone, along during the transport. This is how a true epidermofascioosteoplastic treatment is performed.

At this time the distraction system based on the oblique wires or on the hook-shaped intramedullary wire is removed and the tibial fragment is fixed to an additional ring by two cross transverse wires, in order to enable a more effective interfragmentary compression and to obtain consolidation (Figs. 7, 8). Knee and ankle kinesitherapy and muscle strengthening are started immediately, and standing and walking start a few days after the operation. Weight bearing is allowed soon in the case of wire fixation and is allowed after the distraction phase in the bent wire technique.

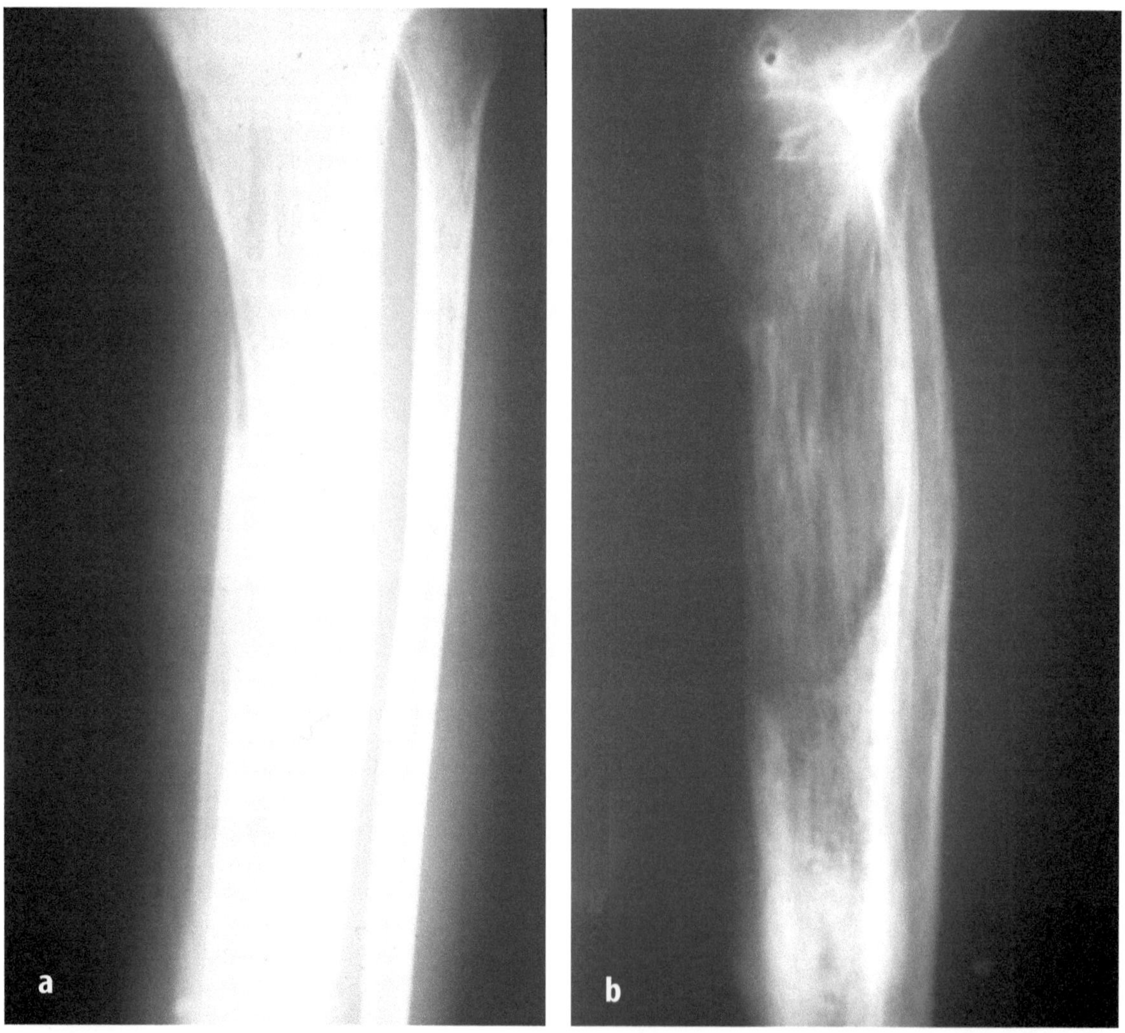

Fig. 7a, b. Same case as in Fig. 1. X-rays at the removal of the compression-distraction device (after 16 months), with corticalization of the regenerate and callus formation at the docking site

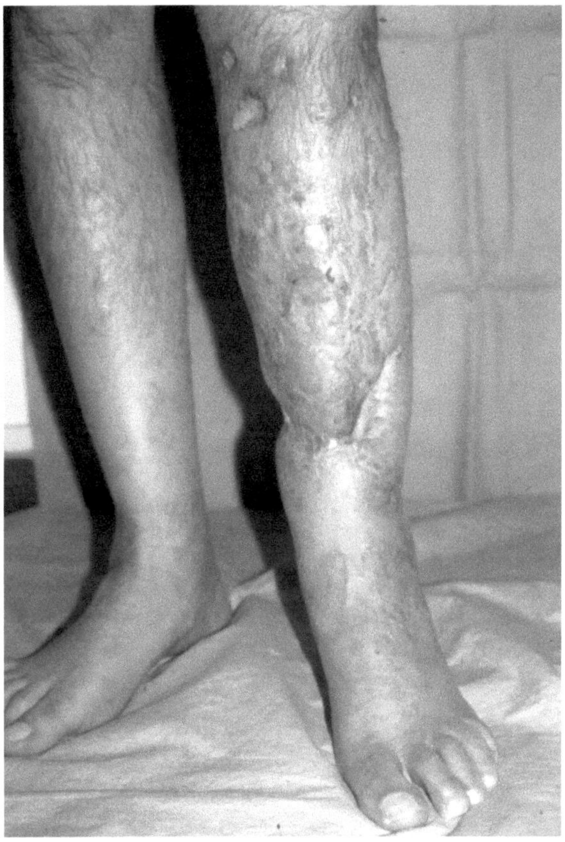

Fig. 8. Same case as in Fig. 1. Clinical features at the end of treatment show complete soft tissue reconstruction

Patients and Methods

In all, 220 infected nonunion were treated (eight humeral, 26 femoral, and 186 tibial); of the patients 131 were males and 89 females. Four humeral nonunions were type 1 and four were type 2 of the Umiarov classification [1]. Of the femoral nonunions 16 were of type 1, six were of type 2, and four were of type 3. There were 81 tibial nonunions of type 1, 28 of type 2, 23 of type 3, and 54 of type 4.

Our indications are based on the Umiarov principles of treatment [1]. Therefore the treatment of types 1, 2 and 3 was similar to that for corresponding non-infected nonunion, with the addition of accurate *débridement* and specific antibiotic therapy.

In all, 101 nonunions were classified as type 1; 54 patients were male and 47 female, and the average age was 35 (range 26–61). Type 2 included 38 patients, aged from 30 to 63 (average 38).

The 27 patients with type 3 nonunion (15 male and 12 female) were 33 years old on average (range 24–54).

Patients with infected type 4 nonunion underwent epidermofascioosteoplastic surgery. Average age was 36 years (range 24–57 years); 47 of these patients were male, seven female.

Of the patients who already had other kinds of surgery, 35 had previously had two operations, 14 had had three operations, and five had had four operations. Time from trauma to the epidermofascioosteoplastic treatment was between 5 and 27 months, with an average time of 10 months. In all cases, cultures were positive for Staphylococcus and in 16 cases also for *Pseudomonas aeruginosa.*

At the time of operation, the tibial bone resection was from 6 to 18 cm, with an average of 9.5 cm. In all patients the Ilizarov apparatus was used with the oblique wires technique, but in two patients, in whom a multilevel bone transport was performed, the technique with transverse wires was employed. In five cases, an autoplastic bone graft was necessary to obtain consolidation at the docking site (Figs. 9–15).

Results

After surgery, all patients were clinically, radiologically, sonographically, and bacteriologically controlled (Figs. 16–23). Treatment lasted from 4 to 8 months for type 1, 5 to 9 months for type 2, and 6 to 11 months for type 3 infected nonunions. In Umiarov classification type 4 infected nonunions, the healing time was 7–18 months (average 10 months). No intraoperative complications were observed.

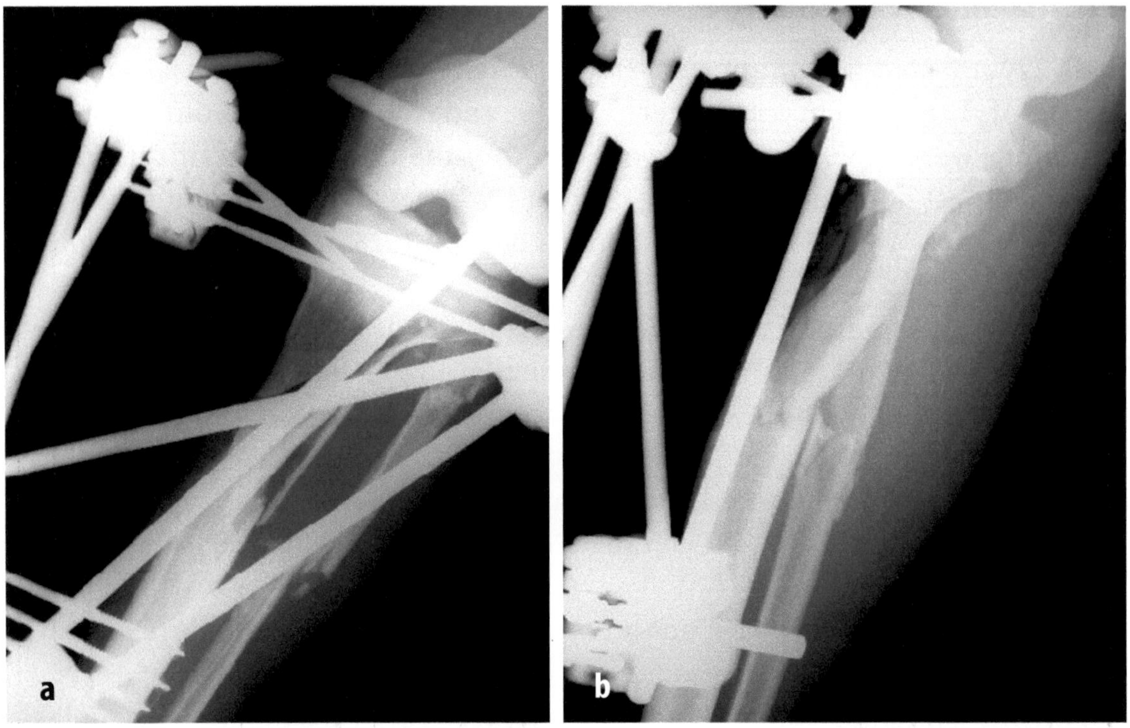

Fig. 9a, b. X-ray of an infected nonunion of the proximal left tibia with bone and soft tissue loss in a 25-year-old man previously treated with external fixation by means of a Hoffmann II device

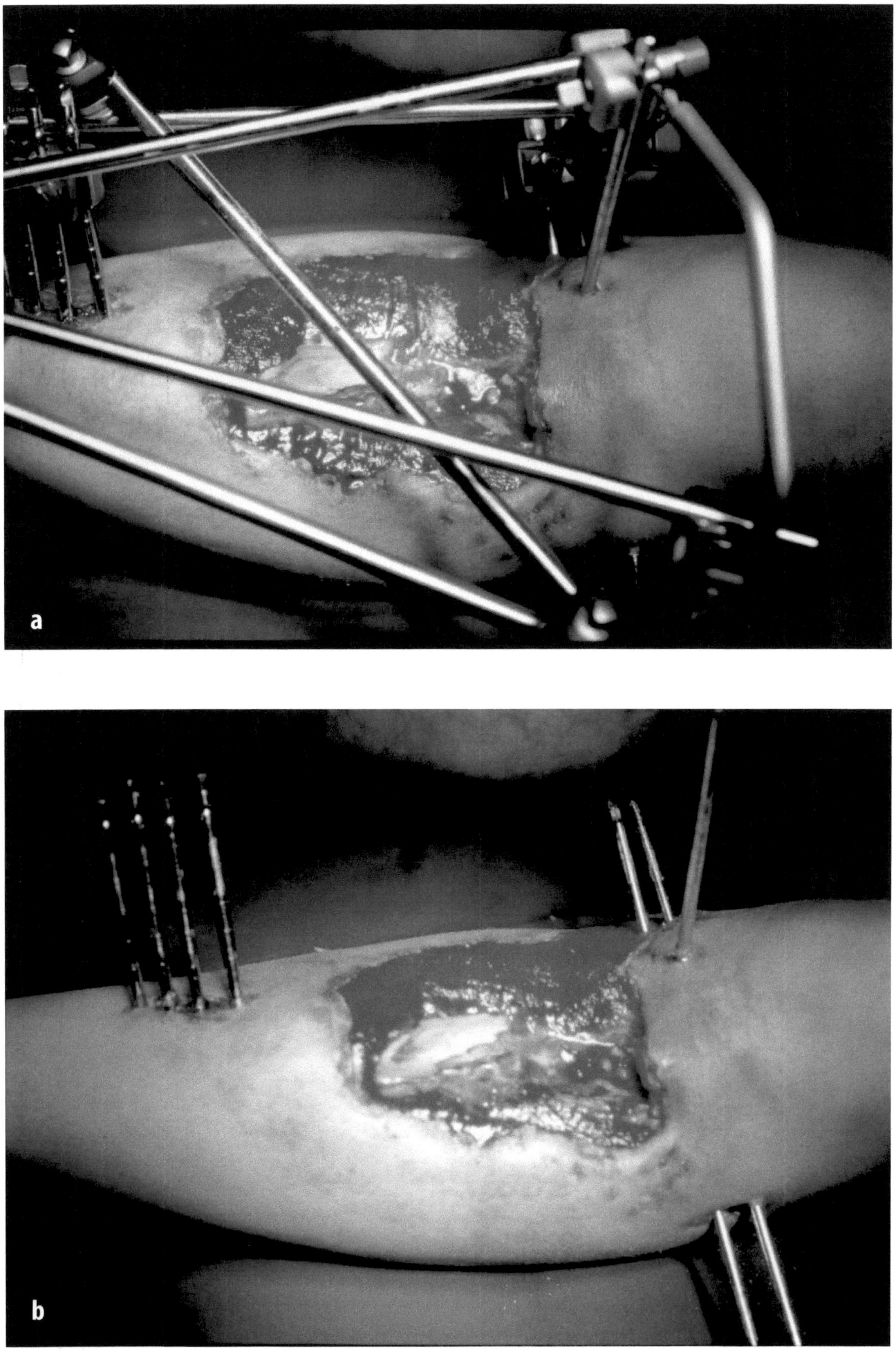

Fig. 10a, b. Same case as in Fig. 9. Clinical features of the large bone and soft tissue loss

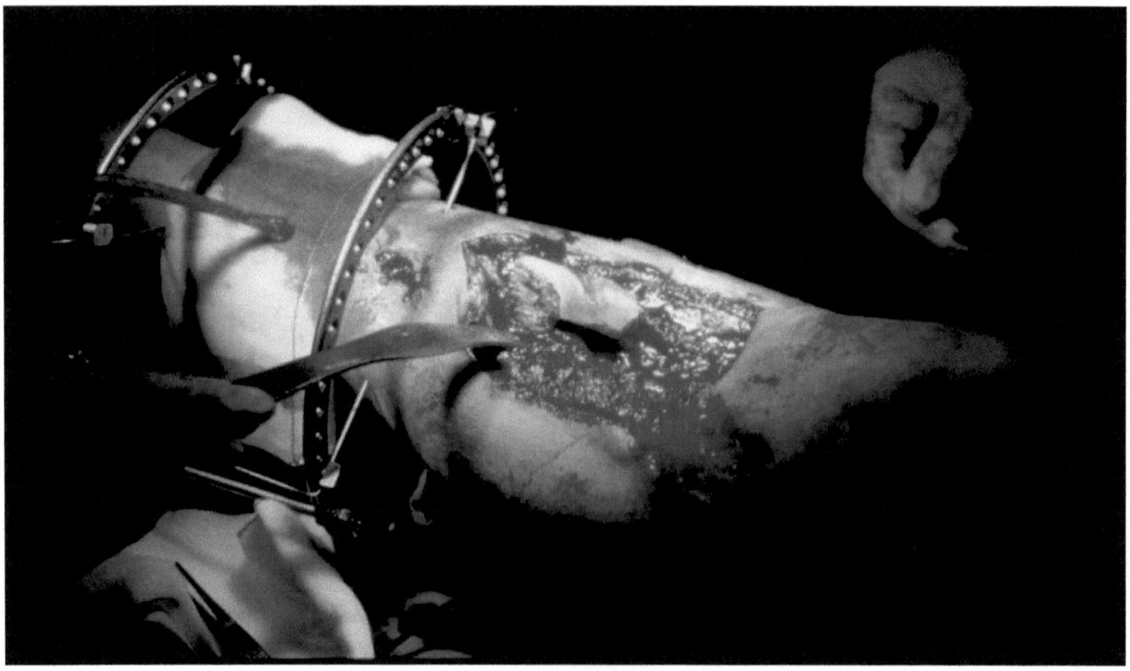

Fig. 11. Same case as in Fig. 9. Treatment with Umiarov's technique. After distal tibial corticotomy, excision of the infected proximal tibial segment (length: 12 cm) and soft tissues is performed

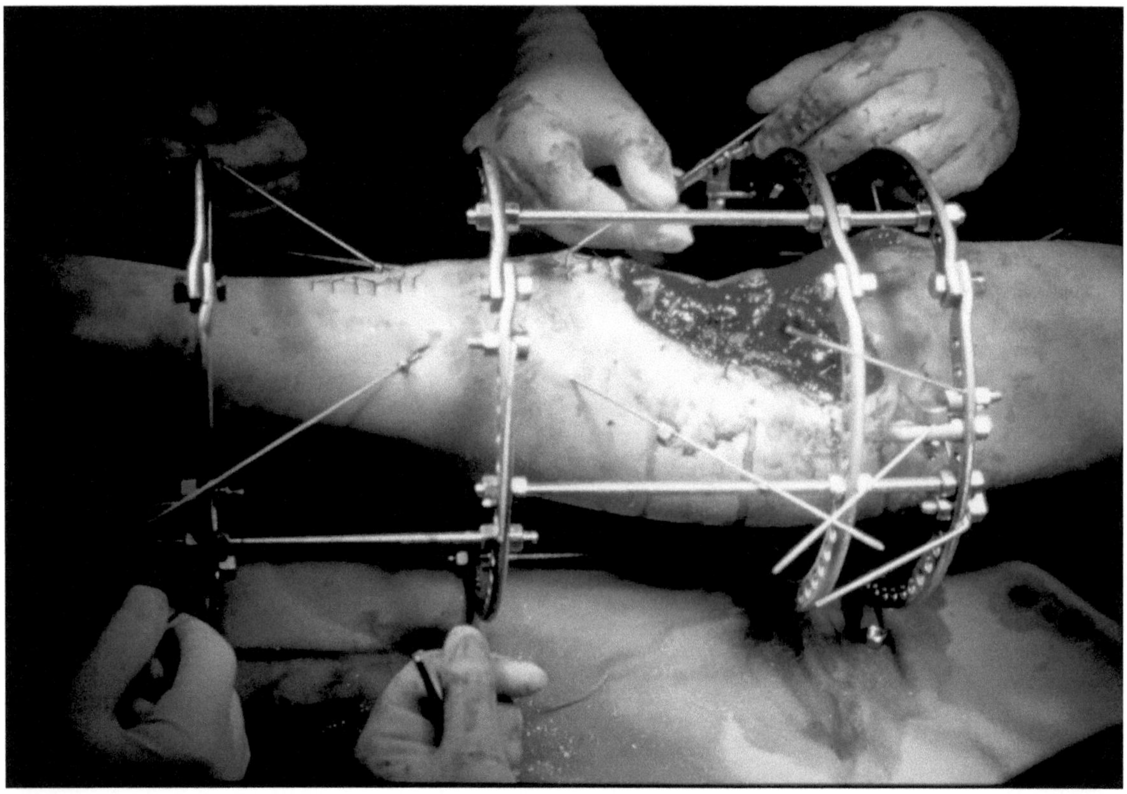

Fig. 12. Same case as in Fig. 9. The mounting of the Ilizarov device with oblique wire traction system is completed. The wound is kept open

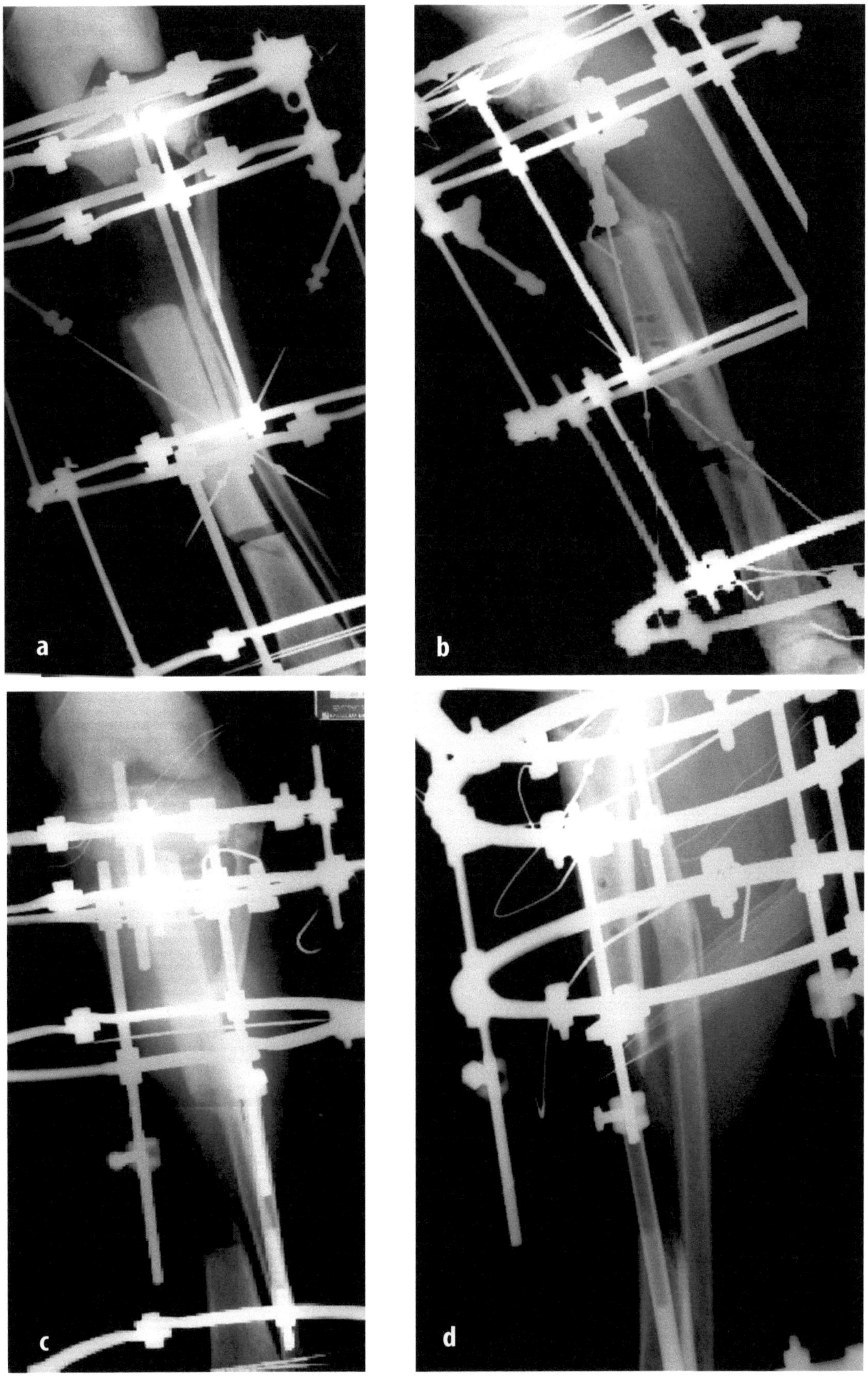

Fig. 13a, b. Same case as in Fig. 9. **a, b** X-rays at the beginning of the bone and soft tissue transport. **c, d** X-rays at the end of the bone and soft tissue transport

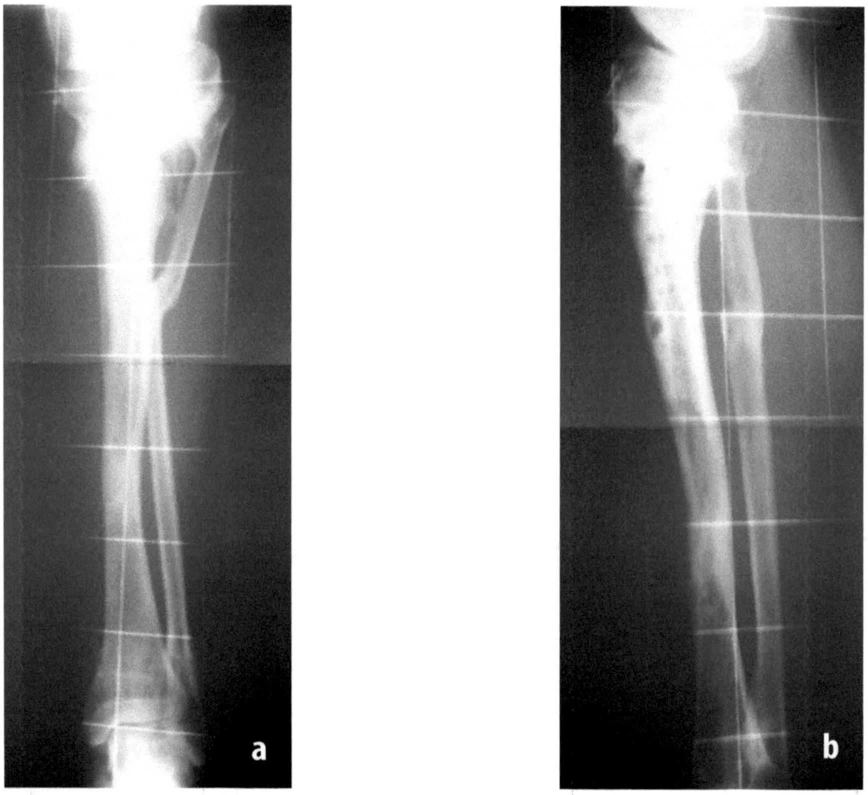

Fig. 14a, b. Same case as in Fig. 9. X-rays at the removal of the circular external fixation device (after 12 months)

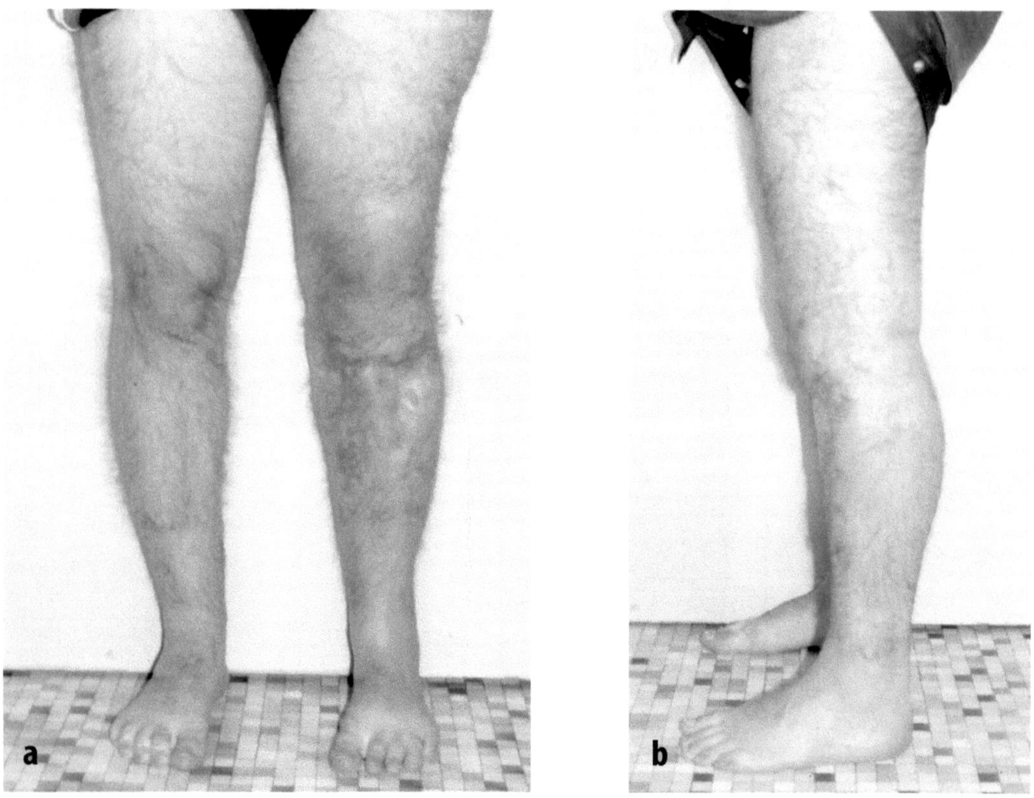

Fig. 15a, b. Same case as in Fig. 9. Clinical features at the end of treatment show a good soft tissue reconstruction

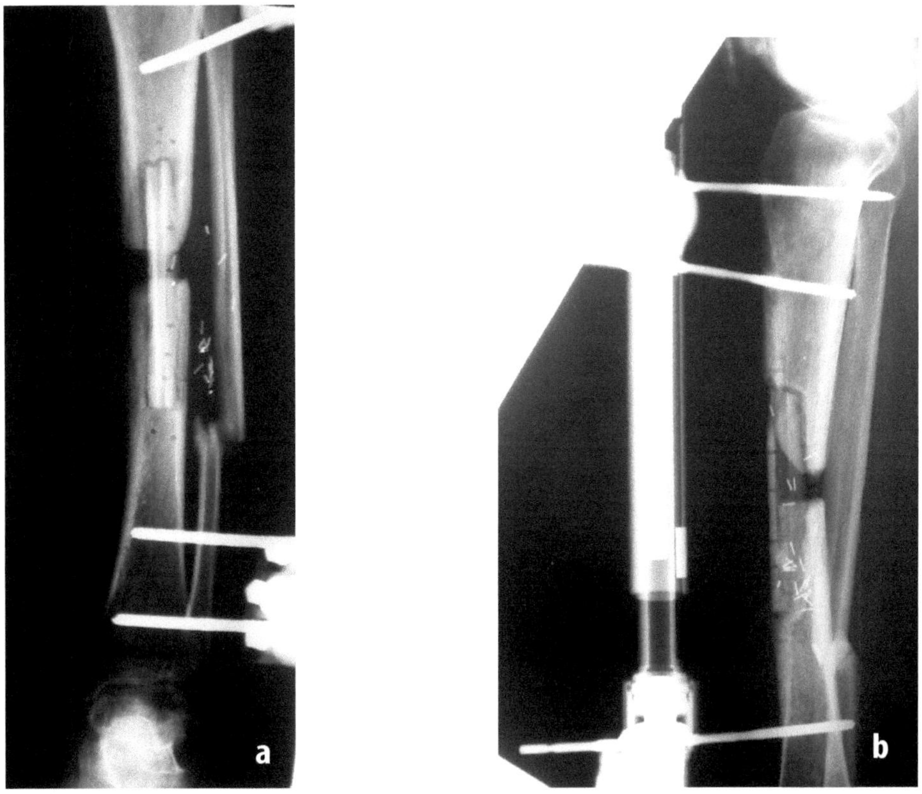

Fig. 16a, b. X-rays of an infected nonunion of the left tibia with bone and soft tissue loss in a 30-year-old woman previously treated with vascularized fibular bone graft and stabilization by means of an axial external fixator

During the follow-up, one patient, who was treated by epidermatofascialosteoplasty, died 40 days after operation due to pulmonary embolism. Five patients developed a superficial infection at one or two wire sites: the infection was successfully treated with a local dressing and general antibiotic therapy.

In 21 cases breakage of one or two wires was observed. This complication required wire substitution in 16 cases.

The overall results, divided into bone results and functional results, were evaluated according to the Paley classification [17]. In type 4 infected nonunions in particular the infection was eliminated, bone and soft tissue were reconstructed, and the postoperative rehabilitation period was shortened.

An apparently paradoxical feature is the absence of fair results in the treatment of the most severe cases (type 4 of the Umiarov classification), which showed only excellent and good outcome and the infection eradicated in all cases. This "anomaly" is explained by the operative technique, which completely removes all the infected and necrotic tissues and involves further complete sterilization of the nonunion site (Table 2).

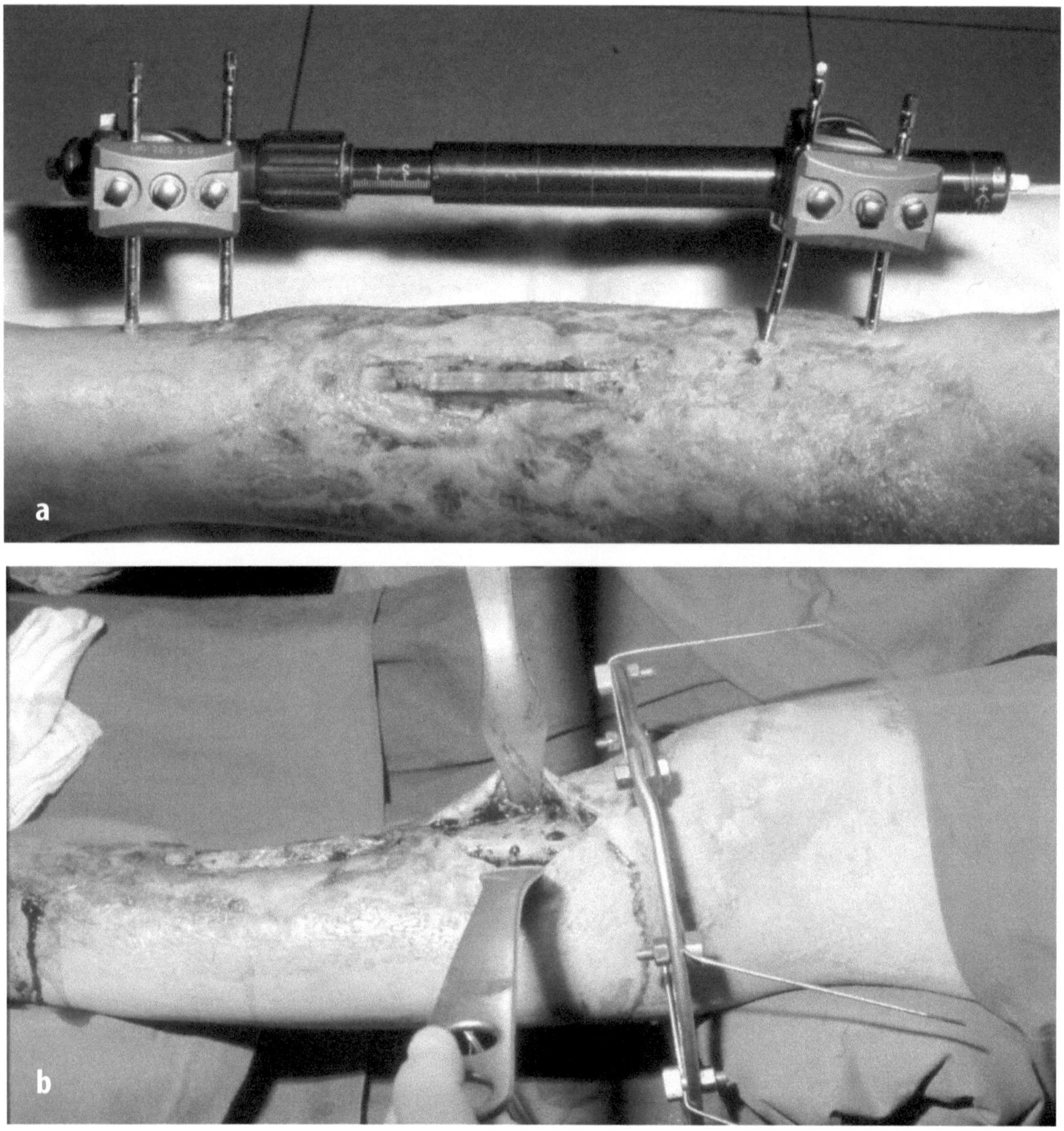

Fig. 17a, b. Same case as in Fig. 16. **a** Clinical features of the completely exposed and necrotic fibular graft. **b** Treatment with the Umiarov's technique: proximal tibial corticotomy is performed

Table 2. Bone and clinical results

	Bone results			Functional results	
	Excellent	Good	Fair	Excellent	Good
Type 1	44	53	4	51	44
Type 2	14	15	9	20	18
Type 3	7	9	11	14	13
Type 4	21	33	-	26	28

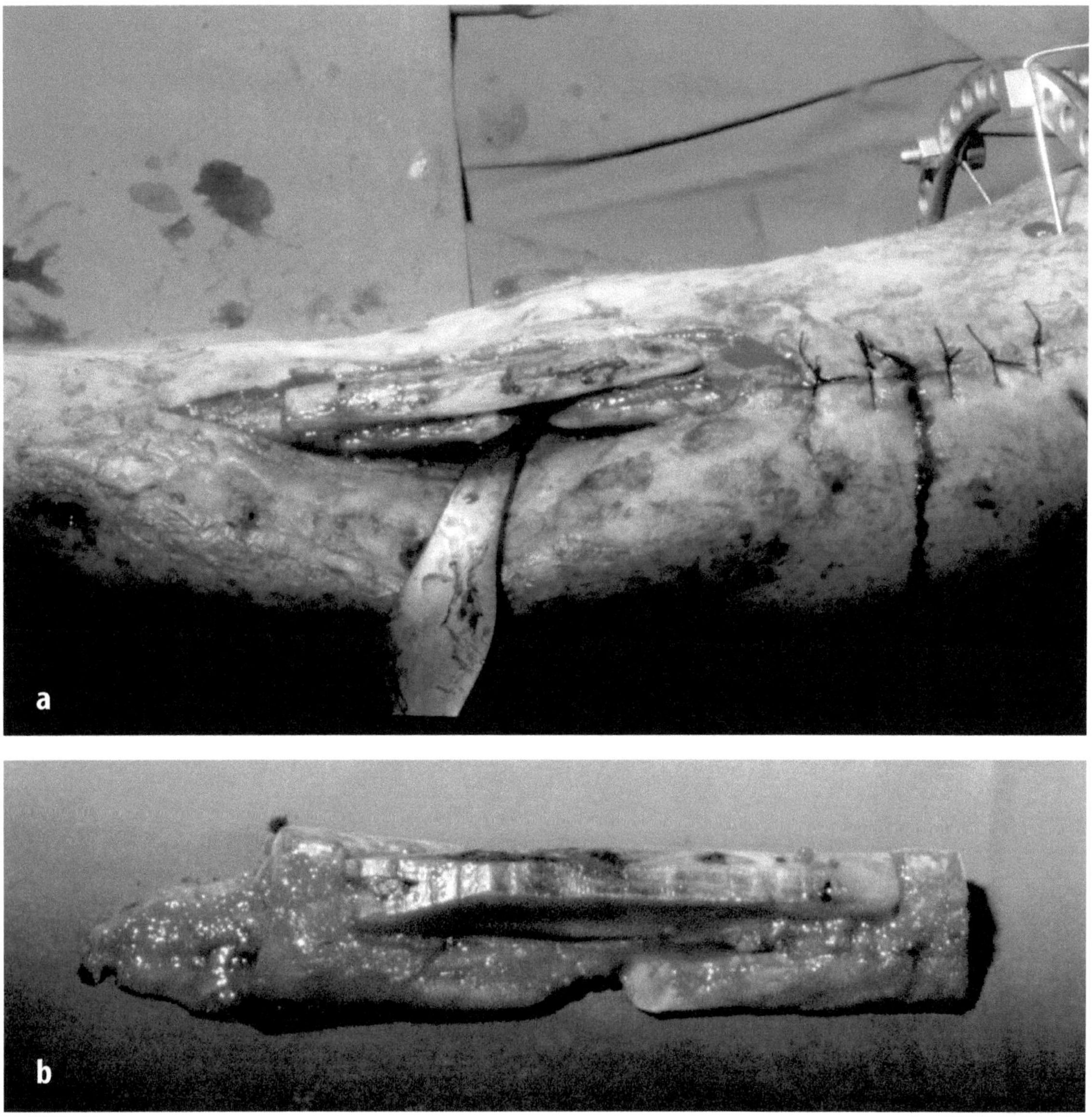

Fig. 18a, b. Same case as in Fig. 16. **a** Excision of the infected tibial segment (with the necrotic fibular graft) and the infected and necrotic soft tissues. **b** The resected bone (length: 15 cm)

Discussion

An optimally performed *débridement* is, in Gustilo's opinion [7], the most important part of the treatment of open fractures.

In the same way, the radical removal of the necrotic and infected parts of both bone and soft tissues represents the most important element for the success of treatment by compression-distraction technique in severe, infected nonunions of the tibia. This highly aggressive approach to the problem, which is reminiscent of the guidelines for state-of-the-art surgical therapy of bone tumors, is the key to understanding the effectiveness in the outcomes with these methods.

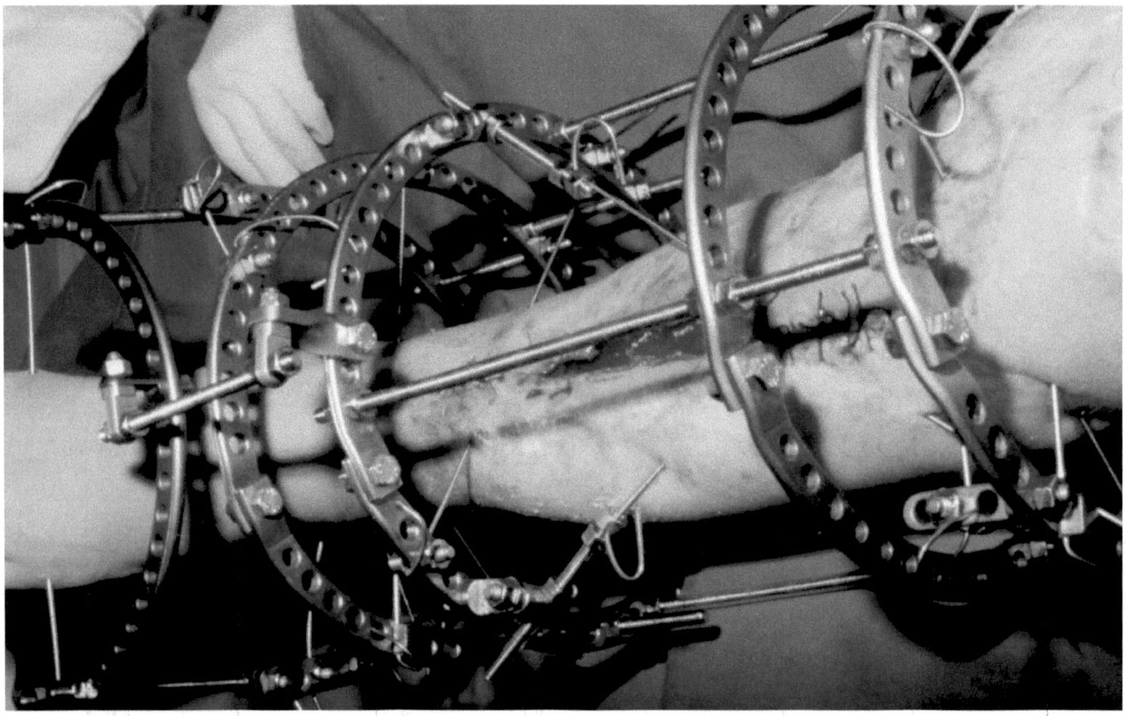

Fig. 19. Same case as in Fig. 16. The mounting of the compression-distraction apparatus is completed. The wound is kept open

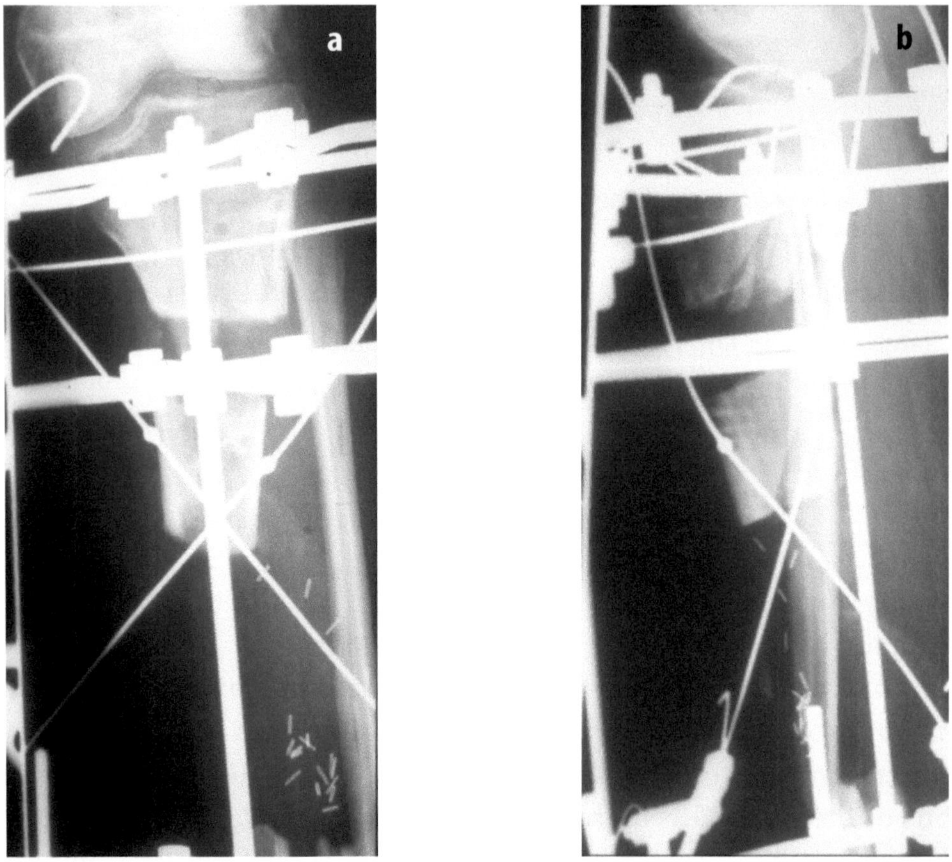

Fig. 20a, b. Same case as in Fig. 16. X-rays 30 days after the beginning of the bone and soft tissue transport

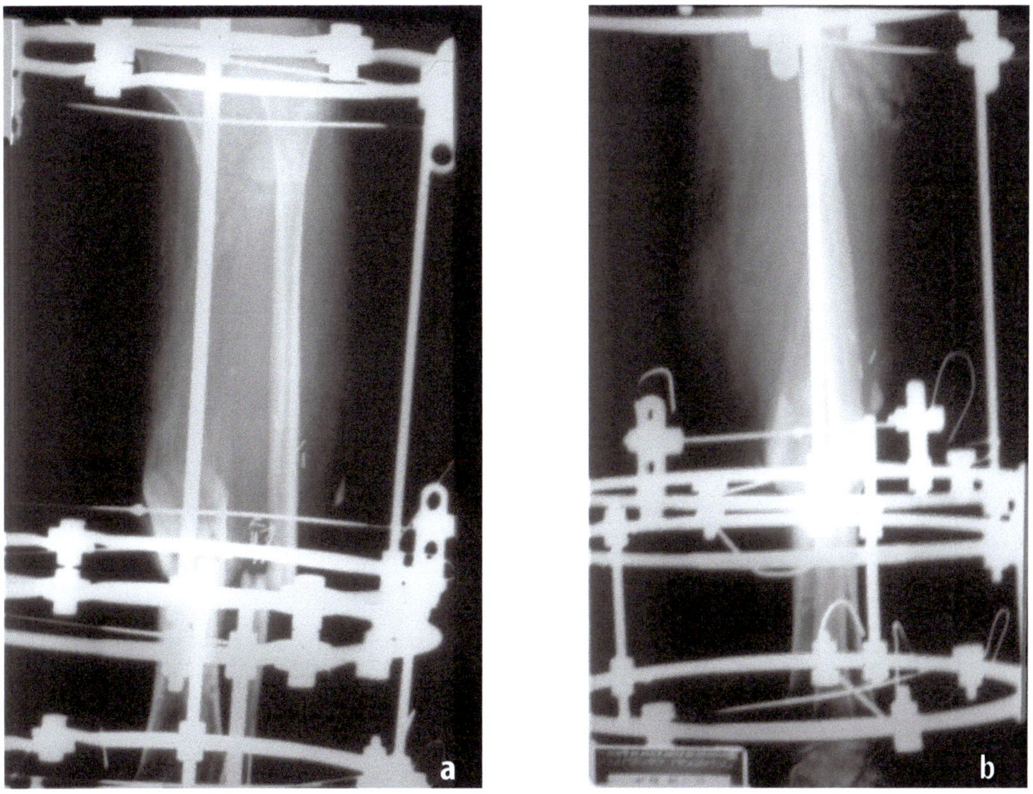

Figs. 21a, b. Same case as in Fig. 16. X-rays at the end of the transport

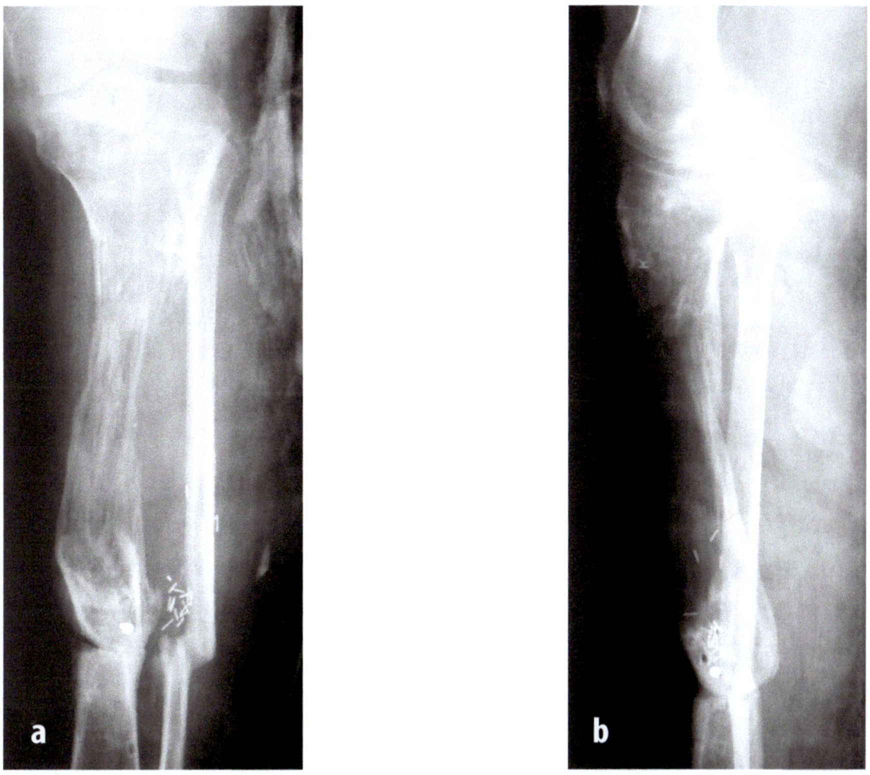

Fig. 22a, b. Same case as in Fig. 16. X-rays at the removal of the compression-distraction apparatus (after 14 months), with good proximal corticalization of the regenerating bone and callus formation at the docking site

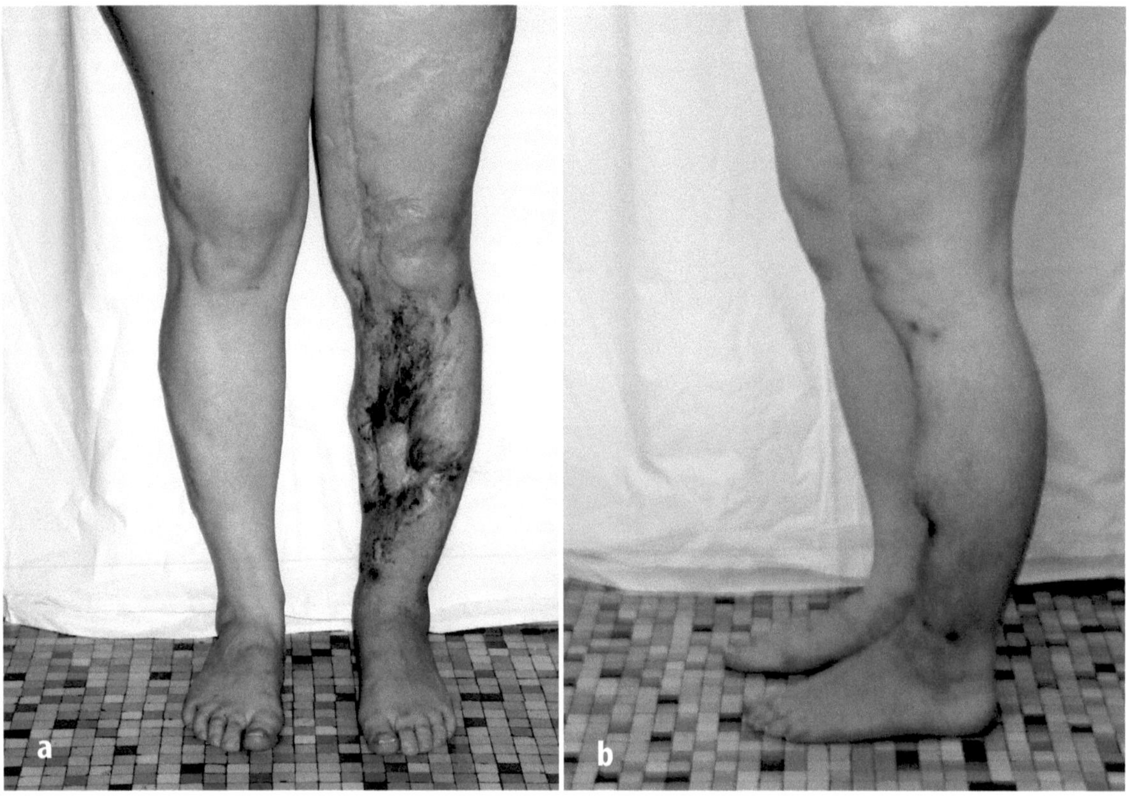

Fig. 23a, b. Same case as in Fig. 16. Clinical features at the end of treatment, with satisfactory soft tissue reconstruction

It is evident that only with the development of gradual distraction techniques and the knowledge of distraction osteogenesis can extremely large resections be performed (up to 18 cm in a patient treated at the Department of Orthopaedics and Traumatology of the University of Pavia), reasonably assuming that the large bone segments will gradually be regenerated through a metaphyseal corticotomy and further distraction. Many Authors limit the bone resection to 3–12 cm, over which a reconstructive technique should not be performed (as reported by Prokuski and Marsh [5]), but we disagree with this opinion.

Since it is a particular form of compression-distraction osteosynthesis, the osteotomy produces a significant improvement in vascularization in all the bone segments and has a stimulating effect on the dystrophic soft tissue even in such cases. The overall treatment time is prolonged and directly depends on the width of the resection. It was quite surprising, though, that in almost all cases, patients well tolerated the fixator over the entire treatment period, while maintaining good joint function.

This is one of the main arguments in support of employing the circular external fixation systems rather than the axial fixators. Actually, the stability of the circular external device allows weight bearing on the operated limb from the first few days after the operation. Furthermore, during the entire treatment period, the fragment positions can be easily modified according to therapeutic needs.

With regard to the tolerability, morbidity of soft tissues is low, even in cases of bone transport over many centimeters, which is possible with the oblique wires; however, the use of transverse screws, which is necessary when axial fixators are employed, produces deep lesions in soft tissues during the transport.

These advantages are obtained not only by using the Ilizarov system, but with all external circular fixation systems. Umiarov himself performed epidermatofascialosteoplasty in more than 300 patients using the Volkov-Oganesian circular external device [32].

An alternative to this method is represented by the compression-distraction osteosynthesis with "acute shortening" of the bone segment (to get close and compress the fragment immediately) and further lengthening by means of a distractional corticotomy [5, 33–36]. In our opinion this technique produces satisfactory results but has some disadvantages, related to the negative psychological effect on the patient, the possible limitations of articular function, difficulty walking in the early stages of treatment, and the possible damage to soft tissue produced by a shortening of many centimeters.

The multilevel bone transport technique, suggested by Moussa [36] and cited by Paley [18] as "ipsilateral" compression-distraction osteosynthesis, is very smart and aims to obtain "multiple" simultaneous distractions by dividing the fragment into many parts in order to shorten the treatment period. The assembly is very complex, due to the multiple transfixion areas of the soft tissues, but seems to be surprisingly well tolerated by the patient (the patient must be highly motivated and selected for this kind of treatment).

Finally, some other methods employed to shorten the treatment period have been described: docking site stimulation with autoplastic spongy bone graft, bone marrow injections, decortication, association with internal osteosynthesis by intramedullary nailing, electric or magnetic stimulation, ultrasound stimulation, and use of bone growth stimulating factors (bone demineralized matrix, bone morphogenetic protein, and osteoblast cells cultures).

A strong opinion on the true effect of these stimulating techniques is premature, however, considering the few cases reported. The bifocal or multifocal osteosynthesis techniques are particularly complex and compelling for the patient and the surgical team. However, they are an effective option in the management of infected nonunions and, in experienced hands, provide results that previously were absolutely unthinkable.

References

1. Umiarov GA (1986) Classification of nonunions of the long bones complicated by infection and principles of treatment. Sborn Trud CITO 30:5–9
2. Mora R, Maccabruni A, Paparella F et al (1991) Classificazione e trattamento delle pseudoartrosi infette. Atti SERTOT 33:205–207
3. Mora R (2000) Tecniche di compressione-distrazione. Amplimedical, Milano
4. Ilizarov GA, Green SA (1992) Transosseous osteosynthesis. Springer, Berlin Heidelberg New York
5. Prokuski LI, Marsh JL (1994) Bone transport in acute trauma. Curr Orthop 8:152–157
6. Bonanni F, Rhodes M, Lucke JF (1993) The futility of predictive scoring of mangled lower extremities. J Trauma 34:99–104
7. Gustilo RB (1989) Orthopaedic infection. Diagnosis and treatment. Saunders, Philadelphia
8. Weiland AJ, Moore JR, Hotchkiss RN (1983) Soft tissue procedures for reconstruction of tibial shaft fractures. Clin Orthop Relat Res 178: 42–53
9. Daniel RK, Taylor G (1973) Distant transfer of an island flap by microvascular anastomoses. Plast Reconstr Surg 68:73–79
10. Perry CR (1999) Bone repair techniques, bone graft, and bone graft substitutes. Clin Orthop Relat Res 360:71–86
11. Papineau LJ (1973) L'excision-greffe avec fermeture retardée déliberée dans l'ostéomyélite chronique. Nouv Presse Med 2:2753–2755
12. Khaleel A, Pool RD (2001) Bone transport. Curr Orthop 15:229–237
13. Lewertowski J.M, Lenoble E, Goutallier D (1993) Comblement des pertes de substances complexes os-parties molles de jambe par corticotomie et régénération osseuse progressive sous fixateur externe d'Ilizarov. Rev Chir Orthop 79[Suppl]:141
14. Volkov M, Bizer V (1969) Homotransplantation of bone in pediatric orthopaedics. Meditsina, Moscow
15. Imamaliev AS (1975) Homoplasty of the articular ends of bones. Meditsina, Moscow
16. Cierny G (1990) Chronic osteomyelitis: results of treatment. AAOS Instr Course Lect 39:495–508
17. Paley D, Catagni M, Argnani F et al (1989) Ilizarov treatment of tibial nonunions with bone loss. Clin Orthop Relat Res 241:146–165
18. Paley D (1990) Treatment of tibial nonunions and bone loss with the Ilizarov technique. AAOS Instr Course Lect 39:185–197
19. Catagni M, Guerreschi F, Cattaneo R (1993) Treatment of chronic osteomyelitis using the method of Ilizarov. Intern J Orthop Trauma 3[Suppl]:92–95
20. Ilizarov GA, Kaplunov AG, Degtyarev VE et al (1972) Treatment of pseudoarthroses and ununited fractures, complicated by purulent infection, with the method of compression-distraction osteosynthesis. Ortop Travmatol Protez 33:4–11
21. Ilizarov GA, Ledyaev VI, Degtyarev VE (1973) Operative and bloodless methods of repairing defects of long bones in osteomyelitis. Vestn Khir 5:55–59
22. Rybacuk OI (1977) Treatment of defects of long bones by the method of compression-distraction. KNIITO, Kiev
23. Morandi M, Zembo MM, Ciotti M (1989) Infected tibial pseudoarthrosis. Orthopaedics 12:497–508
24. Umiarov GA (1982) Epidermato-fascial osteoplasty of tibial defects under conditions of purulent infection. Ortop Travmatol Protez 6:65–66
25. Umiarov GA (1984) Treatment of extensive wounds and bone defects of the tibia by redislocation of skin-fascial-bone transplant. Sborn Trud CITO 28:36–42

26. Umiarov GA (1984) Plastic repair of traumatic defects of the leg in suppurative infections. Khirurgiia 38:132–135
27. Umiarov GA (1985) Repositioning-elongation for infected post-traumatic leg defects. Adv Orthop Surg 9:58–62
28. Mora R, Soldini A, Raschellà F et al (1989) Le traitement des pseudoarthroses infectées du tibia selon la technique d'Umiarov. Z Unfallchir Vers 82:187–190
29. Mora R, Paparella F, Benazzo F et al (1995) Il trattamento delle pseudoartrosi infette di tibia con perdita di sostanza ossea e dei tessuti molli mediante epidermo-fascio-osteoplastica. Minerva Ortop Traumatol 46:453–455
30. Mora R, Pedrotti L, Benazzo F et al (1999) L'epidermo-fascio-osteoplastica nel trattamento delle gravi pseudoartrosi infette di gamba con perdita di sostanza ossea e delle parti molli. Giorn Ital Ortop Traumatol 25 [Suppl. 1]:389–394
31. The Medical Letter (1998) Profilassi antimicrobica in chirurgia. Ital Edition 27:1–6
32. Umiarov GA (1996) Personal communication
33. Sales de Gauzy J, Vidal H, Cahuzac JP (1993) Primary shortening followed by callus distraction for the treatment of a post-traumatic bone defect: case report. J Trauma
34. Sneddon DG (1996) Open tibial fractures treated with acute shortening and simultaneous lengthening. Proceedings of the International Congress on Advances in the Ilizarov Method. Houston (Texas)
35. Lowenberg D, Van der Reis W (1996) Acute shortening for tibia defects. When and where. Techn Orthop 11:210–215
36. Varsalona R (1999) La fissazione esterna ibrida. Proceedings Intern Meeting "Incontri di Traumatologia", Cortina d'Ampezzo
37. Moussa M (1989) Multilevel bone transport. Proceedings of the 3rd International Seminar on the Improvement of External Fixation Apparatus and Methods, Riga

Amputations and Prosthetic Fitting

REDENTO MORA, BARBARA BERTANI, LUISELLA PEDROTTI

Introduction

Bone loss of traumatic origin is more frequent at the lower limb and particularly at the leg, where it is usually associated with soft tissue loss. In these cases the possible therapeutic options must be accurately evaluated (reconstruction and amputation) according to the features of the patient and the lesion [1, 2]. Furthermore, all the alternatives must be explained to the patient before the final decision is madc [3].

Patient features that may suggest amputation are principally: old age, chronic diseases such as diabetes and peripheral arteriopathy, vascular diseases caused by smoking, and inability of the patient to collaborate in the reconstructive program. Features of the lesion that may indicate amputation are represented by: damage of the posterior tibial nerve, injury of the ipsilateral foot, severe vascular lesion, and a severely contaminated lesion.

Various scoring systems were developed in the last few years in order to help in decision making (Mangled Extremity Syndrome Index, Mangled Extremity Severity Score, Predictive Salvage Index, and Limb Salvage Index). However, they did not prove to be practical for clinical application [4, 5].

An amputation may be the only alternative when reconstruction has failed (or is impossible), when the functional result of a reconstruction will probably be poor [6], or when the danger of major operations in elderly patients is too high [3].

It is important to mention that post-traumatic amputations are carried out most frequently in younger adults, while in the 50-to-75-year age group amputations are more related to peripheral vascular diseases.

Concerning the amputation site, it was calculated that approximately 85% of all amputations are performed through the lower limbs [3]. Therefore, considerations expressed in this chapter will deal mainly with amputation and prosthetic fitting of lower limbs.

Amputation Site

Thanks to today's construction technologies, the amputation site has become less important than in the past, and it is now determined by surgical considerations. Historically, amputation levels at the lower limb can be classified [7] as outlined in Table 1.

Table 1. Classification of amputation levels at the lower limb

Amputation site	Levels				
Hip disarticulation					
Thigh amputations	Very short A/K	Short A/K	Medium A/K	Long A/K	Very long A/K
Knee Disarticulation					
Leg amputations	Very short B/K	Short B/K	Medium B/K	Long B/K	
Ankle amputations	Syme amputation	Boyd amputation			

Evaluation Before Prosthetic Fitting

After amputation, a careful evaluation of the general and local clinical features helps decide which kind of prosthesis is the most appropriate for that patient to achieve the highest level of autonomy and the most complete integration into the familial and social network, and to set a specific rehabilitation program that is planned by a team composed of the orthopaedic surgeon, psychologist, technician, and physiotherapist. This evaluation is essentially based on three elements: the patient's general condition, the condition of the stump, and the condition of the opposite limb [8].

Patient's General Condition

Evaluation of the patient's general condition is mandatory to obtain detailed information on problems that may obstruct or impede rehabilitation. This includes information about limited physical resources and impaired function of one or both upper limbs. Concerning the former problem, it is important that the prosthesis be light and safe during ambulation (to reduce as much as possible the mental effort in using it and to avoid falling).

Concerning the latter problem, an impaired function of the upper limbs (caused by trauma or chronic disease) can make rehabilitation difficult.

Condition of the Stump

A preprosthetic treatment must sometimes be planned in order to maintain or improve the articular, muscular, and cutaneous situation and to regularize the stump itself. Moreover, the choice of the most appropriate socket for the prosthesis is fundamental.

An optimal stump should have these features: good articular range of movement, good muscle trophism, good skin condition, efficient blood and lymphatic circulation, and absence of pain. Another fundamental element is the stump length, which determines the choice of prosthesis and the type of socket.

In thigh amputations a distal rather than a proximal amputation site is desirable, and the bone stump should be well covered by soft tissue, without tension. At the leg site, in transtibial amputations, the ideal level is 12–24 cm from the knee joint. The minimum utilizable stump length is 4 cm, provided that the patellar tendon insertion is preserved.

Condition of the Opposite Limb

The opposite lower limb provides fundamental support for a limb with a prosthesis. Therefore, its condition is important to define the duration and the methods to be used in the rehabilitation program. These are determined by a number of circumstances (presence of fractures or nonunion, joint diseases, and neurological diseases such as diabetic neuropathy or sequelae of ictus cerebri).

Prostheses

The Evolution of Prostheses

The technological evolution of prostheses for the lower limb was slow. Until the end of the 1970s, prostheses were built almost exclusively by the exoskeletal method, also called the "traditional" method, since most components were made of wood. It is interesting to remember that, in the same period, electromechanical prostheses with myoelectric control were already available for the upper limbs.

Only since the 1980s, with the development of new and sophisticated materials (aluminium alloys, titanium alloys, and carbon fibers) and components with functional features and thanks to the integration of electronics, was it possible to significantly improve the performance of prostheses, built with the so-called endoskeletal (or skeletal-modular) method. Therefore, modern prostheses enable recovery of both the function and autonomy damaged by amputation significantly better than in the past.

Features of Prosthesis Manufacturing

Prostheses for the upper limb can be classified as follows: passive prostheses (e.g., cosmetic hands), lightweight and simple to use, and active prostheses.

There are three kinds of active prostheses: myoelectric prostheses, activated by electric signals produced by muscular contraction; kinematic prostheses, activated by bodily energy; and hybrid prostheses, which combine a myoelectric control of the hand function and a kinematic control of the elbow function.

The main components of a prosthesis for the lower limb are: socket, liner (interface between the skin and the socket), knee (in prostheses for tight amputation), adapters, feet, and cosmetic finishing [9]. Lower limb prostheses are built in two different ways, as previously underlined: the exoskeletal (or traditional) method and the endoskeletal (or skeletal-modular) method. The exoskeletal method has now almost been completely abandoned. This kind of prosthesis is strong, lasting, and requires little maintenance but it cannot generally satisfy the functional needs of patients today. The endoskeletal method is the method mainly employed currently. The prosthesis has a carrying structure, inserted between socket and prosthesic feet. Moreover, it has an adjustable alignment system at the knee and foot level.

Prosthetic knees are classified on the basis of the mechanical or electronic control of flexion and extension. Knees with mechanical control have some limitations because they require continuous control by the patient. This kind of knee may be monofunctionally articulated (polycentric or friction-driven), monofunctional with a manual locking device, or polyfunctional (polycentric or friction-driven), with higher speed and safety. In prosthetic knees with electronic control, the device that generates the movement is controlled by a microchip. This kind of knee offers higher performance than a mechanical knee with regard to speed and safety.

Two kinds of prosthetic feet can be produced: rigid (without energy return) and dynamic (with energy return).

Thank to these innovations, the components of prostheses can be assembled quickly, they are modular (providing easy interchangeability of the modules, and mainly of the articulations), the components can be easily aligned to obtain the best setting, they are light, and a wide range of components are built in different materials.

Particular prosthesis types are:

- Junior prostheses, which can be employed from 10-12 months of age and must be periodically replaced due to growth (on average every 8–10 months).
- Geriatric prostheses, characterized by lightness and safety, due to the poor physical resources and the frequent coexistence of collateral diseases in these patients.
- Bath prostheses, fit for immersion into water. These are endoskeletal prostheses provided with a "filling tank", which can be filled with water or emptied through two holes in the upper portion and in the lower portion.

Rehabilitation Program

A fundamental component of this kind of treatment is rehabilitation, which aims to recover an adequate ambulation in a physiological way. The rehabilitation program is planned in two steps: the preprosthetic treatment and training to use the prosthesis.

The preprosthetic treatment must be started as soon as possible and includes: contracture prevention, stump handwraps (to reduce the postoperative edema), physiotherapy (including respiratory gymnastics, upper limb reinforcement, healthy limb physiotherapy, and stump physiotherapy).

Training to use the prosthesis is composed of a starting phase of exercises while waiting for the prosthesis to be delivered and a second phase of learning the right technique to wear it. The next steps include assisted ambulation with a walking device, nonassisted ambulation with a walking device, ambulation with two crutches, ambulation with one crutch, and free ambulation.

References

1. Prokuski LL, Marsh JL (1994) Bone transport in acute trauma. Curr Orthop 8:152–157
2. Mora R, Pedrotti L, Bertani B, Tuvo G (2003) Le perdite di sostanza ossea nel traumatizzato. Proceedings of the 16th Congress OTODI, Vieste
3. Crenshaw AH (1987) Delayed union and non-union of fractures. In: Crenshaw AH (ed) Campbell's Operative Orthopaedics, 7th edn. Mosby, St. Louis
4. Bonanni F, Rhodes M, Lucke JF (1993) The futility of predictive scoring of mangled lower extremities. J Trauma 34:99–104
5. Mora R (1998) Fissazione esterna: metodiche chirurgiche nel trattamento delle fratture esposte. Inquadramento e classificazione. Proceedings of the 9th Congress CIOD, Capri

6. Hulnick A, Highsmith C, Boutin FJ (1949) Amputations for failure in reconstructive surgery. J Bone Joint Surg Am 31:639–647
7. Wilson AB Jr (1967) Classification of amputations by level. Artif Limbs 2:1–16
8. Verni G, Ammaccapane A (2003) La protesizzazione delle amputazioni della gamba. Tecnica Ortop Intern 63:13–27
9. Ossur Prosthetic Product Catalog (2005). Ossur, Reykjavik

Antibiotic Therapy

Anna Maccabruni, Redento Mora

Introduction

The aim of appropriate treatment for chronic osteomyelitis is not only to heal the infection and prevent any possible relapse, but also to restore satisfactory vascularization and viability in the surrounding tissues and functional recovery of the limb.

First surgical treatment is required to completely excise the sinus tract and remove necrotic bone tissue (both superficial and next to the medullary canal) and the infected soft tissues [1–5]. The goal of surgery is to keep only healthy and viable tissues around the primary site of infection; necrotic tissues should be excised until the bone bleeds (so-called "paprika sign") [2, 6].

When infection affects a wide area, local *débridement* creates a large bone defect, called "dead space", which, due to the poor vascularization, represents an optimal site for infection persistence and development; moreover, it compromises the stability of the entire bone segment. Therefore, appropriate medical and surgical management of the "dead space" is mandatory to stop the infection and restore the bone integrity [7].

Antibiotic Therapy

In a non-negligible rate of cases, the cultures of material aspirated from the sinus tract do not offer reliable information about the microorganisms actually responsible for the bone infection (owing to the frequent risk of contamination from skin saprophytic bacteria). Thus, it is very important that cultures are prepared from biological specimens collected from deep inside the infected site during the operation in order to more clearly identify the pathogens and to test the drug sensitivity of the isolated colonies [8, 9].

At the time of surgery, it is useful to start an antibiotic therapy with cephalosporins (usually effective against gram-positive and many gram-negative bacteria, except for *Pseudomonas aeruginosa*) and continue this until the culture results are available.

The definitive antibiotic therapy is then based on the results of the culture and antibiograms of the isolated pathogens, according to the available data concerning drug toxicity, tissue kinetics, and bone antibiotic levels (Table 1).

Table 1. Antibiotic diffusion in the bone tissue

Good	Fair	Poor
Rifampin	Cephalosporins	Penicillins
Macrolides	Phosphomycins	Aminoglycosides
Lincosamides	Carbapenems	
- Lincomycin	- Imipenem	
- Clindamycin	- Meropenem	
Fluoroquinolones		
Glycopeptides		
- Vancomycin		
- Teicoplanin		

It has been demonstrated that the highest ratio between bone and serum concentrations is obtained with the administration of clindamycin; subsequently, nafcillin and oxacillin, among the semi-synthetic penicillins, and cephalothin and cefamandole, among the cephalosporins, should be given; then vancomycin, teicoplanin, rifampin, trimethoprim-sulfamethoxazole, and gentamicin follow [10]. The antibiotic or antibiotics chosen (whose combination should exploit their synergistic properties) should be administered at the highest therapeutic doses for not less than 4–6 weeks.

The average duration of antibiotic therapy as established by *in vivo* studies for revascularization of bone tissue after surgical *débridement* is almost 4 weeks. Longer treatment periods (6 months or more) through both intravenous and oral administration did not prove to be more effective for either infection healing or reducing relapses rates [11, 12].

Drugs should be administered intravenously in the first weeks to obtain high concentrations as soon as possible in tissues that are still damaged and to limit further spread of infection.

Among the bacteria, staphylococci are the most common. They are characterized by the ability to express, once they come in contact with proteinous bone components, specific membrane receptors (adhesins) with which they bind to bone and cartilaginous tissues [13].

Another important element in staphylococcal osteomyelitis development is the formation of the glycocalyx, a thin membrane able to encapsulate bacterial colonies and defend them from the phagocytic host response and from the action of most antibiotics [14, 15].

Staphylococci, as well as other pathogens, can elude the defensive response by the host, entering osteoblasts and osteocytes. Here they can survive for long periods, adapting their metabolism as needed. In this regard, it has been recently demonstrated, by means of several *in vitro* experiments, that necrotic osteoblasts could release *S. aureus* that was still alive and able to infect other cells.

Today, the most common problem in the management of chronic staphylococcal osteomyelitis is *S. aureus* methicillin resistance (MRSA), whose biochemical basis is the presence of a penicillin-binding protein with low affinity to beta-lactamic antibiotics inside the pathogens.

Data concerning MRSA rates are cause for considerable concern: whereas these rates are quite low in Northern European countries (0.1% in Denmark, 5% in Germany), in Central and Southern Europe they are much higher (30% in France, 33% in Spain, 34% in Italy). Even more significant results come from MRSA rates related to colonies of coagulase-negative staphylococci.

In clinical practice, bacterial methicillin resistance is a cross resistance to all beta-lactamic derivates; therefore, antibiotic therapy in staphylococcal bone infection should be based, as first choice, on glycopeptides. They have proven to be highly effective against almost all gram-positive aerobic pathogens. Among these, vancomycin (which can be administered intravenously at a dosage of 1 g every 12 h) represents the drug of choice [16]; among the possible side effects are phlebitis at the site of infusion and flushing of the face, neck, and thorax, with burning pain (so-called "red man syndrome"), which is more common after fast drug infusion and probably due to histamine release associated with local hyperosmolarity rather than representing a real intolerance reaction.

The presence of macular-papular or erythematous eruptions on the skin, due to drug hypersensitivity and which is reversible after administering antihistaminic or steroid drugs, is described in 4%–5% of cases [16].

An important adverse reaction to vancomycin is neurotoxicity, which is manifested by a permanent auditory nerve damage with hearing loss.

Nephrotoxicity was relatively common in the past, due to the use of unpurified drug preparations, but is now uncommon; however, renal function must be accurately monitored during the vancomycin treatment, especially if other nephrotoxic drugs are used at the same time.

In cases of vancomycin intolerance, teicoplanin is the most effective alternative; its antimicrobic range and mechanism of action are similar to that of vancomycin; however, it is distinguished by the low toxicity and the very prolonged half-life time, which allows once-daily administration.

In the treatment of chronic osteomyelitis, teicoplanin is usually administered at a dose of 400 mg/day (400 mg every 12 h in the first day).

In recent years, linezolid, a bacteriostatic synthetic antibiotic of the Oxazolidinones class, has proven to be effective (at a dose of 500 mg twice daily intravenously) in serious infections by Gram-positive pathogens (MRSA colonies, coagulase-negative staphylococci, and penicillin-resistant *S. pneumoniae*). Linezolid can reach a very high concentration in lung parenchyma, skin, and soft tissues. Although data concerning its use in chronic osteomyelitis are still limited, it might represent an effective therapeutic tool in bone and joint infections caused by multi-resistant staphylococci [17].

For the medical management of the less common chronic osteomyelitis caused by penicillin-susceptible *S. aureus*, the antibiotic of choice should first be penicillin G (at a dosage of 4,000,000 I.U. every 6 h); alternatively first-generation cephalosporins (cefazolin at a dosage of 2 g every 6 h; cephalothin at a dosage of 1 g every 6 h; cephalotin at a dosage of 1g every 6 h until 1–2 g every 4 h in most severe infections), clindamyicin (at a dosage of 600 mg every 6 h), or vancomycin (at a dosage of 1 g every 12 h) could be used.

When beta-lactamase producing staphylococcal colonies (penicillin G resistant) are present, semi-synthetic, hydrolysis-resistant penicillins must be given (among these: nafcillin – not available in Europe – at a dosage of 1–1.5 g every 4-6 h, or flucloxacillin – which belongs to isoxazolyl penicillin –); alternatively, a first-generation cephalosporin can be employed.

The therapeutic approach to bone and joint infections caused by streptococci (usually beta hemolytic streptococci of groups A and B, and pneumococci) is still based on penicillin G; available alternative choices are clindamyicin and macrolides (erythromycin at a dosage of 500 mg every 6 h) or vancomycin.

Second-generation quinolones (ciprofloxacin and ofloxacin) usually are not very effective in streptococcal infections, which are susceptible to third-generation levofloxacin or fourth-generation trovafloxacin, characterized by high efficacy even against anerobes [18].

Among the gram-negative pathogens most commonly involved in chronic osteomyelitis, *Haemophilus influenzae*, Enterobacteriaceae (*Escherichia coli, Klebsiella, Enterobacter, Proteus, Serratia*), and *Pseudomonas aeruginosa* are predominant.

Infections by Enterobacteriacee can be successfully treated with quinolones (ciprofloxacin at initial dosage of 400–750 mg every 12 h intravenously) or third-generation cephalosporins (ceftriaxone at a dosage of 2 g daily; cefepime at a dosage of 2 g every 12 h).

After intravenous administration, ceftriaxone reaches very high serum levels and reaches the bone tissue in 10%–20% of serum concentration; the long half-life in serum and bone allows the dosage schemes of only once-daily administration to be adopted, which can be easily be followed by patients even at home.

As for *Pseudomonas aeruginosa* osteomyelitis, the susceptibility of these microorganisms to antibiotics is extremely unpredictable, even if limited, and should be evaluated on a case-by-case basis: an appropriate therapeutic approach should be based on ceftazidime (at a dosage of 2 g every 8 h) associated with an aminoglycoside (in single or multiple daily administration) for the first 2 weeks of treatment.

Imipenem (at a dosage of 500 mg every 6 h); a combination of piperacillin (at a dosage of 4 g every 8 h) and tazobactam (at a dosage of 500 mg every 8 h); or a combination of cefepime and aminoglycosides (for the first two weeks of treatment) can represent a good therapeutic choice [19]. Gram-negative anaerobic pathogens (mainly *Bacteroides fragilis*) play a very important role in bone and joint infections associated with conditions of poor vascularization or located close to bedsores or deep diabetic ulcers.

The most effective antibiotics against these pathogens are clindamycin (at a dosage of 600 mg every 6 h), a combination of amoxicillin and clavulanic acid (at a dosage of 2 g every 8 h), or metronidazole (at a dosage of 500 mg every 8 h).

Management of the "Dead Space"

As already emphasized, an adequate therapeutic approach to chronic osteomyelitis should include, alongside systemic antibiotic therapy, sterilization of the dead spaces created during the surgical *débridement* of the infected site.

To this aim it is possible to install locally slowly releasing devices containing antibiotics [20–25].

The choice of antibiotic depends on formulation, *in vitro* activity against the isolated pathogen, and stability at high temperatures: aminoglycosides (gentamicin and tobramicin) are the most widely employed antibiotics, because of their high resistance to heat; other available drugs are cefazolin, vancomycin, ciprofloxacin, and clindamycin [20].

The highest peak in drug release is obtained in the first 24 h after implantation and is maintained for about 28 days (1 week in the case of vancomycin); at the end of this period the device must be removed.

The first nonbiodegradable material used as a delivery vehicle for depot antibiotics was gentamicin-loaded PMMA (polymethylmethacrylate), available both as amorphous material or pearls, named Palacos and Septopal, respectively). Here, it is possible to obtain high antibiotic levels in the bone tissue independently of the vascularization grade of the tissue itself.

An important limitation in using such material is represented by the pathogen's susceptibility to gentamicin; moreover, since the nonbiodegradable device must be removed after some weeks, further hospitalization for a secondary procedure is required.

To eliminate these problems, alternative biodegradable materials for delivery of depot antibiotics have been evaluated, including protein-based materials, bone graft materials and substitutes, and synthetic polymers.

Protein-based materials are made of collagen sponge (composed of tendinous tissue of bovine origin, sterilized, and incubated with gentamicin) that releases the drug during collagen degradation by macrophage collagenase, offering a bone drug concentration that is higher but not as lasting as that obtainable with PMMA.

Ceramic hydroxyapatite pearls impregnated with gentamicin are an interesting kind of bone graft substitute. They are not only an antibiotic reserve but even represent a source of calcium, which can be used during the healing process; because the hydroxyapatite is gradually replaced by the new bone, using these kinds of implants avoids further reconstructive operations.

Among the biodegradable synthetic polymers, which allow an optimal antibiotic release, are the lactic acid synthetic polymers in the shape of pearls made of polylactide, polyglycolide, or poly-DL-lactide. Polymers of a higher molecular weight, usually combined with quinolones, release higher drug dosages, favoring very high concentration rates compared to minimal inhibitory concentration (MIC), and degrade in about 30 days.

In cases in which the osteomyelitic site is small and the bone defect is limited, it is possible to implant computerized micropumps for direct delivery of antibiotics (clindamycin and amikacin) into dead spaces, for periods lasting from 3 to 7 months [21, 22].

A particular situation is that of atrophic, infected bone nonunions and loss of soft tissue treated with the compression-distraction techniques. In these cases, in fact, the dead space created by the radical resection of the necrotic and infected bone tissue is gradually filled by the formation of new bone through the methods of bifocal or plurifocal osteosynthesis, without the need for bone grafts.

Moreover, because it is a radical resection in "oncologic way" which leads to infection eradication with consequent sterilization of the dead space, there is no need for prolonged antibiotic treatments.

Hyperbaric Therapy

Hyperbaric therapy is a useful complement to medical therapy in chronic osteomyelitis, mainly in patients already surgically treated and suffering relapse in spite of repeated antibiotic therapies [26]. The results of many clinical studies demonstrate that, in a high number of cases of infected osteomyelitis refractory to other types of treatment, the hyperbaric therapy was decisive. Therefore, it is difficult to precisely define the role this kind of treatment plays in chronic osteomyelitis management, since the result in each case strictly depends on variables involving not only the patient's general condition and the kind of surgery performed, but also vascularization of the bone segment and how aggressive the pathogen is and how susceptible it is to the drug [27]).

In experimentally infected animal models, hyperbaric therapy has been shown to be able to heal medullary infections by *Staphylococcus aureus*, probably through the elevation and restoration of oxygen tension at the medullary canal site and therefore as a result of an improvement in physiologic phagocytotic mechanisms [28].

Even infections by anerobes and microaerophilic pathogens (which do not have enzyme patterns such as superoxide-dismutase and catalase, indispensable in the degradation of toxic process by oxygen radical) can profit from oxygen therapy; in particular an improvement in local oxygen pressure can promote healing of *Clostridium perfrigens* infection, improving phagocytotic mechanisms at the PMN leukocyte level.

In animal experimental trials it has also been demonstrated that hyperbaric therapy employed simultaneously with antibiotic treatment in chronic osteomyelitis by *Pseudomonas aeruginosa* can improve the effectiveness of antibiotic drugs such as aminoglycosides, vancomycin, and quinolones, whose activity is reduced in conditions of low oxygen tension as occurs in long-standing bone infections [29].

Bone healing mechanisms are accelerated by oxygen treatment with 100% oxygen at 2–3 atmospheres, administered 1–2 h per a day.

If oxygen tension in bone is maintained below these values (as occurs during osteomyelitis), fibroblast, osteoblast, osteoclast, and macrophage activity are reduced and tissue reconstruction is delayed; in contrast, prolonged exposure to a too-high oxygen pressure produces a functional acceleration in fibroblast function, which results in deposition of thick but structurally weak collagen tissue [30].

References

1. Clerny G, Mader JT (1983) The surgical treatment of adult osteomyelitis. In: Evarts CMC (ed) Surgery of the musculoskeletal system. Churchill Livingstone, New York, pp 15–35
2. Clerny G (1990) Chronic osteomyelitis: results of treatment. AAOS Instr Course Lect 39:495–508
3. Lazzarini L, Mader JT, Calhoun JH (2004) Osteomyelitis in long bones. J Bone Joint Surg Am 86:2305–2318
4. Lew DP, Waldwogel FA (2004) Osteomyelitis. Lancet 364:369–379
5. Parsone B, Strass E (2004) Surgical management of chronic osteomyelitis. Am J Surgery 188[Suppl]:57–66
6. Simpson AH, Deakin M, Latham JM (2001) Chronic osteomyelitis.The effect of the extent of surgical resection on infection-free survival. J Bone Joint Surg Br 83:403–407
7. Mader JT, Ortiz M, Calhoun JH (1996) Update on the diagnosis and management of osteomyelitis. Clin Pediatr Med Surg 13:701–724
8. Mackowiak PA, Jones SR, Smith JW (1978) Diagnostic value of sinus tract cultures in chronic osteomyelitis. JAMA 239:2772–2775
9. Perry CR, Pearson LR, Miller GA (1991) Accuracy of cultures of material from swabbing of the superficial aspect of the wound and needle biopsy in the preoperative assessment of osteomyelitis. J Bone Joint Surg Am 73:745–749
10. Boselli E, Allaouchiche B (1999) Diffusion osseuse des antibiotiques. La Presse Med 40:2265–2276
11. Hedstrom SA (1974) The prognosis of chronic staphylococcal osteomyelitis after long-term antibiotic treatment. Scand J Infect Dis 6:35–83
12. Mader JT, Shirtliff ME, Bergquist SC, Calhoun J (1999) Antimicrobial treatment of chronic osteomyelitis. Clin Orthop Relat Res 360:47–65
13. Johansson A, Fleck JL, Svensson O (2001) Collagen and fibronectin binding in experimental staphylococcal osteomyelitis. Clin Orthop Relat Res 382:241–246
14. Mayberry-Carson KJ, Tober-Meyer B, Smith JK et al (1984) Bacterial adherence and glycocalix formation in osteomyelitis experimentally induced with Staphylococcus aureus. Infect Immun 43:825–833
15. Ellington JK, Harris M, Webb L et al (2003) Intracellular Staphylococcus aureus. A mechanism for the indolence of osteomyelitis. J Bone Joint Surg Br 85:918–921
16. Watanakunakorn C (1982) Treatment of infections due to methicillin-resistant Staphilococcus aureus. Ann Intern Med 97:376–378
17. Rayner CR, Baddour LM, Birmingham MC et al (2004) Linezolid in the treatment of osteomyelitis: results of compassionate use experience. Infection 32:8–14
18. Ernst ME, Ernst EJ, Klepser ME (1997) Levofloxacin and Trovafloxacin: the new generation of fluoroquinolones? Am J Health Syst Pharm 54:2569–2584
19. Stengel D, Bauwens K, Sehouli J et al (2001) Systematic review and meta-analysis of antibiotic therapy for bone and joint infection. Lancet Infect Dis 1:175–188
20. Wininger DA, Fass RJ (1996) Antibiotic-impregnated cement and beads for orthopaedics infections. Antimicr Agents and Chemother 40:2675–2679
21. Perry CR, Pearson RL (1991) Local antibiotic delivery in the treatment of bone and joint infections. Clin Orthop Relat Res 263:215–226
22. Perry CR, Davenport K, Vossen MK (1988) Local delivery of antibiotics via an implantable pump in the treatment of osteomyelitis. Clin Orthop Relat Res 226:222–230

23. Nelson CL (2004) The current status of material used for depot delivery of drugs. Clin Orthop Relat Res 427:72–78
24. Zalavras CG, Patzakis MJ, Holtom P (2004) Local antibiotic therapy in the treatment of open fractures and osteomyelitis. Clin Orthop Relat Res 427:86–93
25. McLaren AC (2004) Alternative materials to acrylic bone cement for delivery of depot antibiotics in orthopaedic infections. Clin Orthop Relat Res 427:101–106
26. Greensmith JE (2004) Hyperbaric oxygen therapy in extremity trauma. J Am Acad Orthop Surg 12:376–384
27. Davis JC, Heckman JD, DeLee JC et al (1986) Chronic non-hematogenous osteomyelitis treated with adjuvant hyperbaric oxygen. J Bone Joint Surg Am 68:1210–1217
28. Mader JT, Brown GL, Guckian JC et al (1980) A mechanism for the amelioration by hyperbaric oxygen of experimental staphylococcal osteomyelitis in rabbits. J Infect Dis 142:915–922
29. Mader JT, Adams KR, Sutton TE (1987) Infectious diseases: pathophysiology and mechanisms of hyperbaric oxygen. J Hyperbaric Med 2:133–140
30. Mainous EG (1982) Osteogenesis enhancement utilizing hyperbaric oxygen therapy. HBO Review 3:181–185

Rehabilitation

Luisella Pedrotti, Gabriella Tuvo, Barbara Bertani, Redento Mora

Introduction

Many patients successfully treated with circular external fixation for nonunions or infected nonunions continue to complain of limited joint function at the end of treatment [1–4]. Joint stiffness can affect both upper and lower limbs and quite frequently occurs in the knee after the application of a circular external fixator at the femur [5]. Knee stiffness frequently develops after femoral traumatology and can occur after a fracture of the femoral shaft has been treated conservatively or surgically or after a treatment for nonunions: it has been reported in 6.5% of cases treated with dynamic internal fixation [6], in 45% after axial external fixation [7], and in 27% of cases after circular external fixation [8].

Factors Leading to Joint Stiffness

The care of soft tissues is fundamental in order to avoid joint stiffness during a treatment with circular external fixation: any tension in the soft tissue caused by bone fixation elements, longitudinally and transversely, should be avoided. When tension is generated longitudinally, normal muscular contraction can be impaired, giving rise to local inflammation; when tension is applied transversely, the venous and lymphatic drainage can be affected, causing soft tissue edema that can aggravate the initial condition.

Joint stiffness is the result of intraarticular adherence, periarticular fibrous tissue, muscular contracture in patients treated with distraction osteogenesis [9]. All joint structures are progressively involved: bone, cartilage, synovium, capsule, and ligaments [10]. The muscular contracture is related to the tension induced by distraction (muscles that are more frequently involved are biarticular muscles, which cross two joints: sural triceps in leg lengthening and muscles of the posterior compartment of the thigh in femoral lengthening) and to transfixion of muscles, fascial plane, tendons, capsule, and ligaments by transosseous screws or wires [11].

Prevention and Treatment

When treating nonunions of long bones (by definition not an urgent treatment), it is crucial to plan a good rehabilitation program to minimize the side effects related to this technique. The correct prevention and treatment of joint stiffness should start before surgery and continue after the orthopaedic treatment: a specific rehabilitation protocol should be adapted to the individual case. Therefore, four rehabilitation phases can be identified: preoperative, operative, early postoperative, and late postoperative phases.

During the *preoperative phase* the patient should be carefully evaluated and at the same time the orthopaedic and rehabilitation staff should plan the treatment. This evaluation should take account of the patient's personality and his or her capability to tolerate the treatment: this aspect is frequently neglected but it is crucial in order to optimize the result of the treatment. These consultations should be conducted with the patient and his relatives with the aim of complete understanding of the advantages and disadvantages of the proposed treatment and the more frequently occurring complications, discomfort, expected duration, and characteristics of the rehabilitation plan. The orthopaedic staff should have a good knowledge of this type of treatment, enough time, and a high level of experience; moreover, the treatment should be given in close collaboration with the rehabilitation staff, who will care for the patient during and after the orthopaedic treatment. The rehabilitation treatment during the preoperative period includes active and passive exercises for muscular lengthening (stretching) with the aim of obtaining the maximum elasticity, combined with exercises to control muscular contraction and relaxation and exercises to strengthen the muscles.

During the *operative phase* (under the care of the orthopaedic staff), any maneuvers that can prevent or reduce, insofar as possible, joint stiffness (mainly at the knee, when an external fixator is applied at the femur) should be put into effect. The joint should be maintained in a correct position when screws and wires are applied near the joint (the fixation elements should be inserted through the flexor muscles with the knee in complete extension and through the extensors muscles with the knee flexed). Transfixion of muscular-tendineous-fascial structures and capsular-ligamentous structures should be avoided when the fixation elements are applied at the femur. Near the knee, three different types of fixation have been proposed other than classical fixation with two crossed wires in a transverse plane [12]: fixation with one screw in the coronal plane [13]; fixation with wires crossed in the coronal plane [14]; and fixation with two nontransfixing wires in the transverse plane, inserted obliquely from posterior to lateral and from posterior to medial [15]. The device should be assembled with screws and wires placed near the frontal plane of the limb, whereby placement of bone fixation elements crossing with an angle of more of 60° should be avoided, and using, when required, variants of the classical assembly ("nonstandard" configurations) in order to maximize the tolerability of the device and the patient's compliance, and to maintain stability.

During the *early postoperative phase* an active and passive mobilization associated with early load bearing and assisted ambulation (in case of nonunion of the femur or tibia) can reduce adherences and can improve the muscular strength. Light massages to reduce the pain and some vascular gymnastics to improve venous return and at the same time reduce the risk of thromboembolic adverse events are useful in this phase [16].

During the *late postoperative phase*, when knee or ankle contracture tends to evolve during the treatment, it is important to position elastic bands, an orthosis, or a rigid sole fixed with elastics to the external fixator itself. When distraction osteogenesis is planned, requiring at first a phase of gradual distraction (1 mm per day) and then a phase of bone consolidation and corticalization of the regenerating bone (that takes generally twice the time of the first phase), the main objective, when the treatment is performed at the femur, is to maintain normal motion of the knee, which tends to reduce its flexion and extension [16].

The rehabilitation treatment for joint mobilization and muscular strenghtening should be kept in place. Ambulation should be allowed at first with partial loading, using canes, and at the end, without any restrictions. Periodically, a dressing should be applied to the skin around screws or wires. Adherences or impalements of muscles, fascia, or tendons should be treated through joint mobilization to maintain a good motion of all these structures. To prevent or to treat the joint stiffness, several mechanical devices positioned at the affected segment can be used: Continuous Passive Motion (CPM) machines or dynamic splints such as "Dynasplint" that apply a constant strength during flexion and extension of the joint by means of an adjustable dynamometric springs [11].

After removal of the circular external fixator, having verified that the bone callus or the regenerating bone is healing well, rehabilitation treatment should be intensified with the aim of completely restoring the joint ROM, correcting postural deformities, and improving load bearing and ambulation. In very few cases, significant stiffness of the knee joint might persist. In these patients, a conservative treatment (passive mobilization) or surgical application of a dynamic fixator such as "Compass Universal Hinge System" (Smith

& Nephew) or "Stiff Elbow Fixator" (Orthofix) must be applied. Less frequently, the Judet procedure of arthromyolysis can be performed [5, 17].

Conclusion

Joint stiffness is quite common after the application of an external fixation device and can affect all joints to various degrees. In particular, knee stiffness is a frequent complication after circular external fixation for femoral nonunions, having a multifactorial cause, depending on the level at which the femoral nonunion occurs: soft tissue transfixion by screws and wires (causing a mechanical stiffness) and progressive muscular fibrosis. An appropriate kinesitherapy during the postoperative period, based on continuous cooperation between orthopaedic surgeons and physiotherapists, is crucial in order to maximize the functional result of the orthopaedic treatment.

References

1. Marsh DR, Shah S, Elliot J et al (1997) The Ilizarov method in non-union, malunion and infection of fractures. J Bone Joint Surg Br 79:273–279
2. Maini L, Chadha M, Vishwanath J et al (2000) The Ilizarov method in infected nonunions of fractures. Injury 31:509–517
3. Lerner RK, Esterhai JL, Polomano RC et al (1993) Quality of life assessment of patients with posttraumatic fracture nonunion, chronic refractory osteomyelitis, and lower extremity amputation. Clin Orthop Relat Res 295:28–36
4. Barker KL, Lamb SE, Simpson AH (2004) Functional recovery in patients with nonunion treated with the Ilizarov technique. J Bone Joint Surg Br 86:81–85
5. Mora R (2000) Tecniche di compressione-distrazione. Amplimedical, Milano
6. Mercuri M, Boriani S, Jure FD et al (1995) G.K. femore. Serie multicentrica con riferimento alle complicazioni. Atti del 6° Congresso CIOD, Sesto di Pusteria
7. Alonso JE, Geissler W, Hughes JL (1989) External fixation of femoral fractures. Clin Orthop Relat Res 241:83–88
8. Jacchia GE, Pavolini B, Ciampalini L et al (1993) Le fratture del terzo medio-inferiore di femore trattate con fissatori esterni. Atti del 24° Congresso OTODI, Cernobbio
9. Ceciliani L, Mora R, Di Castri U et al (1995) Fissazione esterna in traumatologia e rigidità. Giorn Ital Ortop Traumatol 21[Suppl. 1]:346–350
10. Akeson WH , Amiel D, Abel MF et al (1987) Effects of immobilization on joints. Clin Orthop Relat Res 219:28–37
11. Paley D (1991) Problems, obstacles and complications of limb lengthening. In: Bianchi Maiocchi A, Aronson J (eds) Operative principles of Ilizarov. Williams and Wilkins, Baltimore
12. Ilizarov GA, Green SA (1992) Transosseous osteosynthesis. Springer, Berlin Heidelberg New York
13. Volkov M, Oganesian O (1987) External fixation: joint deformities and bone fractures. International University Press, Madison
14. Pavolini B (1996) X crossing wires in the distal tibia. Techn Orthop 11:208–209

15. Herzenberg JE, Scheufele LL, Paley D et al (1994) Knee range of motion in isolated femoral lengthening. Clin Orthop Relat Res 301:49–54
16. Iorio L, Forte R, Spinelli R et al (1990) Problemi di riabilitazione. Giorn Ital Ortop Traumatol 16[Suppl. 1]:222–228
17. Ghisellini F, Ceffa R, Fortina A et al (1995) Trattamento della rigidità di ginocchio mediante artromiolisi secondo Judet. Giorn Ital Ortop Traumatol 21[Suppl. 1]:333–338

Prevention of Venous Thromboembolism

Luisella Pedrotti, Redento Mora, Giovanni Battista Galli, Gabriella Tuvo

Introduction

Venous thromboembolism (VTE), which can present clinically either as deep venous thrombosis (DVT) or as pulmonary embolism (PE), is observed quite frequently, often complicating surgery. In orthopaedic and trauma surgery it has been estimated that, without anti-thrombotic prophylaxis, the rate of DVT was 45%–57% (23%–26% proximal) in total hip replacements, 40%–84% (9%–20% proximal) in total knee replacements, and 45%–50% in proximal femoral fractures [1-3]. An accurate evaluation of the incidence of VTE in patients with lower limb fractures or soft tissue injuries is difficult at the present time, due to the lack of research on this topic. A reliable estimate of VTE incidence in lower limb fractures is 6%–45 % (4%–8% proximal). Exact data on the frequency of VTE in upper limb fractures are not available; nevertheless, the risk of PE in conjunction with DVT of the upper limb is considerable. With regard to the injuries of the soft tissues, such as tendons, it has been calculated that the DVT rate in these injuries is about 50% of the rate in bone injuries [3].

DVT must be rapidly diagnosed, not only in order to establish a suitable therapeutic strategy in the acute stage but also to prevent relapses and further complications. Without adequate and rapid medical treatment, the risk of relapse seems to be 40% in the first month after the primary event and 10% during the second and the third month [4].

Since a possibly fatal PE can follow DVT, it is mandatory that the clinical clues of such a disease not be underestimated. Edema, more or less associated with skin color alterations and pain (described sometimes as cramp and sometimes as heaviness and which increases upon local pressure) actually are not signs or symptoms specific for DVT; in fact, they can obscure a vascular disease of different origin, for example, superficial thrombophlebitis, lymphedema, or vasculitis. They can also be the expression of orthopaedic diseases such as stretching, muscular, or tendon ruptures or rupture of a synovial cyst [5].

However, these symptoms become increasingly significant in the presence of risk factors predisposing to thrombotic events by themselves.

Risk Factors

Among the so-called permanent risk factors (i.e., risks always present even without clinical evidence) are congenital factors such as anti-thrombin III, protein C, and protein S deficits. Anti-thrombin III deficit seems to be related more to venous thromboembolic risk than the two others. Homozygous carriers of protein C or protein S deficit are susceptible for severe clinical diseases, such as porpora fulminans, whereas heterozygous carriers can suffer DVT episodes before 45 years of age even at uncommon sites such as upper limb veins.

Other congenital risk factors include mutation of the Leiden factor, which is responsible for protein C-activated resistance, and mutation of prothrombin G20210A, which determines a 30% increase in circulating prothrombin.

Age, neoplasms, anti-phospholipid antibodies, and previous episodes of DVT represent permanent, acquired risk factors.

Moreover, in some clinical cases the thromboembolic risk is hardly detectable, such as in cases of hyperhomocysteinemia, hyperfibrinogenemia, and an increase in factor VIII, IX, and XI levels.

Among the most easily detectable transient risk factors are surgery (mainly orthopaedic surgery or neurosurgery), multiple trauma, prolonged immobilization, pregnancy, and oral contraceptive use [4].

Instrumental Diagnosis

If clinically suspected, especially in patients in whom these factors have been detected, further investigations are indispensable for a detailed diagnosis and an appropriate therapy. The significance of the investigations depends on the anamnestic and clinical data in combination with the evidence for risk factors: an accurate study of these parameters is required for a precise diagnosis and appropriate therapeutic procedure.

By scoring the symptoms, clinical signs. and other possible diagnoses the patient can be classified as being at clinically low, medium, or high risk for DVT [5–7].

Venous Doppler Ultrasonography (DUS), hematological investigations, and contrast venography are the instrumental investigations commonly used for diagnosis. A different role is played by impedance plethysmography, angio-CT scan, and angio-MRI.

DUS, which demonstrates the venous system through high-resolution ultrasonography, is the most universally accepted test for the diagnosis of proximal DVT of the lower limbs [8]. This examination is fast, inexpensive, and, most importantly, harmless, and because of these features it can be repeated soon, if necessary. In this test the probe is put on the common femoral vein, at the inguinal ligament level. Then it is moved distally along the superficial femoral vein path; at the back of the knee joint, the popliteal vein is followed until it trifurcates into anterior and posterior tibial veins and peroneal vein.

The venous areas are examined with the patient in different positions. The diagnostic criterion is the lack of compressibility of the vein's lumen under probe pressure: if the vein is compressible, its walls collapse and it does not contain a thrombus. Venous compressibility, better detectable in transverse scans, is difficult to perform at some sites (superficial femoral vein in the Hunter canal and deep femoral vein) for anatomic reasons. However, the introduction of color Doppler and power Doppler ultrasonography has improved the diagnostic accuracy even at those sites. The quality of the examination at distal sites closely depends on the operator and on employing adequate instruments.

For hematological investigation in suspected DVT the D-dimer levels are evaluated (products of stabilized fibrin degradation) [9]. A high level of D-dimers is nevertheless not highly specific for thrombosis since it can be detected in many other conditions, too (neoplasm, IMA, infections, and surgery). Therefore the levels of those substances is more significant for excluding thrombosis when the value is normal rather than confirming it when the value is high.

Contrast venography is performed by injecting contrast medium into a superficial vein of the back of the foot. Then, numerous radiograms of the limb are taken in different positions [8, 10]. An alternative procedure uses a tourniquet at the limb root, making it possible to adminster a lower quantity of contrast medium. Compared with the other technique, however, it is less accurate in visualizing gastrocnemius veins and anterior tibial and deep femoral veins.

The presence of a thrombosis is identified by a defect in lumen filling, evident in each projection. The sensitivity of this technique is 100% for lesions of 0.5 cm or more in diameter. In spite of the high resolution and accuracy of this procedure, venography has many limitations, related to the cost and the invasiveness of the technique, which can also be painful and involve complications.

Immediate side effects, whose incidence varies according to the contrast medium concentration and quality, are mostly minor reactions such as nausea, vomiting, and itching, sometimes associated with skin reactions; less frequently systemic complications such as anaphylactic reactions occur, which can cause heart arrest. Some cases of PE developing during venography have been reported, due to thrombus mobilization. The delayed side effects include postphlebitic syndrome, characterized by pain, warmth, and edema of the proximal calf and which resolve in few days, or a true thrombophlebitis, usually at the leg veins. For these reasons, in spite of the high resolution and accuracy, contrast venography cannot be considered the examination of choice.

Among the instrumental investigations, impedance plethysmography plays a particular role. Plethysmography records blood volume alterations inside the leg veins [11, 12]. The examination is performed by placing electrodes sensitive to this parameter at the site. A tourniquet is then inflated at the limb root to stop the venous blood flow and then deflated to restore the flow. In normal limbs the blood stagnation produced during the early stage creates an increase in blood volume, which rapidly decreases as soon as the tourniquet is deflated. If there is a thrombosis in the thigh, the volume increase is slower because the flow is already congested due to the thrombus and the emptying of the calf will be slower as well.

Plethysmography cannot detect most of the isolated thrombi: its sensitivity was evaluated at 95% in the 1970s and 1980s but now has been reduced to 70%. Therefore this technique has now been almost completely abandoned [5].

From the radiological point of view, angio-CT scan and angio-MRI play a very important role because they offer undoubted advantages to traditional phlebography. With these techniques, sites formerly difficult to investigate can be visualized, reducing side effects thanks to the very low quantity of contrast medium employed and obtaining very good results in terms of sensitivity and specificity. The limitations of these techniques are related to costs and high radiation exposure of the angio-CT scan [4].

As already mentioned, the choice of the instrumental investigation and its predictive value change according to the combination of clinical data and evidence of risk factors. In patients showing signs and symptoms of DVT, the first choice is DUS. If findings are positive, a diagnosis is made and it is necessary to initiate adequate therapy. If the DUS findings are negative, clinical data are not significant, and there are no associated risk factors, this examination must be repeated within 5–7 days if symptoms get worse. It is important to remember that a distal DVT becomes proximal in 30% of cases in about 1 week, and thus it can be better assessed by DUS. If, otherwise, clinical evidence is strong and associated risk factors are present, the use of an aggressive means of investigation such as phlebography is justified from the start because it provides a definite diagnosis.

Whereas phlebography, due to its typical features, is performed just once, DUS can be repeated to monitor DVT development until total vessel recanalization or stabilization of the thrombus dimensions has been achieved.

These data are important to determine the duration of anticoagulant therapy; moreover, they are indispensable in cases of suspected DVT relapse, which should be documented by the presence of a new thrombus (in case of a previously negative DUS) or by increased dimensions (of at least 4 mm) of a known thrombus [4].

Therapy

Once DVT is diagnosed, adequate therapy must be established as quickly as possible to prevent thrombus enlargement, detaching of emboli, and distant complications. Treatment is based on drugs interfering with coagulative mechanisms such as unfractionated heparin (UH), low-molecular-weight heparins (LMWHs), oral anticoagulants, and use of fibrinolytics and caval filters [4]: the two latter methods will not be discussed here.

Unfractionated heparins are composed of a heterogenic mixture of polysaccharide chains of different molecular weights of between 6,000 and 30,000 Daltons. Heparin directly interferes with coagulation, by locking a plasmatic factor (ATIII) and therefore inactivating the FXa and FIIa (thrombin) [13]. The two main activities of UH are performed by polysaccharide chains of different length: low-molecular-weight chains in particular are enough to obstruct FXa action, while heavier molecular chains are required to inhibit thrombin.

The anticoagulative effect, monitored by the aPTT dosage, is obtained when scores are 1.5–2.5 times the basal rate. LMWHs are derived from heparin digestion by chemical or enzymatic means and have a relatively low molecular weight, between 3,000 and 8,000 Daltons [14]. Their anticoagulative effect is a result of a link with ATIII producing an anti-Xa effect similar to that of heparin. However, because of the different molecular weights, they have a reduced anti-IIa activity.

LMWHs have a limited plasmatic protein link, which improves their bioavailability at low doses, makes the anticoagulant action predictable, and enables a once daily administration, without monitoring.

The use of LMWSs, even if prolonged, is associated with a lower rate of plateletpenia and osteoporosis than the use of unfractionated heparin. These features are common to all LMWHs, although they differ in average molecular weight, specific anti-Xa and anti-IIa activity, and anti-Xa and anti-IIa rate.

Oral anticoagulants interfere with vitamin K metabolism, inactivating the vitamin K-dependent coagulation factors (II-VII-IX-X). The most commonly used drugs of this family are warfarin and acenocumarol, which have different pharmacokinetics but not different clinical effects. Although oral administration makes these drugs easy to use, the individual variability in anticoagulative effect requires accurate and prolonged monitoring and exact therapeutic adjustment of the drug. The prothrombin time (PT) must be determined, which is sensitive to the reduction of only three of the four vitamin K-dependent coagulative factors, but not to factor IX variations.

Since the therapeutic effect is evident when all the factors are inactivated, variations in PT are not a reliable measure of anticoagulant efficacy in the early stages of therapy. Moreover, its value can vary according to the reagent employed in the laboratory test. This problem was resolved by the introduction of a standardized system called INR (International Normalized Ratio). In most cases, therapy is considered effective at INR values of between 2.0 and 3.0 [6, 15].

DVT therapy is based on the inhibition of coagulation mechanisms. Since oral drug efficacy is evident a few days after beginning treatment, the antithrombotic effect is initially obtained with simultaneous heparin administration and then maintained until the therapeutic anticoagulant levels have been reached (INR 2–3); heparin is generally administered for 5–7 days.

Until recently, heparin was given intravenously with frequent aPTT dosages; that is why DVT therapy was performed exclusively under hospitalization in the past and was only continued at home after therapeutic dosages had been reached.

Since the efficacy of UH and LMWHs has been demonstrated to be similar, the therapy can also be given to patients at home in the early phases of DVT, using subcutaneously administered LMWHs until INR therapeutic levels have been reached using the oral anticoagulant drug [15].

The therapy must be continued for a variable period of time (depending on whether it is the first episode or a relapse, and on the presence or absence of risk factors), but for at least 3 months and at most 12 months, or forever in cases of relapsing idiopathic DVT or in individuals with persistent risk factors.

In some exceptional cases, in which it is impossible to use oral anticoagulant therapy, LMWHs at therapeutic dosage are employed for the period mentioned above. DVT therapy is crucial to prevent immediate and delayed complications such as PE and fatal PE, relapses, and postphlebitic syndrome.

Prophylaxis

Prophylaxis is as important as therapy itself. Epidemiological studies, which have demonstrated the high incidence of the disease, and the fact that the disease is silent in the early stages represent the rationale for prophylactic measures in patients at risk.

In orthopaedic surgery prophylaxis consists of early mobilization, use of elastic stockings with graduated compression, and intermittent pneumatic compression. Such measures can represent the only prophylaxis in some kinds of surgery, but more invasive orthopaedic surgery requires drug therapy [6, 15].

LMWHs are very effective in reducing the risk of DVT, with a lower risk of major bleeding than UH [16]. A major bleeding is clinically evident and associated with a decrease of at least 2g/dl of hemoglobin and requires blood transfusion. It may be subperitoneal or intracranial or located in critical organs, or it causes death of the patient.

A minor bleeding such as epistaxis or macrohematuria is not associated with the features mentioned above.

Various LMWH belong to a homogeneous drug group, but differ from each other in molecular weight, bioavailability, and antiXa-IIa rate. These differences determine their differing efficacy and safety profiles.

Studies conducted on the use of LMWHs in orthopaedic surgery have shown them to be superior to UH in reducing both thromboembolic events and major bleedings; however, definitive data to help distinguish between the different LMWHs are lacking. Some clinical randomized trials defining symptomatic DVT relapse as an endpoint compared safety and efficacy of subcutaneously administered enoxaparin and nadroparin with intravenous UH in patients affected by proximal DVT. In both cases LMWHs were demonstrated to be as effective and safe as UH. Reviparin sodium and parnaparin also showed good efficacy and clinical tolerance. The dosages are different according to the molecule and (in some cases) to the weight.

Among the new anti-thrombotic drugs, those that were most highly developed in clinical phase III trials are fondaparinux (synthetic pentasaccharide, which specifically links anti-thrombin, improving its Xa factor inhibition capacity) [17], and the oral thrombin inhibitors (synthetic molecules, among which the most studied is melagatran, a direct inhibitor of thrombin active site, can be administered orally every 12 h at fixed dosages) [18].

Fondaparinux can be administered subcutaneously; it has a plasmatic half-life of about 17 h and thus can be given daily. Specifically, among the drugs commonly used, fondaparinux can be given for prophylaxis but does not seem to be indicated for DVT long-term therapy. Here, melagatran seems to be more promising [19].

A discussed problem is the duration of administration, particularly in patients who have undergone subarachnoidal anaesthesia. The American College of Chest Physicians (ACCP) recommendations [2] call for particular attention to patients whose history reveals coagulation alterations or bleeding risk factors. In these patients, in case of spinal anesthesia, anti-thrombotic administration may cause hematoma and bleeding that may lead to neurological deficits (sometimes permanent).

Since the risk seems to be related mainly to the procedures of placing and removing the catheter, regional anesthesia should be considered for both pre-

and postoperative prophylaxis, provided that the time of drug administration is far enough from such manuevers.

As for the duration of prophylaxis, it is necessary to remember that some patients may develop a DVT after discharge. Therefore, it is useful to continue the prophylaxis for a sufficient time and corresponding to the kind of surgery [19].

According to the most recent recommendations of the American College of Chest Physicians [2], in patients who are candidates for a total hip replacement or total knee replacement, prophylaxis must be started with LMWHs at full dosage 12 h before surgery or 12–24 h after surgery, or 4–6 h after surgery at half dosage and at full dosage from the day after.

An alternative may be to start the administration of fondaparinux 6–8 h after surgery or the administration of vitamin K antagonists, whose dosage must maintain the INR at 2.0–3.0, in the preoperative period or on the evening of the day of surgery.

As for the prophylaxis duration, there is near consensus that it must be continued until the patient can move by himself, i.e., for a period of about 4–6 weeks.

For the so-called minor orthopaedic surgical procedures, which involve patient immobilization, guidelines are not as accurate; in any case, there are sufficient indications to suggest the use of LMWHs for at least 2 or 3 weeks or until the patient can move by himself [2].

Finally, even respecting the guidelines, it would be useful for all clinics to develop personal multisubject operative procedures, based on wise preoperative study of the patient and in consideration of all the possible human and technical resources to optimize the diagnostic-therapeutic course.

References

1. Kujath P, Spannagel U, Habscheid W (1996) Incidence and prophylaxis of deep vein thrombosis in outpatients with injury of the lower limbs. Haemostasis 23[Suppl. 1]:20–26
2. Geerts WH, Pineo GF, Heit JA et al (2004) Prevention of Venous Thromboembolism. Chest 126[Suppl]:338–400
3. Agnelli G, Cimminiello C (2004) Linee guida per la profilassi del tromboembolismo venoso in ortopedia e traumatologia. SIOT, Roma
4. SIAPAV, SISET, SIDV-GIUV, CIF (2000) Linee guida per la diagnosi e il trattamento della trombosi venosa profonda. Minerva Cardioangiol 48:199–275
5. Hirsh J, Agnelli G (1993) Tromboembolismo venoso. Guida alla diagnosi, profilassi e trattamento. Il Pensiero Scientifico Editore, Roma
6. Molina E (2002) Patologia tromboembolica venosa: prevenzione e trattamento con un'eparina a basso peso molecolare, la nadroparina. How Why Med 5:12–18
7. Palareti G, Genovese U, Marra A (2003) Profilassi del tromboembolismo venoso in ortopedia. Aspetti clinici e medico-legali. Passoni, Milano

8. Leizorovicz A, Kassai B, Becker F et al (2003) The assessment of deep vein thrombosis for therapeutic trials. Angiology 54:19–24
9. Bernardi E, Prandoni P, Lensing AW et al (1998) D-dimer testing as an adjunct to ultrasonography in patients with clinically suspected deep vein thrombosis: prospective cohort study. BMJ 317:1037–1040
10. Rabinov K, Paulin S (1972) Roentgen diagnosis of venous thrombosis in the leg. Arch Surg 104:134–144
11. Agnelli G, Cosmi B, Ranucci V et al (1991) Impedance plethysmography in the diagnosis of asymptomatic deep vein thrombosis in hip surgery. A venography-controlled study. Arch Intern Med 151:2167–2171
12. Kahn SR, Joseph L, Grover SA et al (2001) A randomized management study of impedance plethysmography vs. contrast venography in patients with a first episode of clinically suspected deep ven thrombosis. Thromb Res 102:15–24
13. Prandoni P (2000) Terapia e prevenzione secondaria della trombosi venosa profonda. In: Prandoni P (ed) Terapia e prevenzione della malattia tromboembolica venosa. Piccin, Padova, pp 43–107
14. Hirsh J, Levine MN (1992) Review. Low molecular weight heparin. Blood 79:1–14
15. Agnelli G, Moia M (2001) Terapia antitrombotica. Media Med, Milano
16. Lassen ML, Borris LC, Christiansen HM et al (1989) Low molecular weight heparin in the prevention of thromboembolism in elective hip replacement. Thromb Haemost 62[Suppl. 1]:398
17. Eriksson BI, Lassen MR (2003) Duration of prophylaxis against venous thromboembolism with fondaparinux after hip fracture surgery. Arch Intern Med 163:1337–1342
18. Gustafsson D, Antonsson T, Bylund R et al (1998) Effects of melagatran, a new low molecular weight thrombin inhibitor, on thrombin and fibrinolytic enzymes. Thromb Haemost 79:110–118
19. Planes A, Vochelle N, Darmon JY et al (1996) Risk of deep-venous thrombosis after discharge in patients having undergone total hip replacements: double blind randomised comparison of enoxaparin versus placebo. Lancet 348:224–228

Section V

Future Directions

Future Perspectives: Computer-Assisted Surgery

Pier Paolo Raguzzi, Redento Mora

Introduction

The use of external circular fixation in the management of recent injuries and fracture complications (malunions and nonunions) involves two possible major disadvantages, which are related to each other:

1. Difficulty in the correction of displacements or deformities (simple or combined)
2. Exposure to multiple doses of radiation because an image intensifier must be used frequently.

Integrating computer technologies into surgical procedures, known as computer-assisted surgery (CAS), represents an important way to reduce these problems.

Since the mid 1970s, CAS has emerged as an accepted and clinically appropriate alternative to traditional surgery. Hundreds of articles on the subject have been published in peer-reviewed medical publications in the form of case reports, retrospective reviews, clinical studies, and randomized clinical trials. Though CAS has been described in the medical literature under a variety of terms, including "image-guided surgery", "surgical navigation", "surgical simulation", and "3-D computer surgery", the studies have collectively shown that CAS has:

- Revolutionized operating room procedures;
- Enhanced preoperative planning;
- Improved intraoperative effectiveness and efficiency;
- Increased the speed of postoperative recovery;
- Improved clinical outcome.

Computer-assisted surgery is now part of the "consensus view of the near future" and one of the more interesting applications is navigation: orthopaedic surgeons will probably receive the most significant benefits by using this technology.

With CAS surgeons can perform "minimally" invasive surgery with "maximum" accuracy [1]. As already mentioned, one of the most rapidly developing applications of CAS is computer-assisted orthopaedic surgery (CAOS). Technologies are being developed and introduced that will greatly influence how orthopaedic surgery is planned, simulated, and performed [2]. The community of orthopaedic surgeons, medical technology engineers, and computer scientists are working together to develop:

- Interactive and patient-focused preoperative planning processes that enhance the surgeon's performance and operating procedure and increase successful postoperative patient outcomes;
- Precise, less invasive, smart tools and sensors to reduce intraoperative trauma for patients, increase surgical efficiency, and improve postoperative patient recovery [3].

At the present time, navigation – in the broad sense of the word – is indispensable in orthopaedic surgery and mainly in trauma surgery.

Radiography, in the form of standard C-arm fluoroscopy, is the oldest and the most often employed kind of orthopaedic and trauma surgery navigation. This technique has several important limitations: imaging is only available in one plane at a time, and significant operating room time is unavoidably expended while the C-arm is positioned to supply views in multiple planes. Moreover, x-rays expose both surgeon and patient to significant radiation doses, even if trauma surgeons tend to underestimate the risk of radiation exposure [4–6].

The advantages of surgical navigation systems include the capability of providing real-time guidance during surgical procedures, not only in the biplanar position seen on x-rays but also in three dimensions, while reducing radiation exposure to the surgeon and patient.

CAS navigation involves the creation of a "virtual patient", which allows the computer to give feedback on positioning and anatomy to the surgeon. All the available systems of surgical navigation have some common features:

- Placement of surgical tracking arrays on both the operative site and the instruments;
- Tracking of the arrays by a tracking sensor overlooking the surgical field.

There are two kinds of arrays: active arrays (frames containing IR emitting diodes) and passive (or reflective) arrays [7]. All systems, however, can differ according to the type of anatomical information and the input methodology [8, 9].

One system type is based on preoperative imaging. In this system, the preoperative planning is based on the processing of images obtained by CT scan. This system is expensive and time-consuming and exposes the patient to additional irradiation.

A second type is based on intraoperatively obtained images. With this system, images are acquired with an operating room C-arm fluoroscope, provided by a special targeting device containing two elements: IR emitting diodes and a calibration grid. A disadvantage of this system is that several fluoroscopic shots are required prior to the beginning of the surgery.

The third type, the imageless system, does not require preoperative or intraoperative images. During surgery, a series of landmarks are collected and transmitted to the computer, which then morphs this information into a virtual patient. Presently, this particular technology is mainly applied in joint surgery. The main disadvantage of this method is the difficulty in obtaining some registration points.

Skeletal Trauma

In surgery for skeletal trauma, exact reduction and stabilization are required for long bone fractures. These operations can be performed by means of fluoroscopy or CT-based navigation [9–11]. These classical techniques have traditionally required large surgical exposure of the deep structures of the pelvis, which can be associated with significant complications, including:

- Significant blood loss;
- Infection;
- Lengthy operative times;
- Neurovascular complications.

The majority of these complications are related to the surgical exposure itself rather than to the initial traumatic injury. As a result, surgeons have sought less invasive alternatives to conventional treatment methods.

In particular, VectorVision trauma software (BrainLAB, Heimstetten-Munich, Germany) offers intuitive navigation on bony structures based on real-time fluoroscopic images. Surgical instruments can be tracked in real-time, allowing surgeons to transfer onscreen planning to the OR table with uncompromised precision. This dedicated CAS solution for trauma surgery addresses a broad variety of trauma indications, including long bone, hip, acetabular, and shoulder fractures. VectorVision trauma software delivers first-pass accuracy, creating a chance to significantly decrease operation length as well as reducing radiation exposure for both surgeon and patient. This software offers virtual fluoroscopy, enabling the visualization and manipulation of images across different planes simultaneously, reducing the total number of images needed for surgery.

The system can independently track bone fragments in real-time and provide quantitative data on relative leg-length and rotation. This can improve the precision of bone reduction procedures and applications of internal or external fixation devices without requiring additional images, in cases of fractures, malunions, and nonunions.

The virtual planning of intramedullary nailing, fixation plates, and interlocking screws can bring a new level of accuracy to determining optimal size and position. A dedicated software workflow makes navigated femoral nailing and sacroiliac screw placement user-friendly and efficient. Crowl and Kahler [12] found that procedures conducted with a navigation system were less invasive, as surgeons performed successful closed reduction and fixation with these types of fractures. They reported that:

- The average preoperative and postoperative displacements were 12.0 and 2.4 mm, respectively.
- No patient suffered a loss of reduction during his or her recuperation.
- There was a considerable reduction in radiation exposure (both for the patient and surgeon) when using virtual fluoroscopic surgical navigation compared to CT-guided or standard fluoroscopic technique.
- No patients experienced infection, significant blood loss, or neurological or visceral injury.

For the treatment of long bone fractures, VectorVision trauma provides several features facilitating the complex process of restoring the limb axis as well as controlling rotational alignment. The semi-automatic segmentation allows the display of bone fragments independently and tracks their movements in real time.

Procedure

The surgeon must follow some simple steps to use the BrainLAB CAS system in an OR procedure. The first step is attaching two reference arrays to the proximal and distal end of the long bone. These reference arrays allow the system to track the two segments independently and they remain attached for the whole OR session. They have different geometries: the proximal one is a T-star shape and the distal one a Y-star in order to differentiate the two for the purpose of tracking.

The reference arrays carry three disposable, reflecting spheres that function as passive markers. BrainLAB system uses passive marker technology and a freehand toolset during OR session: no cable or footswitch connect the sterile field and the navigation station (Fig. 1).

The C-Arm and the navigation system are connected via cable or via a network: the connection is usually made with a normal coaxial cable and receives analog image data but it is possible to use the new digital connections from new C-Arm models via DICOM III standard connections.

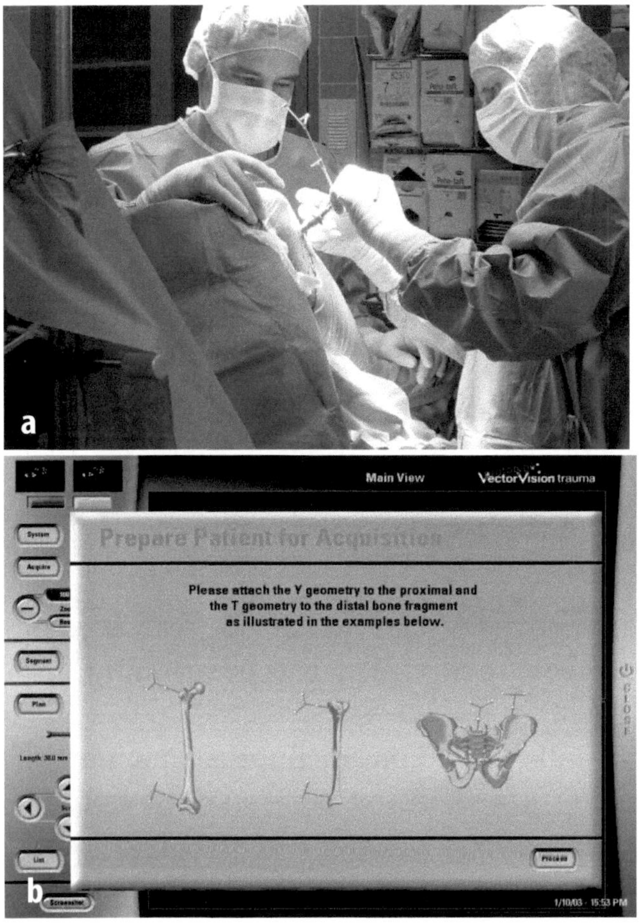

Fig. 1a, b. Attachment of the reference frames to anatomy. Two reference arrays are attached to the proximal and distal ends of the long bone

In order to track the position and the movement of the C-arm, a Fluoro Registration Kit is attached to the C-arm of the image intensifier (Fig. 2).

The second step is image acquisition. A small number of fluoroscopic images are acquired, in anterior/posterior and lateral views, by means of the Fluoro Registration Kit. An additional fluoroscopic image in oblique view can be acquired if necessary.

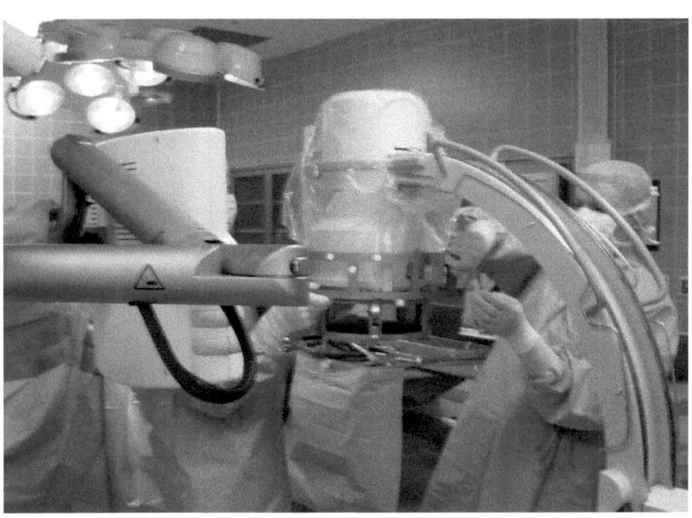

Fig. 2. Attachment of the calibration target to C-arm. A Fluoro Registration Kit is attached to the C-arm of the image intensifier

Images are calibrated and can be used during the entire surgical treatment, because they are constantly updated according to patient movements (Fig. 3).

After the image acquisition, the bone fragment "segmentation" is performed to enable independent tracking and interactive manipulation of the fragments. The segmentation process consists of defining both the axis of the proximal and distal fragments and several "docking points" (paired points depending on the configuration of the fracture or nonunion region) to facilitate the rotational alignment (Fig. 4).

After the anatomical axes and "docking points" have been defined, the bone reduction can be carried out or the deformity surgically corrected.

The software displays in real time the movements of the fragments and the deviations from the target position, using arrows and planes in order to line up the green areas and planned fluoroimages (Fig. 5).

The bone fixation elements (of an internal or external device) can then be inserted. The system allows the surgeon to pre-plan the positioning and direction of the fixation elements (Fig. 6).

Bone fixation elements can be virtually placed on the fluoroscopic images and their optimal direction can be determined. In the same way, the optimal screw length can be calculated (Fig. 7).

The surgical drill is equipped with a special navigation adapter and calibrated. Then the software can guide the surgeon to the planned target by displaying the fixation element position relative to the fluoroscopic images (Fig. 8).

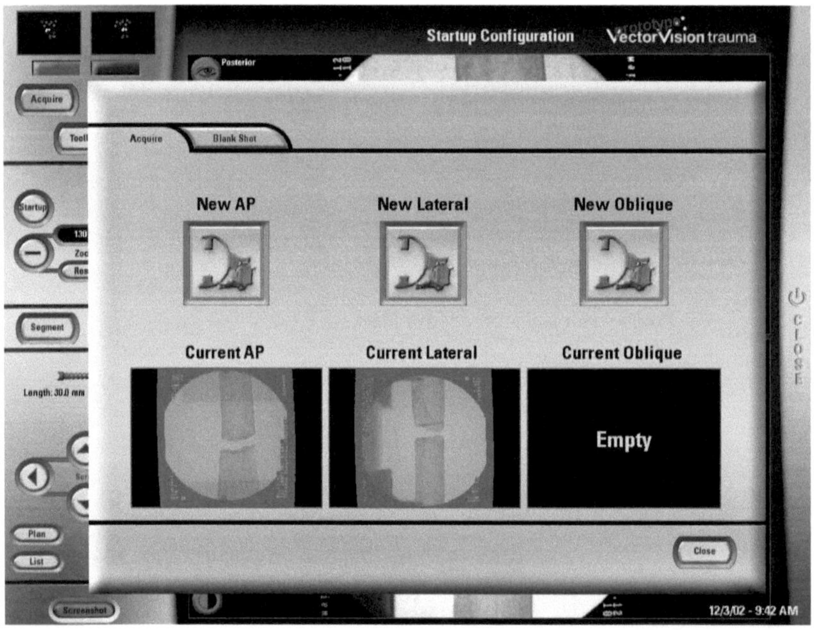

Fig. 3. Image acquisition. Fluoroscopic images in anteroposterior, lateral, and oblique views are acquired and calibrated

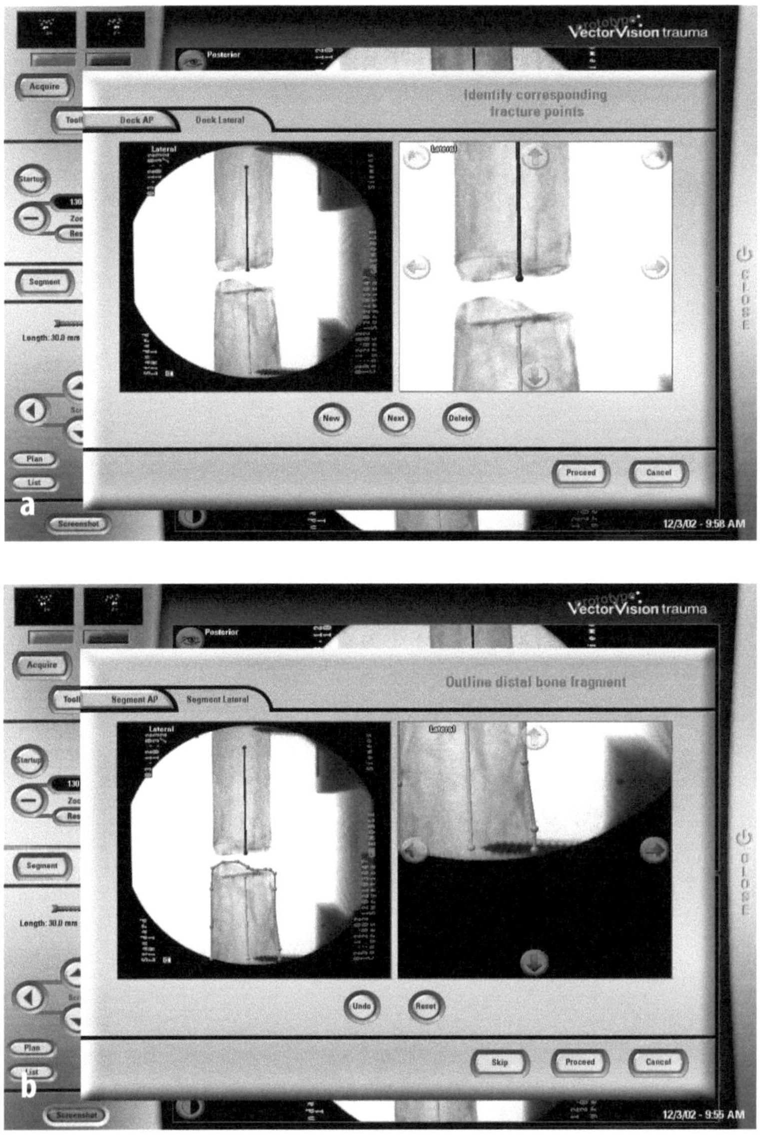

Fig. 4a, b. Bone fragments segmentation process. Definition of axes and docking points

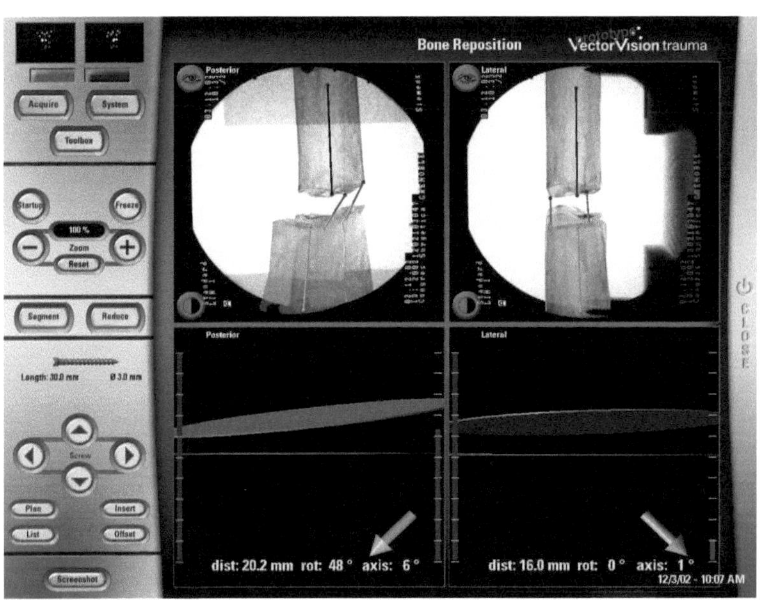

Fig. 5. The movements of the fragments and the deviations from the target position are displayed

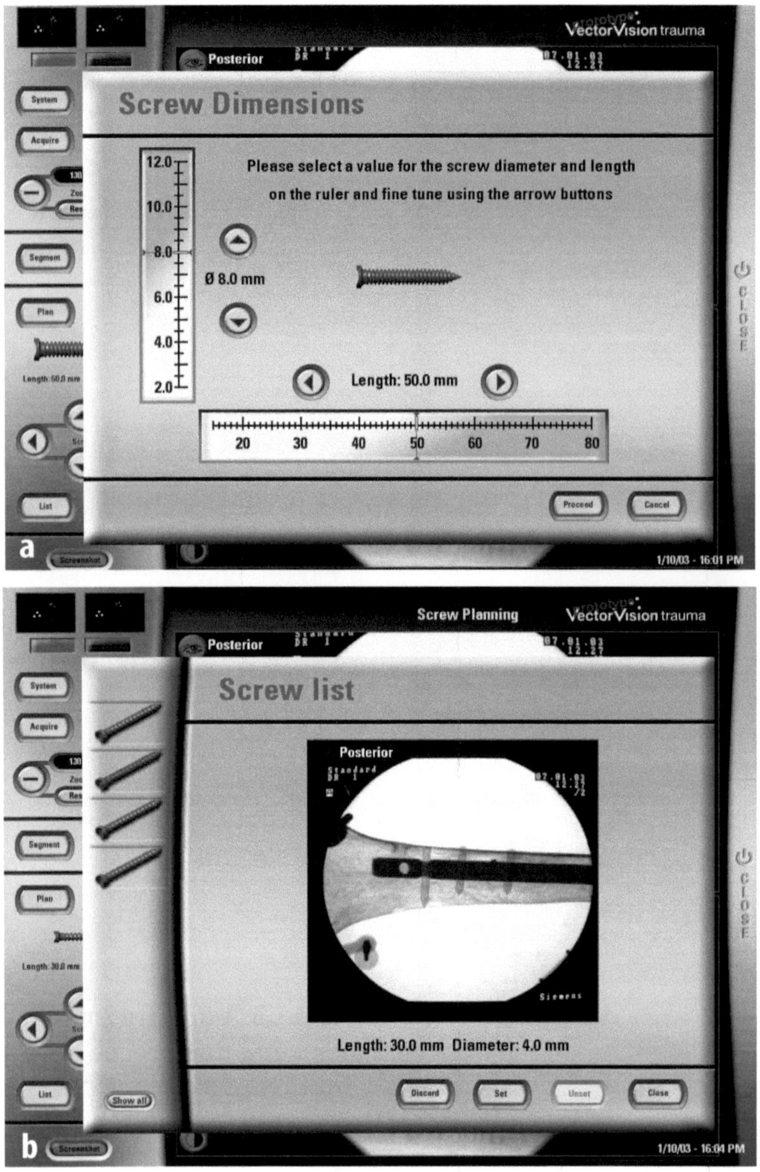

Fig. 6a, b. Planning and insertion of the bone fixation elements

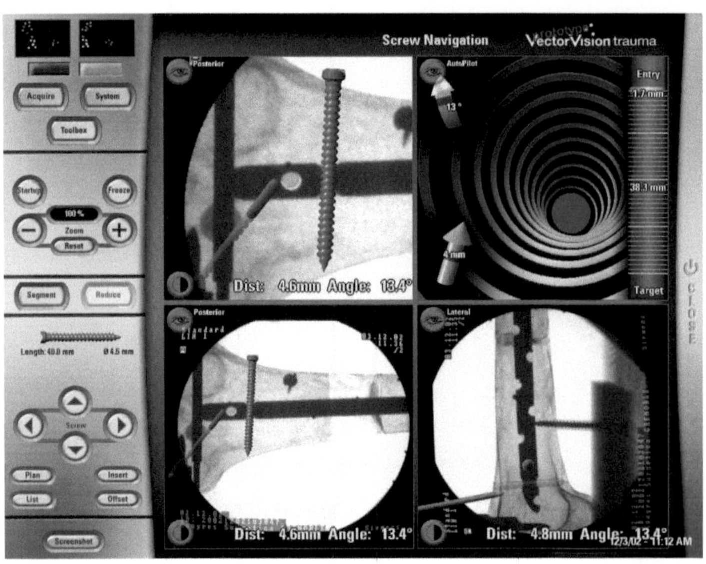

Fig. 7. Determination of the proper direction of bone fixation elements

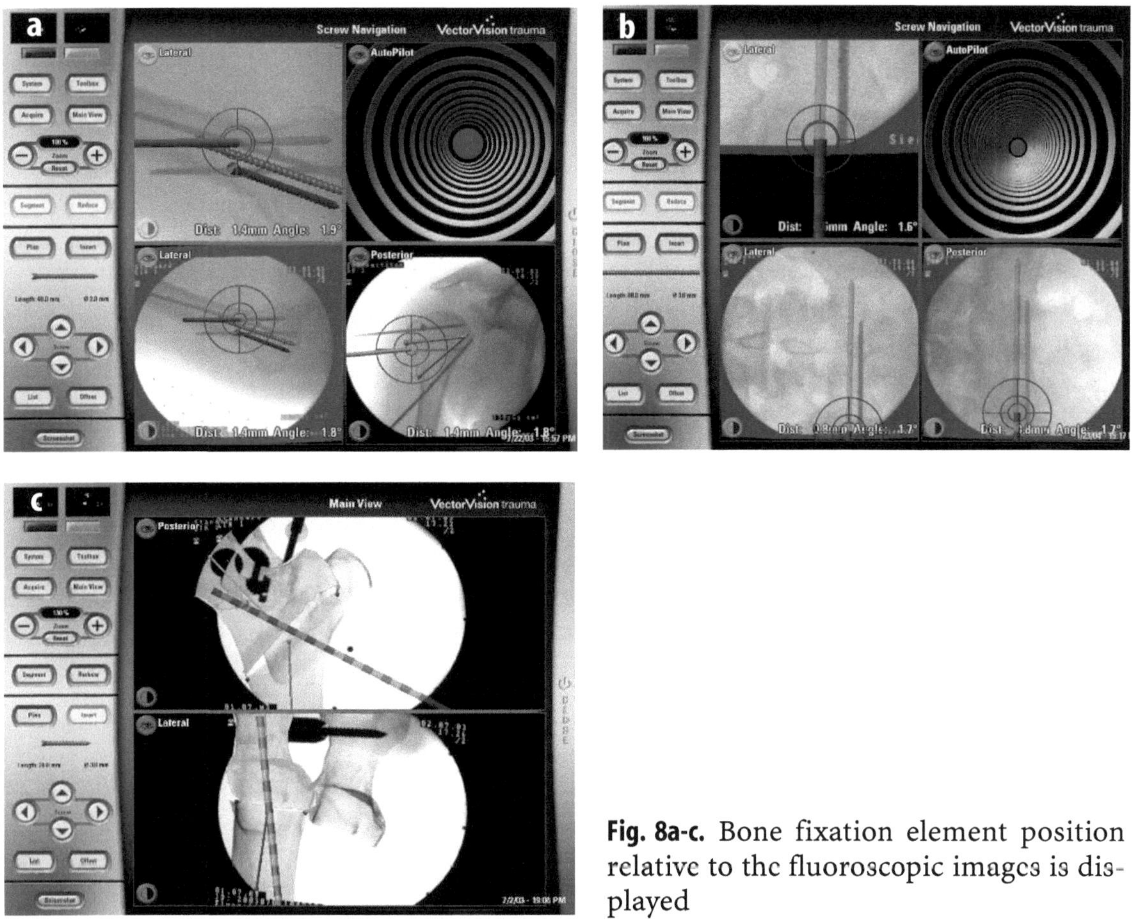

Fig. 8a-c. Bone fixation element position relative to the fluoroscopic images is displayed

Conclusion

One of the main advantages of the circular external fixation methods is that displacement and residual deformities can be corrected even after the apparatus has been assembled. Using this computer-assisted surgery the required corrections and adaptations can easily be carried out without any radiation exposure risk. Indeed, the x-ray exposure is more than 10 times lower than by traditional techniques.

References

1. Liebergall M, Mosheiff R, Segal D (2003) Navigation in orthopaedic trauma. Oper Techn Orthop 13:64–72
2. DiGioia AM, Jaramaz B, Colgan BD (1998) Computer assisted orthopaedic surgery. Image-guided and robotic assistive technologies. Clin Orthop Relat Res 354:8–16
3. Dvorak D (2004) Orthopaedic sector. In: AdvaMed Annual Report. AdvaMed, Washington DC
4. Sanders R, Koval KJ, DiPasquale TG et al (1993) Exposure of the orthopaedic surgeon to radiation. J Bone Joint Surg Am 75:326–332

5. Mehlman CT, DiPasquale TG (1997) Radiation exposure to the orthopaedic surgical team during fluoroscopy: "How far away is far enough?". J Orthop Trauma 11:392–398
6. Kahler DM (2004) Image guidance. Clin Orthop Relat Res 421:70–76
7. Schep NWL, Broeders IA, van der Werken C (2003) Computer assisted orthopaedic and trauma surgery. State of the art and future perspectives. Injury 34:299–306
8. Harwood D (2004) When MIS and CAS come together: role of CAS in hips. Proceedings of the International Meeting: Current technologies and future perspectives in total joint arthroplasty, Cannes
9. Joskowicz L, Milgrom C, Simkin A et al (1998) A system for computer-aided image-guided long bone fracture surgery. Computer Aided Surg 3:257–263
10. Hofstetter R, Slomczytowski M, Krettek C et al (2000) Computer-assisted fluoroscopy-based reduction of femoral fractures and antetorsion correction. Computer Aided Surg 5:311–325
11. Grutzner PA, Vock B, Kowal J et al (2001) Computer aided reduction and fixation of long bone fractures. Proceedings of the 1st Annual Meeting on Computer Assisted Orthopaedic Surgery (CAOS). Davos, Switzerland
12. Crowl AC, Kahler DM (2002) Closed reduction and percutaneous fixation of anterior column acetabular fractures. Computer Aided Surg 7:169–178

Method of Unified Designation of External Fixation

Leonid N. Solomin

Introduction

External fixation is a high-tech procedure in the treatment of patients with orthopaedic and traumatologic profiles. Consequently, the type of transosseous elements (K-wires, S-screws, half-pins) and their levels and their passing positions, the levels of the external supports of the fixator, and the biomechanical relationship between the supports must be strictly regulated (standardized) [1, 2]. Text annotations, even accompanied by explanatory figures, are grossly inaccurate because they leave too much room for data interpretation. The resulting three-dimensional image achieved using this computer technique is by far the most precise application; however, it is very expensive and laborious to create models for all situations considered in external fixation.

With a minimal number of symbols, *the method of unified designation of external fixation* (MUDEF) of long bones provides a comprehensive system for the following: the type and the spatial orientation of transosseous elements, the order and the direction of their passing, the form (geometry) and the dimensions of external supports, as well as the biomechanically indicated relationship between the supports, etc. [3]. Additionally, MUDEF provides:

- *A unique possibility of studying the method of external fixation* [4, 5]. Using MUDEF in instructional course lectures, monographs, manuals, and original articles, the entire algorithm of the operation can be accurately recorded and failure of the method avoided due to inaccuracies and mistakes during its implementation.
- *A basis for eliminating pin-induced damage of neurovascular structures.* In Germany, Italy, the USA, and Russia, atlases have been published that identify the schemes of the transverse cuts of the extremities and the designated sectors where it is dangerous to pass K-wires and half-pins. Using the coordinates of the present method in combination with any of the mentioned atlases significantly facilitates the defining of dangerous sec-

tors and safe corridors during surgery [4, 6].

- *Facilitation of routine work* during the recording operations of external fixation with a simultaneous increase in the self-descriptiveness of performed records.
- *Accuracy and comprehensiveness of corresponding consultations (including teleconsultations)* [7]. With MUDEF data for the recommended configuration of an external fixation device for a specific case can be exchanged during online conferencing/consultations.
- Facilitates simultaneous maintenance of *computer databases* with optimal configurations of external fixation devices for different kinds of orthopaedic and traumatological pathological conditions.
- *The possibility of estimating and describing in detail external fixation complications.* For example, pin-tract infections are often seen in external fixation. The use of MUDEF helps define the levels and the projections of those positions where pin-tract infection appears most frequently. The same principle can be used to define the transosseous elements causing pain or limiting the range of motions of the joints, etc.
- *A basis for the unification of scientific research on improving external fixation devices.* The most important characteristics of the devices for external fixation are the possibility to change the spatial orientation of bone fragments (reduction), rigidity of fixation, and to provide extremity function. During development of generally accepted criteria of each characteristic, specific configurations of external fixation devices can be compared by applying MUDEF in order to select the optimal ones.
- *Accuracy in describing a local area* is increased: place of punctures, cuts, installing of the drains, etc.
- Helps *overcome language barriers* among orthopaedic surgeons in different countries and establishes a *universal international code* for describing external fixator constructions.

Symbols Used

In MUDEF standard and additional symbols are used (Table 1).

By applying additional symbols the comprehensiveness and quality of the information is improved while using MUDEF, but it is not mandatory.

Coordinates

MUDEF of long bones is based on the coordinates. With the help of these coordinates each segment of the extremity is divided vertically (into *levels*) and horizontally (into *positions*).

Table 1. The standard and additional symbols

Standard	Additional
Roman numerals from 0 to IX - designation of level of K-wire or S-screw insertion Arabic numerals from 1 to 12 - designation of position of K-wire or S-screw insertion Mark “,” (comma) between symbols of level and position, and between symbols of position and orientation of S-screw insertion Mark “ -” (dash) between symbols of positions in the projection of which K-wire is passed Mark “ ; ” (semicolon and gap) divides the groups of symbols defining the transosseous elements Numerals, indicating corner of insertion of S-screws (in degrees) “( )” - round brackets - define the transosseous elements passed through radial bone, fibular bone Symbols for designation of biomechanically indicated relationship between the supports: —; ←→; →←; —o—; ←o→	For olive K-wire designation using marking of the corresponding position is in bold type Numerals defining order of insertion of transosseous elements Symbol for the defining of external supports - unbroken line below the symbols of transosseous elements united in one external device Symbols for the designation of the type of device for external fixation: - mon.- monolateral - bil.- bilateral - sec.- sectorial - sem.- semicircular - cir.- circular - hyb.- hybrid Symbols for designation of form (geometry) and dimensions of the external supports. For example, - 3/4 defines the circle without section 90°, 1/2 - semicircle, etc. Defining dimensions of the support in millimeters, for example, the diameter of the circle support.

Levels

Vertically each segment of the extremity is divided into eight basic and equally remote *levels*, designated by Roman numerals from I to VIII (Fig. 1). The device presented in Fig. 2 is used for rapid designation of all the basic levels or any individual one.

Positions

Each of the transverse cuts at each of the ten levels is divided into 12 equal sectors (similar to the face of a clock); the sectors are limited by *positions 1 to 12.*

The long axis of the bone is the center of division of each level into 12 positions (Figs. 3, 4).

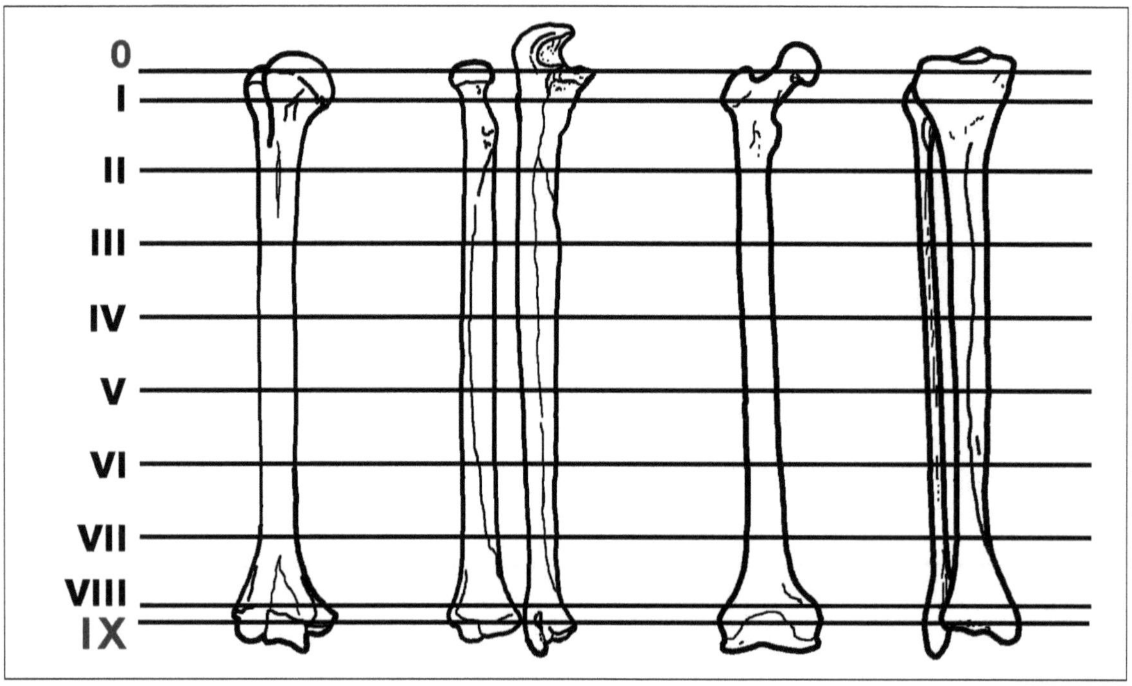

Fig. 1. Division of each segment into levels. Levels **I** and **VIII** are located in the projection of metaphyses of long bones, that is, at the place where the proximal and distal basic transosseous elements are passed, as in the majority of operations on external fixation. On the *shoulder*, level I is the level of the greater tuberculum of the humerus (40 mm distal to acromion) and level VIII the projection of the epicondylus lateralis. On the *forearm*, level I is located in the projection of the collum of radial bone (40–50 mm distal from the apex of the olecranon) and level VIII 30 mm proximally from the apex of the styloid process of the radial bone. On the *femur*, level I is located in the projection of the most prominent lateral part of the greater trochanter and level VIII in the projection of the epicondylus lateralis. On the *shin*, level I is the level of the tibial tuberosity and level VIII the distal tibiofibular syndesmosis. Levels **0** and **IX** located in the projection of the proximal and distal epiphyses of the bones of each segment are rarely used in external fixation. The distance between levels 0 and I (as well as the distance between levels VIII and IX) is less than the distance among the basic levels

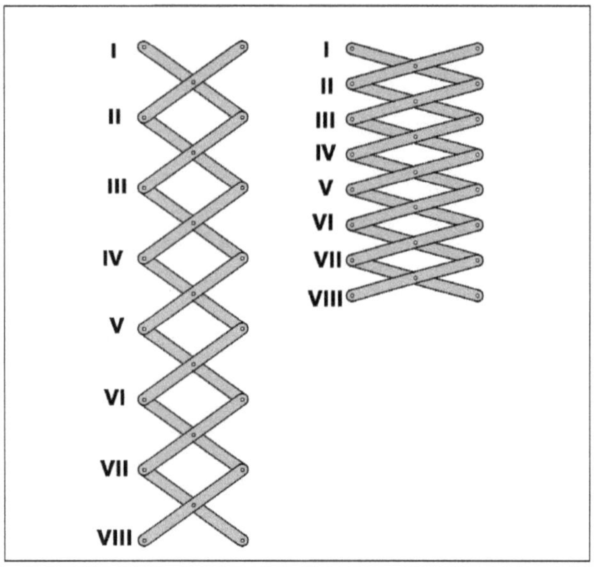

Fig. 2. This device is used for rapid designation of all the basic levels or any individual one. It consists of hinge joints of 14 laths; the dimensions of which are 80x10 mm. During the procedure it is enough to set the marginal joints of the device into the projections of levels I and VIII and the whole segment will be equally divided into eight remote segments. Elastic tape with eight marks of levels can be used for the same purpose

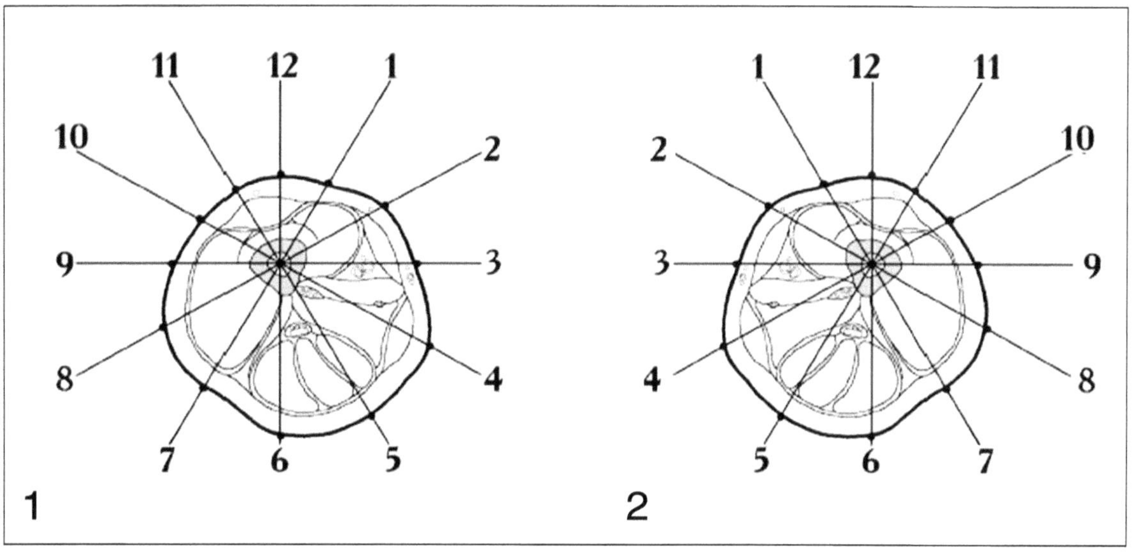

Fig. 3. Designation of positions at level IV of the right (1) and left (2) femurs. Conventionally, position "3" is always located on the *medial* surface of the segment and "12" *anteriorly*. Maintaining this guideline helps avoids failure during the designation of positions on the right and left extremity. According to the topographico-anatomical features of the humerus, the femur positions 2, 3, 4, and 5 can only be imagined theoretically at levels 0 and I (in some individuals at level II due to the constitutional features)

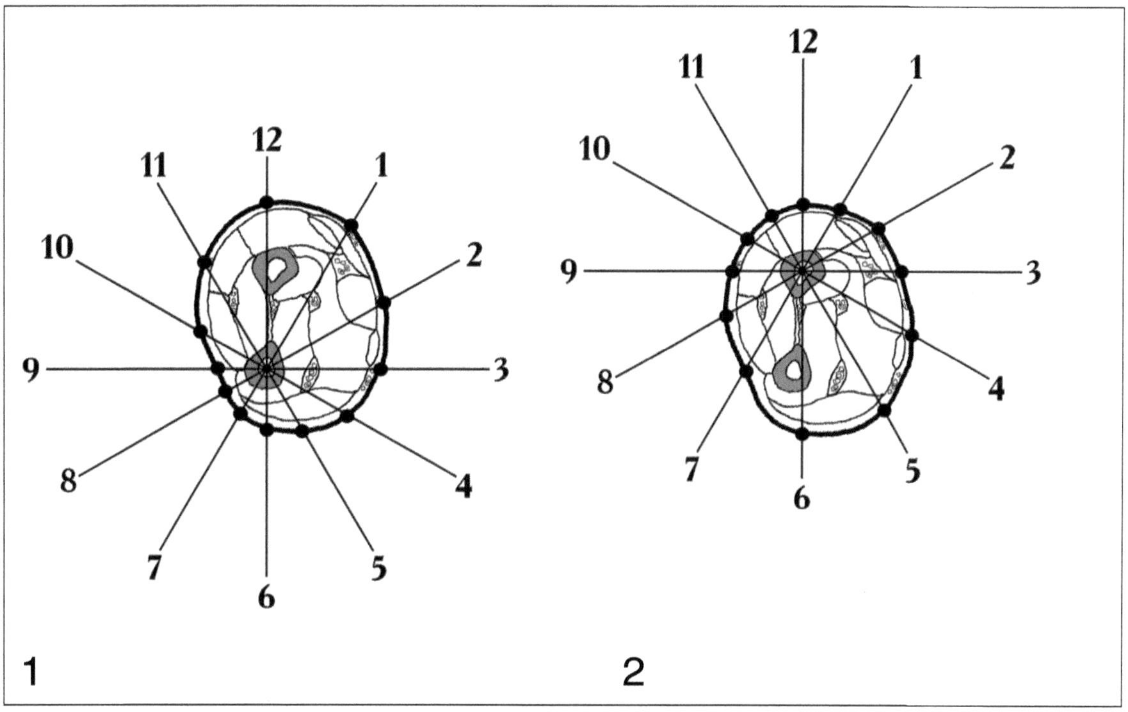

Fig. 4. Designation of positions relative to ulnar (1) and radial (2) bones at level IV of forearm (right forearm, in the middle between supine and prone position). Thus, 24 positions are indicated at each of ten levels of *the forearm and the shin*: 12 positions relative to each bone of the segment

Designation of Transosseous Elements

In MUDEF of the forearm bones, the symbols of transosseous elements installed through *the radial* bone are put into round brackets. To record external fixation of the shin bones, the symbols of transosseous elements passed through *the fibular* bone are put into round brackets.

Transosseous elements introduced between the levels (the position) are designated with the symbol of the level (the position) close to which the transosseous elements are located.

Designation of K-wires

For transosseous elements passed across a segment (for example, K-wires, rods of Steinmann, Kalnberz, etc.) it is necessary to designate two positions that are located at opposite positions with respect to the bone, for example, 3 and 9, 6 and 12, 1 and 7, etc. (Figs. 5, 6). The notation V,2-5 shows that K-wire is out of the bone. These symbols can be used to designate a drain placed at this level in the projection of the mentioned positions.

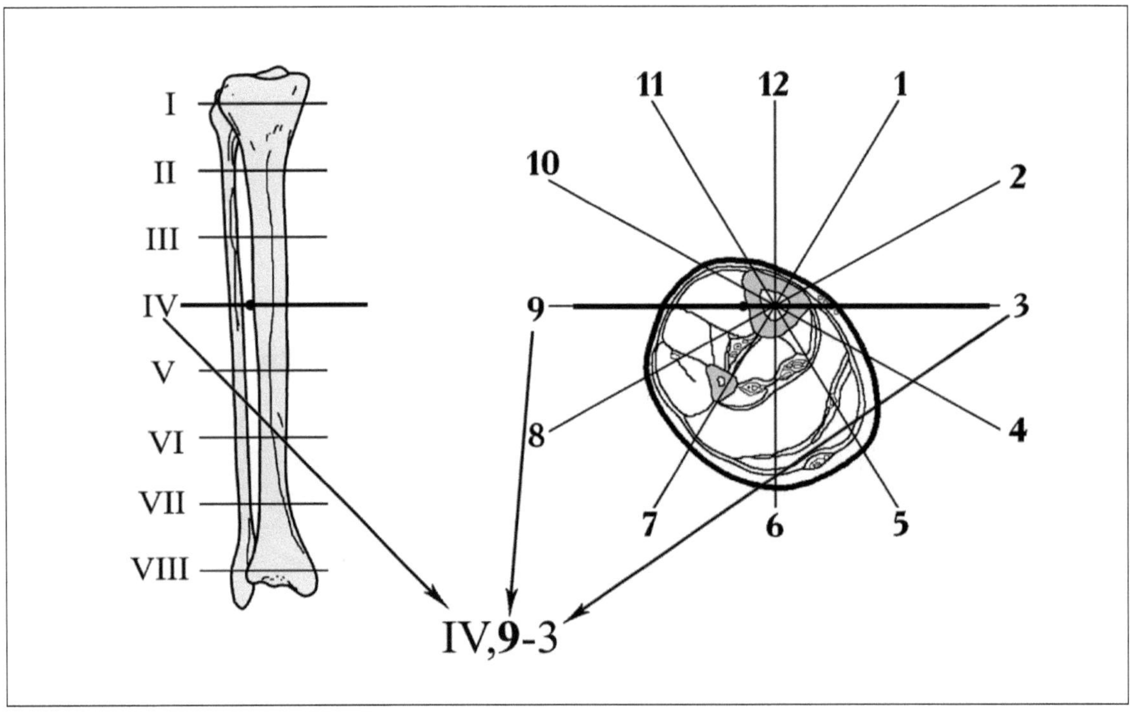

Fig. 5. For designation of K-wires passed *perpendicularly* to the long axis of the segment, the following conditions must be marked: *level* of passing and, after *comma, two positions* through which it was consistently passed. Positions through which the K-wire was consistently passed are divided using *mark* " – ". A K-wire with *an olive* is designated by marking the corresponding position with bold type. This designation is the *clarifying* one. For example, if a K-wire with an olive is passed at level IV in the frontal plane, in a lateral to medial direction, then it is designated: IV,**9**-3

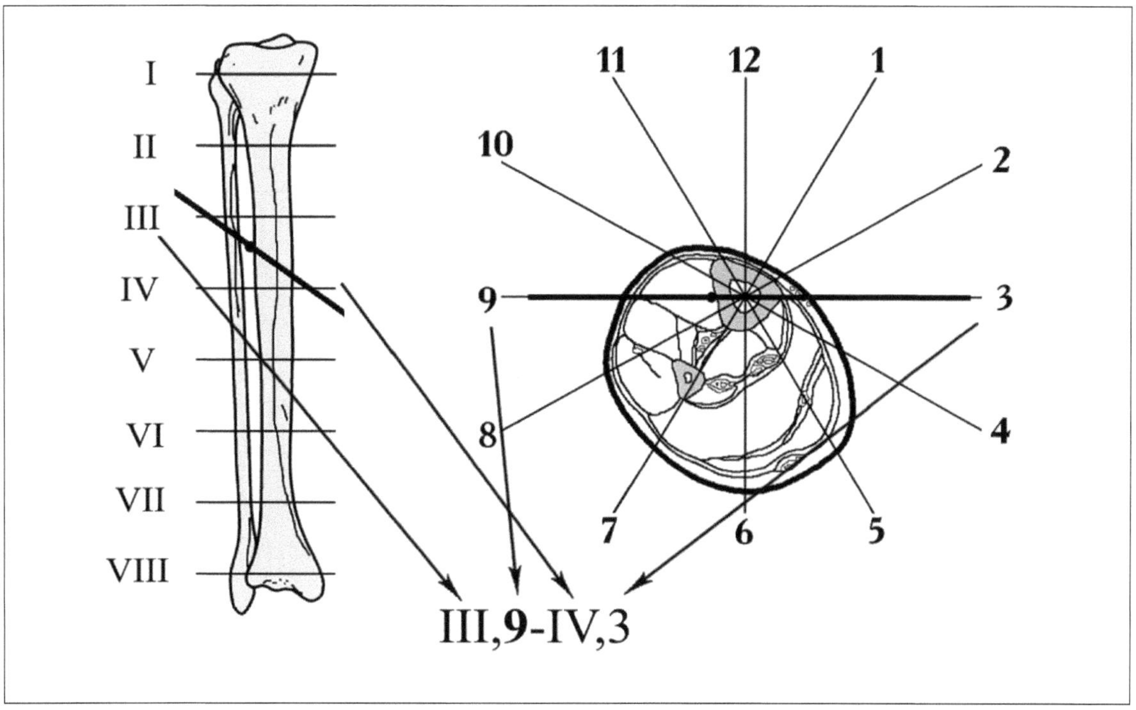

Fig. 6. If a K-wire with an olive is passed *at an angle* to the long bone axis from one level to another (for example, from level III to level IV), from a lateral to medial direction, then it is designated in the following way: III,**9**-IV,3

Several positions of the ulnar and the radial bones on the forearm (the tibial and the fibular bones on the shin) overlap each other. For MUDEF, this circumstance plays a role in the designation of K-wires *passed through both bones* of the forearm or the shin. In this case the same K-wire would have to be designated *twice*: for the part of K-wire passed through the ulnar (the tibial) bone and for the part of the same K-wire passed through the radial (the fibular) bone (Fig. 7).

Another example would be: "K-wire with an olive was passed at level I of the shin, at the side of the fibular bone, in the projection of position 8 and 2". Using MUDEF this text is designated in the standard (a) and clarifying (b) variants in the following way:
-(I,**8**-2)I,8-2 (*a*)
-(I,**8**-2)I,8-2 (*b*)

Designation of S-screws (Half-Pins)

To accurately designate *the console transosseous elements* (S-screws, stiletto-formed, curved rods, half-pins) it is necessary to indicate after the *comma* the following (Fig. 8):

- *Level of* console transosseous element insertion;
- *Position* of its insertion.

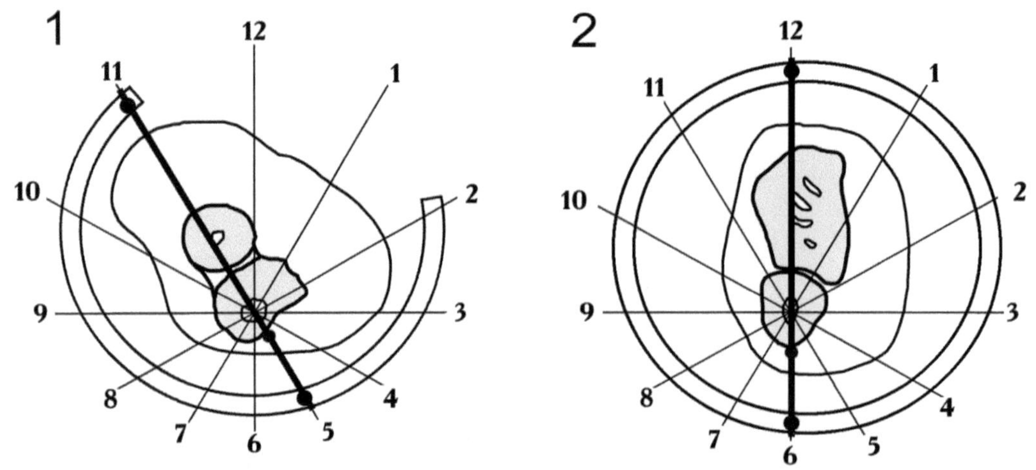

I,5-11(I,5-11) (a) VIII,6-12(VIII,6-12) (a)

I,5-11(I,**5**-11) (b) VIII,**6**-12(VIII,6-12) (b)

Fig. 7. (1) Designation of K-wires passed through both bones of the forearm in standard (*a*) and clarifying (*b*) variants. Positions relative to the radial bone are not shown on the figure. In the middle forearm position (between supine and prone) at the majority of levels (except level I) the ulnar and the radial bones are located one above another. That is why *positions 6* and *12* of both bones are also located one above another. In such a case the sequence of a K-wire with an olive passing at level VIII from the side of the ulnar bone can be represented in the following way (**2**): *position 6* of the ulnar bone → *position 12* of the ulnar bone → *position 6* of the radial bone → *position 12* of the radial bone. Thus, the VIII,**6**-12 designation corresponds to one of K-wire for the ulnar bone. The designation doubling in round brackets (VIII,6-12) shows that the K-wire is passed through the radial bone as well. If a K-wire with an olive is passed at level VIII of the forearm from the side of the radial bone, then it is designated as follows: (VIII,**12**-6)VIII,12-6. The proximal radioulnar joint is not strictly located in the sagittal plane. That is why the common designation for the ulnar and radial bones at level I is axis 5-11 (and not 6-12 as for all other levels). Thus, it is necessary to designate a K-wire with an olive (passed at level I subsequently beginning with the ulnar bone through both bones) as shown on Fig. 7.1. If a K-wire with an olive is passed at the first level of the forearm from the side of the radial bone, it is designated as follows: (I,**11**-5)I,11-5. Note that the symbols of "ulnar" and "radial" parts of K-wire *are not separated* by the symbol "gap"

- *Orientation* of its insertion to the long bone axis. It is accepted that the angle is opened *proximally*.

When the console transosseous element is passed through both bones, it is designated by using the symbol of only one position because the skin is perforated only from one side, for example: VIII,6,90(VIII,6,90) (Fig. 9). This way it differs from the designation of K-wire being passed through both bones (Fig. 7).

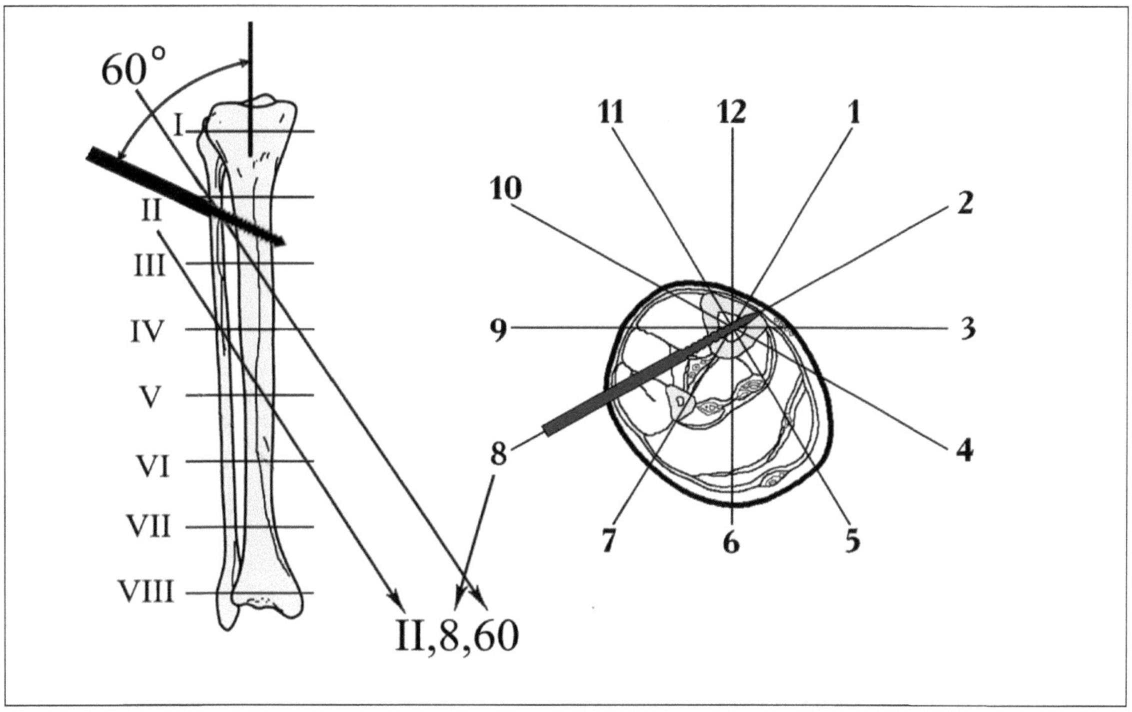

Fig. 8. Designation of S-screw inserted at level II in projections of positions 8, at an angle of 60° to the longitudal axis of the tibia

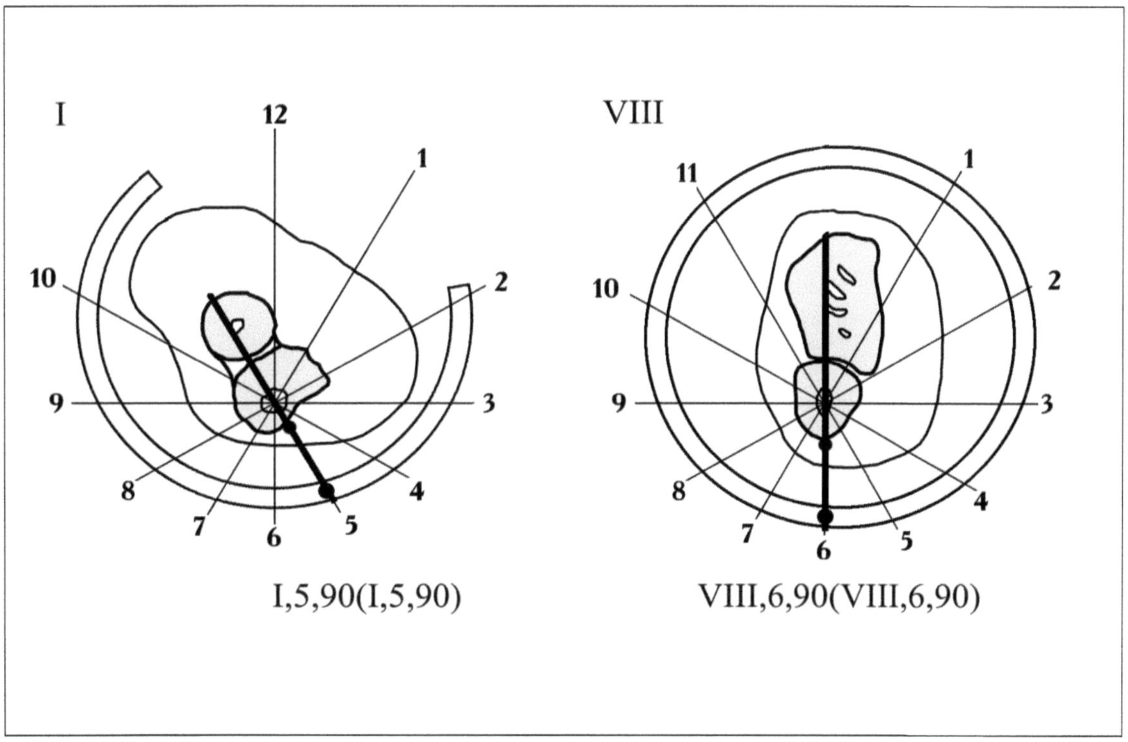

Fig. 9. Designation of half-pins passed through both forearm bones. The positions relative to the radial bone are not shown

Designation of External Support Frame

To encipher *device supports,* the designations of each transosseous element (K-wire, S-screw) fixed to the common support are divided by the marks "semicolon and gap" (Figs. 10, 11).

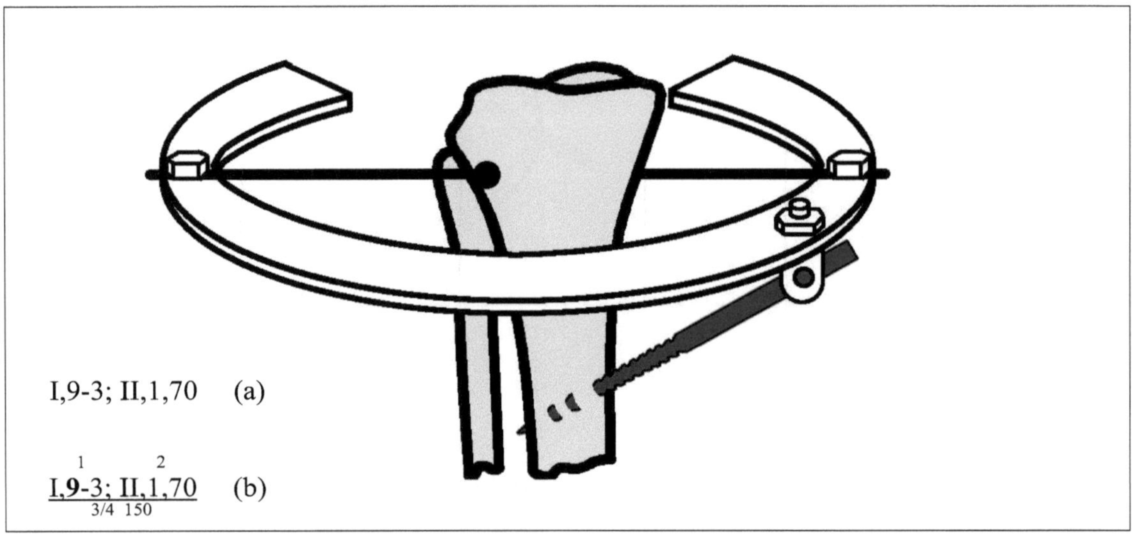

Fig. 10. Designation of hybrid (K-wire – S-screw) support in standard (*a*) and clarifying (*b*) variants. When the additional symbols are used, all the designations of the transosseous elements fixed to the present support must be united below using an *unbroken line*. For the designation of *order* of insertion of transosseous elements (sequence of osteosynthesis performance), the required numeral corresponding to the order of priority of the following transosseous element passing should be indicated above the enciphered designation of K-wires, half-pins. Under the unbroken line the other additional symbols are used, as follows: defining form (geometry) of the support. For example, 3/4 defines the circle without section 90°, 1/2 - semicircle, etc., defining dimensions of the support in millimeters. For example, the diameter of the circle support

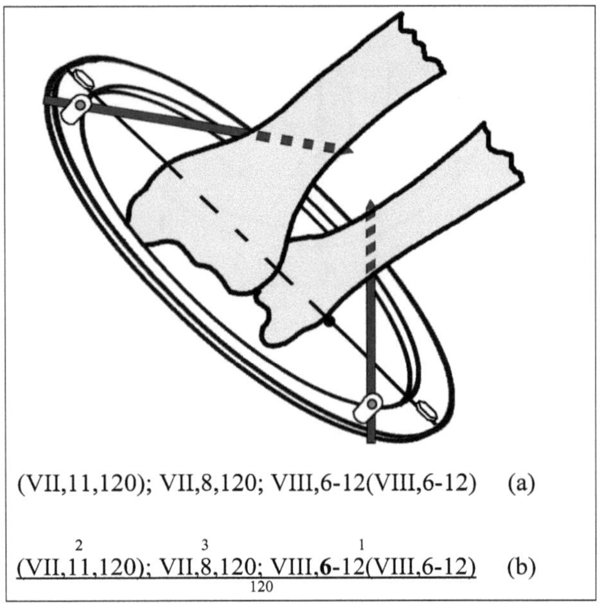

Fig. 11. The support mounted at level VI-II of the forearm in standard (*a*) and clarifying (*b*) variants according to the following text: "K-wire with an olive from the side of the ulnar bone is passed through distal metaphysis of both forearm bones. S-screw is inserted into the radial bone at level VII in the projection of position 11 at an angle 120°. The second S-screw was installed into the ulnar bone at level VII, in the projection of position 8 and at an angle 120° to the long axis of the ulnar bone. All the transosseous elements are fixed to the 120 mm circular support"

Designation of the Whole Device

For designation of the whole device configuration (Figs. 12, 13, 14, 15), symbols representing the recommended *biomechanically* indicated *relationship between them* should be inserted between the symbols of the external supports:

- neutral: ---
- compression: →←
- distraction: ←→
- hinge: —o—
- distraction hinge:←o→

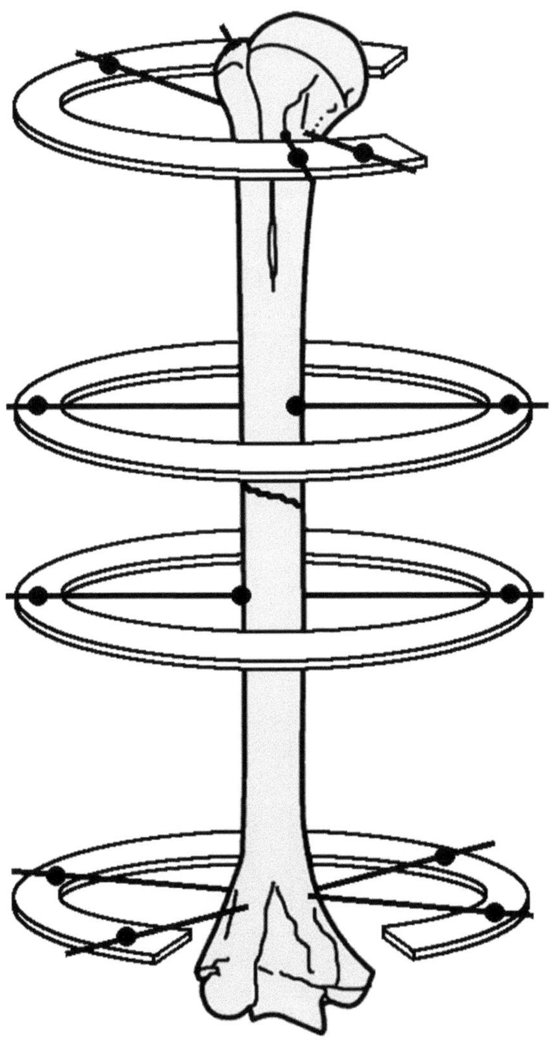

I,1-7; I,11-5 — IV,3-9 →← V,9-3 — VII,8-2; VII,10-4 (a)

$$\frac{\mathrm{I},\overset{1}{\mathbf{1}}\text{-}7;\ \mathrm{I},\overset{2}{11}\text{-}5}{\_\,140}\ \text{—}\ \frac{\mathrm{IV},\overset{5}{\mathbf{3}}\text{-}9}{130}\ \rightarrow\leftarrow\ \frac{\mathrm{V},\overset{6}{\mathbf{9}}\text{-}3}{130}\ \text{—}\ \frac{\mathrm{VII},\overset{3}{8}\text{-}2;\ \mathrm{VII},\overset{4}{10}\text{-}4}{\_\,130} \quad \text{(b)}$$

Fig. 12. Example of MUDEF of humeral bone fracture 12-A3 in standard (*a*) and clarifying (*b*) variants according to the text description: "K-wire with an olive is inserted through the proximal metaphysis of the humeral bone, at a right angle to the long axis of the segment, and oriented at an angle of 75° to the frontal plane, from posterior to anterior. The second K-wire is passed in the same plane as the first one and inserted at an angle 30° to it. Two K-wires are passed through the epicondylar region of the humerus, at right angles to the long bone axis, in the transversal plane, oriented at 30° to each other (the angle in opened outside). The Ilizarov's device is mounted using three supports with a diameter of 130 mm and one (proximal) support with a diameter of 140 mm. In such cases the marginal supports of the device are geometrically mounted as 3/4 of the circle. For reduction of the bone fragments, two K-wires with an olive are inserted in the frontal plane: the first one at the border of the upper and middle thirds of the humeral diaphysis, from medial to lateral direction, the second one at the level of the border of the middle and lower thirds of the segment from lateral to medial. The interfragmental compression is given"

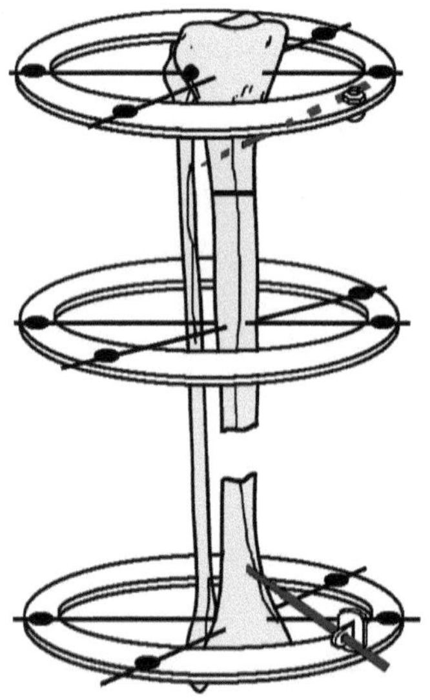

(I,8-2)I,8-2; I,4-10; II,1,60 ←→ IV,2-8; IV,4-10 →← VII,1,120; (VIII,8-2)VIII,8-2; VIII,4-10 (a)

1 2 3 7 8 6 4 5
(I,**8**-2)I,8-2; I,4-10; II,1,60 / 150 ←→ IV,2-8; IV,4-10 / 150 →← VII,1,120; (VIII,**8**-2)VIII,8-2; VIII,4-10 / 150 (b)

Fig. 13. Designation of the bone transport operation (replacement of the tibial defect using the lengthening of the proximal fragment) in standard (*a*) and clarifying (*b*) variants. Note that the designation (1,**8**-2)I,8-2 shows that the olive of K-wire is located on the fibular bone. The designation of K-wire (VIII,**8**-2)VIII,8-2 shows the same

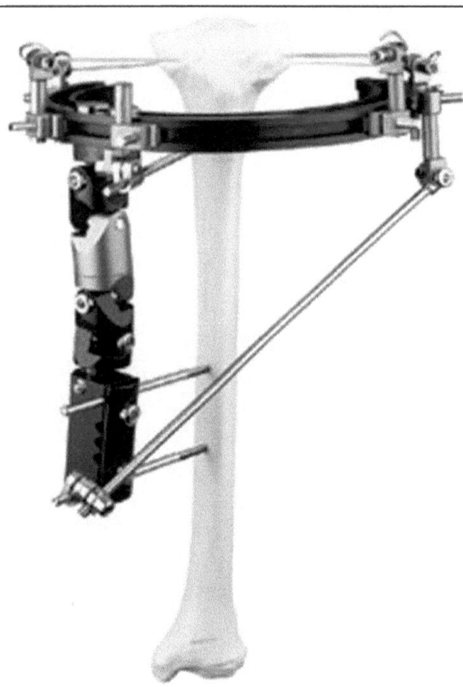

0,3-9; 0,8-2 –_– II,2,90; IV,2,90; V,2,90 (a)

1 2 3 4 5
0,**3**-9; 0,**8**-2 / 2/3 160 –_– II,2,90; IV,2,90; V,2,90 / mon. (b)

Fig. 14. Designation of *Biomed-Merc device* in standard (*a*) and clarifying (*b*) variants

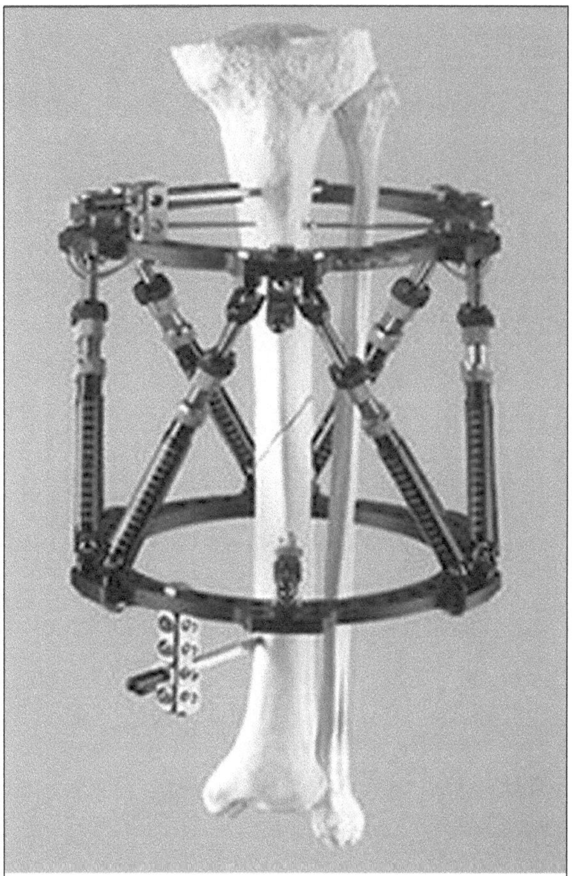

II,1,90; II,9-3; III,12,90 –o– V,12,90; VI,1,90 (a)

$$\underset{150}{\underline{\overset{2}{\text{II,1,90}};\ \overset{1}{\text{II,}\mathbf{9}\text{-3}};\ \overset{3}{\text{III,12,90}}}}\ \text{–o–}\ \underset{150}{\underline{\overset{4}{\text{V,12,90}};\ \overset{5}{\text{VI,1,90}}}}\quad \text{(b)}$$

Fig. 15. Designation of *Taylor Spatial Frame* in standard (*a*) and clarifying (*b*) variants

Additional Data

If necessary, the number of levels and positions can be enlarged, for example, up to 30 levels and 360 positions. The following notations correspond to such conditions: XXII, 162-342; XVIII, 273,65.

If necessary, besides increasing the number of levels and positions, the MUDEF user can apply the additional symbols. They identify the type of the console transosseous element (for example, S-screw, half-pin, hooked rod), the material (from which the external device supports and transosseous elements were made), and the diameter of transosseous elements connecting the supports of the bar, etc. We recommend using the text explanations while designating the transosseous elements introduced into the anatomical formations that are not included in the given schemes as follows:

- Example 1: The phrase "Two mutually crossed K-wires were passed through the acromion of the scapula and fixed in one external support" is designated as "acr.,1-7; acr.,5-11". (acr. - acromion).

- Example 2: The phrase "The half-pin was passed into the posterior surface of the olecranon at an angle 90°" can be designated as "olecr.,6,90".
- Example 3: The phrase "K-wire was passed through the talus in the frontal plane" can be designated as "talus,3-9".

For *the operative record,* then, only the following features of the procedure must be recorded in text form: the operative approach, the characteristics of tissues, and any complications, etc. In the *postoperative period* the comprehensiveness and concrete meaning of the records in the initial medical documentation are perfectly clear as can be seen from the records given for example:

- Additionally the element II,1,60 was passed and fixed to the proximal device support. It is recommended to perform the contralateral compression of the fragments (1 mm per week) using the wire traction device V,9-3.
- Due to the cutting of the soft tissues near to S-screw V,2,90, the screw was changed with K-wire V,4-10.
- The signs of inflammation appeared in the region of K-wire VI,4-10 exit at position 4.

The last two examples illustrate the significant role of MUDEF of long bones in *objectively describing complications.*

The *electronic version* of Method of Unified Designation of External Fixation [1] is located at http://www.aotrf.org/site/metod.html.

References

1. Solomin LN, Kornilov NV, Vojtovich AV, Kondratenko DN (2002) Method of unified designation of external fixation. SICOT/SIROT, 12th World Congress, San Diego, p 603
2. Solomin L, Kornilov NV (2003) Inner contradictions of modern external fixation: causes, significance and ways of their resolution. Minerva Ortop Traumatol 54:57–66
3. Solomin L, Kornilov NV, Wolfson N, Kirienko A (2003) Importance of "Method of unified designation of external fixation". J Bone Joint Surg Br 86[Suppl. 3]:300
4. Solomin LN (2004) Chreskostnij osteosintez [External Fixation] Travmatologija I ortopedija: rukovodstvo dlja vrachej: V 4-h t. Pod red. N.V. Kornilova I E.G. Grjaznuhina. – T. 1, gl. 5. Gippokrat, St. Petersburg, pp 336–388
5. Solomin LN (2005) Osnovi chreskostnogo osteosinteza apparatem G.A. Ilizarova [The Basic Principles of External Fixation Using Ilizarov Device]. Morsar AV, St. Petersburg
6. Barabash AP, Solomin LN (1997) "Esperanto" provedeniya chrskostnykh elementov pri osteosinteze apparatom Ilizarova ["Esperanto" of Passing of Transosseous Elements in Osteosynthesis using Ilizarov's Device]. Nauka Sib Predpriyatiye RAN, Novosibirsk
7. Solomin L, Kornilov V, Shevtsov V et al (2004) Application of "Method of unified designation of external fixation" (MUDEF) in telemedicine. Eur J Trauma 30:42

Subject Index

E

F

G

H

I

J-K

L

M

N

O

P

R

S

T

U

V-W-X